ANDBOOK OF
'DIATRIC
ARDIOLOGY

NDBOOK OF
EDIATRIC
ARDIOLOGY

econd Edition

Jerome Krovetz, M.D., Ph.D.
ofessor, Department of Pediatrics (Cardiology)
iversity of Virginia, Charlottesville

a H. Gessner, M.D.
Professor, Department of Pediatrics (Cardiology)
University of Florida, Gainesville

Gerold L. Schiebler, M.D.
Professor and Chairman, Department of Pediatrics
University of Florida, Gainesville

University Park Press
Baltimore

UNIVERSITY PARK PR
International Publishers in Science, Medicine, and Educa
233 East Redwood St
Baltimore, Maryland 21

Typeset by The Composing Room of Michigan, I
Manufactured in the United States of America
Universal Lithographers, In
and The Optic Bindery Incorporate

Library of Congress Cataloging in Publication Data
Krovetz, L Jerome, 1929–
Handbook of pediatric cardiology, 2d ed.

Includes bibliographies and index.
1. Pediatric cardiology. I. Gessner, Ira H.,
1931– joint author. II. Schiebler,
Gerald 1928– joint author. III. Title.
RJ421.K76 1979 618.9′21′2 79-1092
ISBN 0-8391-1354-4

contents

preface to the second edition

When we decided to revise this *Handbook* we anticipated a quick and easy task. After all, we reasoned, there had been relatively few changes in the field of pediatric cardiology in the last nine years. We would need to revise the sections on surgical results in most of the chapters, since there had been significant improvements in surgery for small infants. We anticipated that it would require at the most a few months of spare time.

As we began to examine the details of what we were going to change we found that there were six entities that we had not discussed in the first edition that warranted separate chapters. Thus we have added chapters on single ventricle, hypertension, atherosclerosis, mitral valve prolapse, hypoplastic left heart syndrome, and hypoplastic right heart syndrome. There were three others that we had discussed briefly that now merited separate chapters of their own: arrhythmias, pericarditis, and problems associated with cyanotic heart disease. It also seemed desirable to include a chapter on a new and exciting diagnostic tool, echocardiography. In order to maintain the handy size of the previous edition, we thought it necessary to reduce our coverage in other areas. For example, the chapter in the first edition entitled "Natural History of Ventricular Septal Defect" was combined with the chapter on Ventricular Septal Defect. We have also eliminated or shortened sections on other subjects that we thought to be of lesser importance.

Although we had anticipated a few of these changes, we were astonished at how many other changes were needed, especially in areas where we thought our notions were relatively stable. In a surprising number of instances we found ourselves saying, in effect, "Did we really say that?" We found that in a number of ways our opinions and handling of even some common anomalies had changed over the years. By the time we finished, there were changes in all except two of the chapters and over a year had elapsed since we started. The number of changes in this revision are testimony to the growth of pediatric cardiology since the first edition of the *Handbook*.

acknowledgments

"For this relief, much thanks."
—Hamlet

The authors would like to acknowledge the aid of several colleagues who reviewed chapters relating to their areas of special expertise and knowledge. In particular we would like to thank Drs. Carlos R. Ayers (Chapter 35, Hypertension), Karen S. Kuehl (Chapter 36, Atherosclerosis), J. Owen Hendley (Chapter 37, Infective Endocarditis), and Thaddeus Kelly (Chapter 41, Connective Tissue Disorders). Our thanks also to Dr. Marius Hubbell for his aid in preparing many of the new illustrations and to Ralph Davis for his excellent typing and his patience with the changes wrought by having three authors.

To Anne, Gerri, and Audrey

PART I
Elements of Cardiology

This section of the Handbook contains materials relating to the basics of heart disease, with the emphasis on congenital cardiac anomalies. Information regarding genetic and teratogenic aspects of congenital heart disease, as well as discussions on cardiac anatomy and the hemodynamics of heart disease, is included.

The latter part of the section concerns the tools available to the physician. We have limited our discussion to those parts of the physical and laboratory examinations that are pertinent to cardiology. The concluding chapter deals with aspects of congestive heart failure.

This section may be read in its entirety, or it may be skipped over at this time and attention directed to the sections on congenital and acquired heart disease. The reader may then refer back to these chapters to gain a further understanding of the parts of the cardiovascular examination as they relate to the descriptions of the cardiac lesions in the latter parts of this book.

chapter 1

ANATOMY OF THE HEART

POSITION AND EXTERIOR APPEARANCE

An understanding of cardiac anatomy includes an awareness of the heart's position within the thorax. Correct interpretation of plain chest roentgenograms as well as angiocardiograms demands this precise knowledge.

As seen in Figure 1, the apex of the heart is directed anteriorly, inferiorly, and to the left. The right border of the cardiac silhouette is made up of the superior vena cava, the right atrium, and the inferior vena cava. The right ventricle does not ordinarily form any part of this border. The left border is formed predominantly by the left ventricle. The left atrium lies in the midline

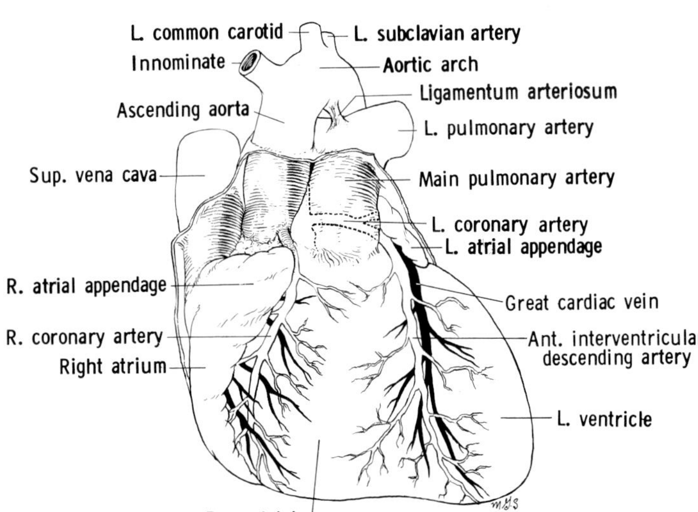

Figure 1. Anterior view of in situ heart and great vessels. The pericardium has been removed and its cut edge is shown reflected from the great vessels. Coronary veins are shown in solid black and coronary arteries in outline.

posteriorly and, because of the short, fixed pulmonary veins, anchors the heart.

The right ventricle is separated from the right atrium by the right atrioventricular groove and from the left ventricle by the anterior interventricular groove. The right coronary artery and the anterior descending branch of the left coronary artery, respectively, lie in these grooves. The coronary sinus lies posteriorly in the left atrioventricular groove.

Figure 1 also illustrates the origin of the pulmonary trunk—it rises anteriorly from the upper left border of the heart. After bifurcating, the right pulmonary artery runs rightward behind the ascending aorta and superior vena cava, and the left pulmonary artery runs directly left and somewhat posteriorly. The aorta originates centrally within the heart, with the aortic valve being inferior, posterior, and slightly to the right of the pulmonic* valve. After the origins of the innominate, the left common carotid, and the left subclavian arteries, the arch of the aorta passes behind the bifurcation of the main pulmonary artery.

Ordinarily, four pulmonary veins—two on either side—enter the left atrium. The right veins pass behind the right atrium to enter the right side of the left atrium and the left veins enter the left side of the left atrium.

RIGHT HEART (Figures 2 and 3)

The superior vena cava enters the right superior portion of the right atrium slightly forward, so that it aims toward the tricuspid orifice. The inferior vena cava enters the lower right atrium in a more medial position, slightly forward and leftward, so that it aims toward the fossa ovalis. Anterolateral to the orifice of the inferior vena cava lies the Eustachian valve, and anteromedial to this is the coronary sinus ostium. The anterior portion of the right atrium is trabeculated and thin walled, as is the right atrial appendage, which extends anteriorly to lie over the root of the aorta.

The atrial septum lies posteriorly and medially. A thin, fibrous depression, the fossa ovalis, is found in the center of the septum, and the muscular portion of the septum forms the limbus fossa ovalis.

The tricuspid valve leaflets are placed anteriorly, posteriorly, and medially. The medial, or septal, cusp lies in close relation to the membranous portion of the ventricular septum.

The inflow portion of the right ventricle is heavily trabeculated. Several papillary muscles attach to the tricuspid valve. The anterior papillary muscle originates from the moderator band and its chordae tendineae attach to the anterior and posterior cusps. The posterior papillary muscle attaches to the

*Pulmonic in this handbook refers to the valve, and pulmonary refers to the lungs. For example, pulmonic insufficiency means regurgitation through the valve, whereas pulmonary insufficiency refers to ventilatory insufficiency of the lungs.

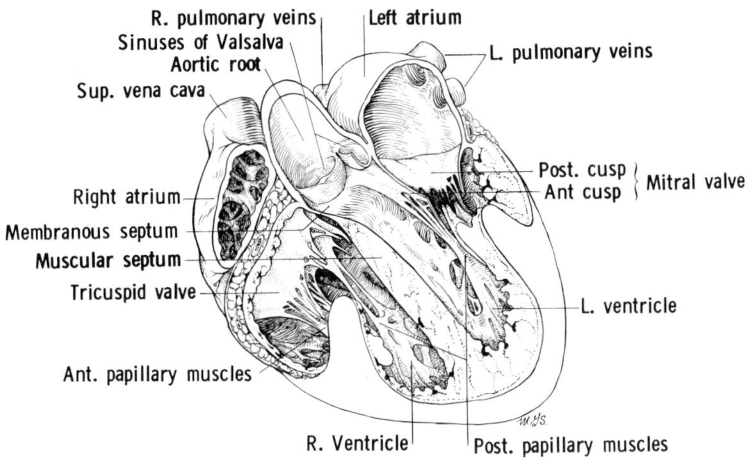

Figure 2. Semifrontal section of the heart. Note the intimate relation of the mitral and aortic valves. Note also the rightward angulation of the membranous portion of the ventricular septum.

posterior and septal cusps. A small, medial papillary muscle arises from the crista supraventricularis at its junction with the septal band and attaches to the anterior and septal cusps.

The outflow tract, or infundibulum, of the right ventricle is a smooth-walled, tubular structure delineated from the inflow portion by four prominent muscular bands: the crista supraventricularis and the parietal, moderator, and septal bands.

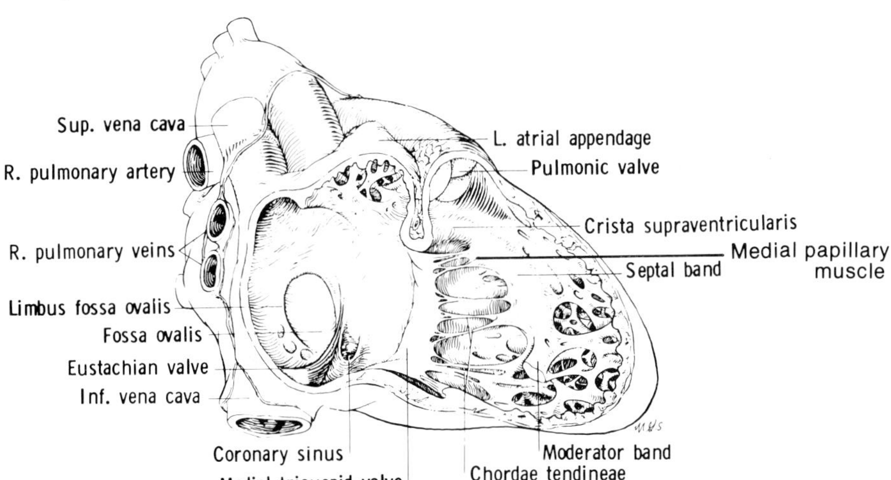

Figure 3. Semischematic view of the opened right side of the heart, illustrating both the right atrium and the right ventricle. Note the heavy trabeculation of the right ventricle in contrast to the smoother left ventricle shown in Figure 4.

The pulmonic valve, which lies at the top of the right ventricular outflow tract, has three cusps: right, left, and anterior.

LEFT HEART (Figures 2 and 4)

The left atrial wall is thicker than the right, and its internal surface is smoother. The left atrial appendage arises superiorly and anteriorly, and extends to the left of the pulmonary trunk to form a small portion of the left upper border of the cardiac silhouette, as viewed *en face*.

The mitral valve consists of two major cusps: a large anterior, or aortic, cusp and a posterior cusp. Usually, two small commissural cusps can also be identified.

The left ventricle has the shape of a megaphone, with the small end forming the apex. The septal surface of the left ventricular cavity is smooth and the free (parietal) wall is trabeculated, although the trabeculae are finer than those in the right ventricle.

Two papillary muscles—the anterior and the posterior—are present. Each attaches via its chordae to both the anterior and the posterior mitral valve cusps.

The ventricular septum is predominantly muscular. It presents a concave surface to the left ventricle and a convex surface to the right ventricle. The small membranous portion is located below the right and posterior aortic valve cusps, as viewed from left ventricle. The medial cusp of the tricuspid valve inserts across the membranous ventricular septum, dividing it into two portions. One portion lies between the left ventricle and the right atrium, the other between the left ventricle and right ventricle. The rightward angulation of the upper part of the ventricular septum forms the floor of the left ventricular outflow tract.

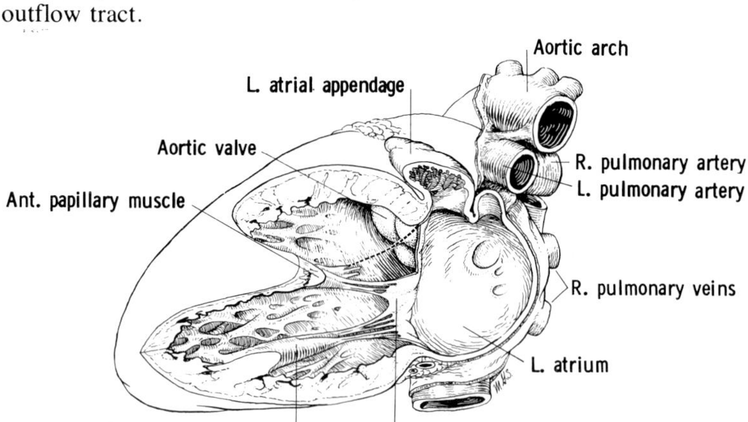

Figure 4. Semischematic view of the opened left side of the heart. A portion of the anterior leaflet of the mitral valve has been cut away (----) in order to view the aortic valve.

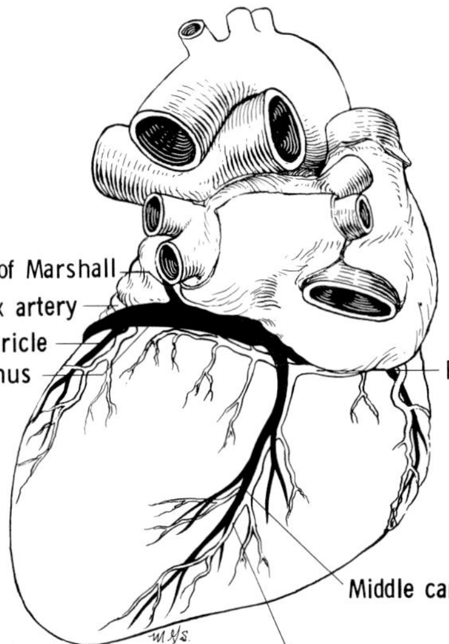

Figure 5. View of diaphragmatic (posterior, inferior) aspect of the heart and great vessels. Coronary vessels are indicated as in Figure 1.

The aortic valve consists of three semilunar cusps: right, left, and posterior. The coronary ostia lie within the sinuses of Valsalva of the right and left cusps. The left posterior cusps are in fibrous continuity with the anterior cusp of the mitral valve.

CORONARY VESSELS (Figures 1 and 5)

The right coronary artery arises from the right aortic sinus of Valsalva. It gives off several branches to the right atrium and right ventricle, including the posterior interventricular descending branch, which runs in the posterior interventricular groove. The left coronary artery originates from the left aortic sinus of Valsalva. It bifurcates within 1 or 2 cm into an anterior interventricular descending artery, which runs in the anterior interventricular groove, and a circumflex artery, which lies in the left atrioventricular groove. The branching pattern of the coronary arteries is subject to a great deal of variation, including an occasional third ostia in the right aortic sinus of Valsalva.

The major coronary veins are the great cardiac vein, the middle cardiac vein, and the posterior vein of the left ventricle. These all enter the coronary sinus from the left atrium, as does the oblique vein of Marshall.

BIBLIOGRAPHY

Netter, F. H. (comp.) 1969. Ciba Collection of Medical Illustrations. Vol. 5, The Heart. CIBA Pharmaceutical Co., Summit, N.J.

chapter 2

EMBRYOLOGY OF THE HEART

Our present knowledge of cardiac embryology is far from complete, especially with regard to the origins of some congenital heart defects. However, this chapter should provide a sound foundation for understanding the more common congenital heart defects.

Formation of the heart necessarily occurs while the heart is carrying out its intended function—pumping blood. The heart is the first organ to achieve functional development, a fact that has intrigued embryologists and cardiologists for some time and that undoubtedly is at least partially responsible for theories suggesting that hemodynamic forces exercise some degree of control on cardiac development. A suggested corollary of this theory is that altered patterns of blood flow may be responsible for abnormal cardiac development, particularly with regard to partitioning events (discussed later in this chapter under "Conversion of the Heart Tube to Final Form"). Blood flow is thought to exert its effect through a molding action on the wall of the primitive cardiac tube, made possible because of the presence of the malleable cardiac jelly.

It is astonishing to realize that the human heart completes its development in 4 weeks, beginning at the end of the third week of gestation. Formation of the heart is complete by the end of the seventh week, at which time the embryo is 25 mm in length and the heart itself is only 3 mm in length.

Growth of the various parts of the heart is not uniform. In general, fibrous or connective tissue components, such as valve annuli, endocardial cushions, truncoconal septa, the aorticopulmonary septum, and the membranous portion of the ventricular septum, complete their development early in embryonic life and thereafter grow relatively little as compared with the muscle mass of the heart (Figure 6). As noted, the heart reaches its adult form by the seventh embryonic week, with subsequent changes taking place only in size. The physical proximity in the adult heart of the great arteries, the septum that separates them, all four valves, and the ventricular and atrial septa is explained by noting that these structures were always intimately related. Their

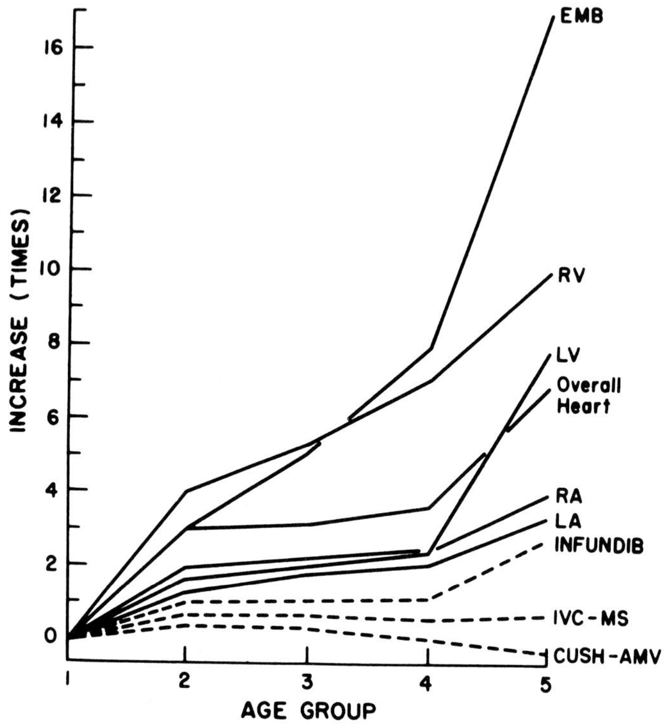

Figure 6. Rate of increase in certain linear measurements during growth of the human fetal heart. Measurements were made from 16 embryos from age groups 2 to 5 (28–50 days).

Key: emb = embryo, RV = right ventricle, LV = left ventricle, RA = right atrium, LA = left atrium, infundib = right ventricular infundibulum, IVC-MS = diameter of the interventricular canal, CUSH-AMV = width of the superior endocardial cushion and a corresponding measurement of the anterior leaflet of the mitral valve in later stages. (From Grant, R. P. 1962. Embryology of the ventricular flow pathways in man. Circulation 25:756. With the permission of the American Heart Association.)

lesser growth, and that of the connective tissue that separates them, serve to maintain their closeness from the time the heart first assumes its complete shape.

The developing cardiovascular system must also prepare for changing conditions that will appear after birth. Prior to birth, the foramen ovale and the ductus arteriosus provide pathways by which blood can bypass the lungs. After birth, these pathways must close rapidly, thus establishing separation of the pulmonary and systemic circulations. A detailed discussion of the anatomy and physiology of the fetal circulation and the changes that take place following birth is beyond the scope of this chapter. A lucid presentation of this material can be found in the first three chapters of Dr. Abraham Rudolph's recent monograph on congenital heart disease (see bibliography).

Most congenital heart anomalies are the results of structural abnormalities that occur in the first 4 to 5 weeks of pregnancy. In certain defects,

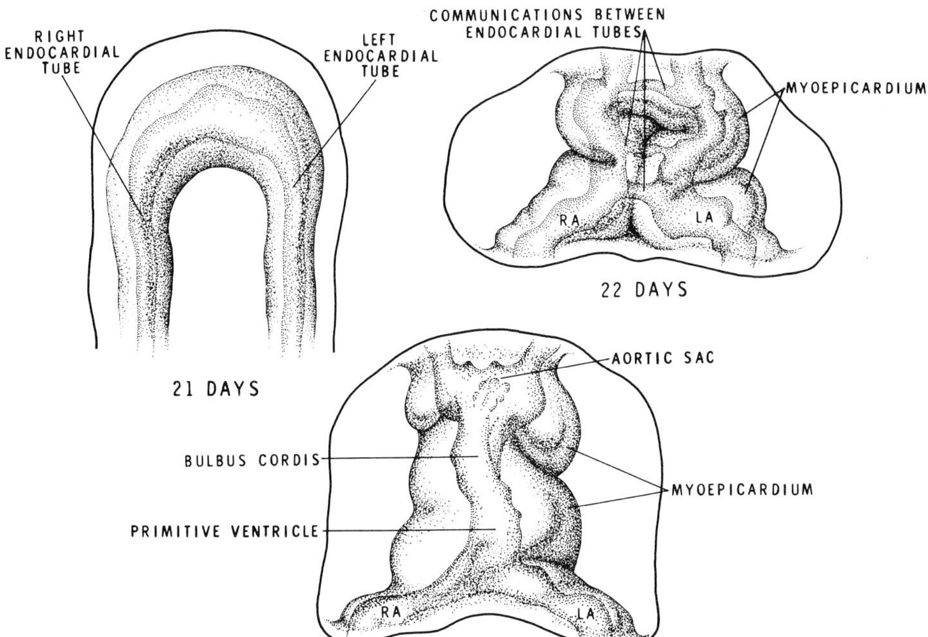

Figure 7. Three stages in the formation of the primary heart tube. Twenty-one days after fertilization, the heart is horseshoe shaped; at twenty-two days, the arms of the horseshoe come together and at their junction the wall breaks down, forming a single lumen; at twenty-three days, the primary heart tube is completed. (Adapted from Van Mierop, L. H. S. 1969. Sections on Anatomy of the Heart: Embryology of the Heart and Congenital Heart Disease. In the CIBA Collection of Medical Illustrations, Vol. 5, Circulatory System, Part 1.)

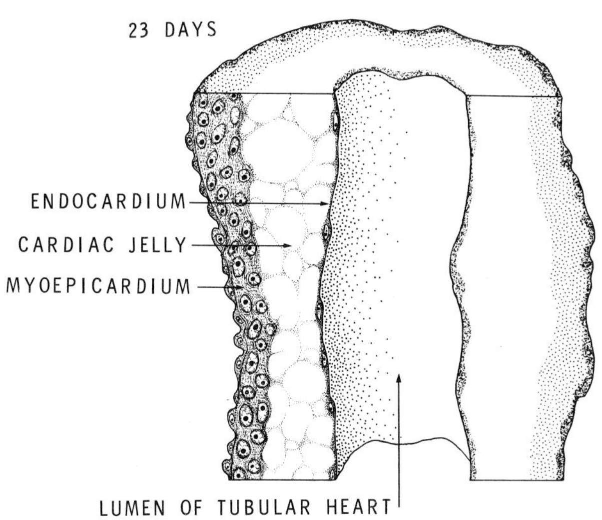

Figure 8. Schematic sagittal section through the 23-day-old heart. Three distinct layers of the wall can be identified; endothelium, cardiac jelly, and myoepicardium.

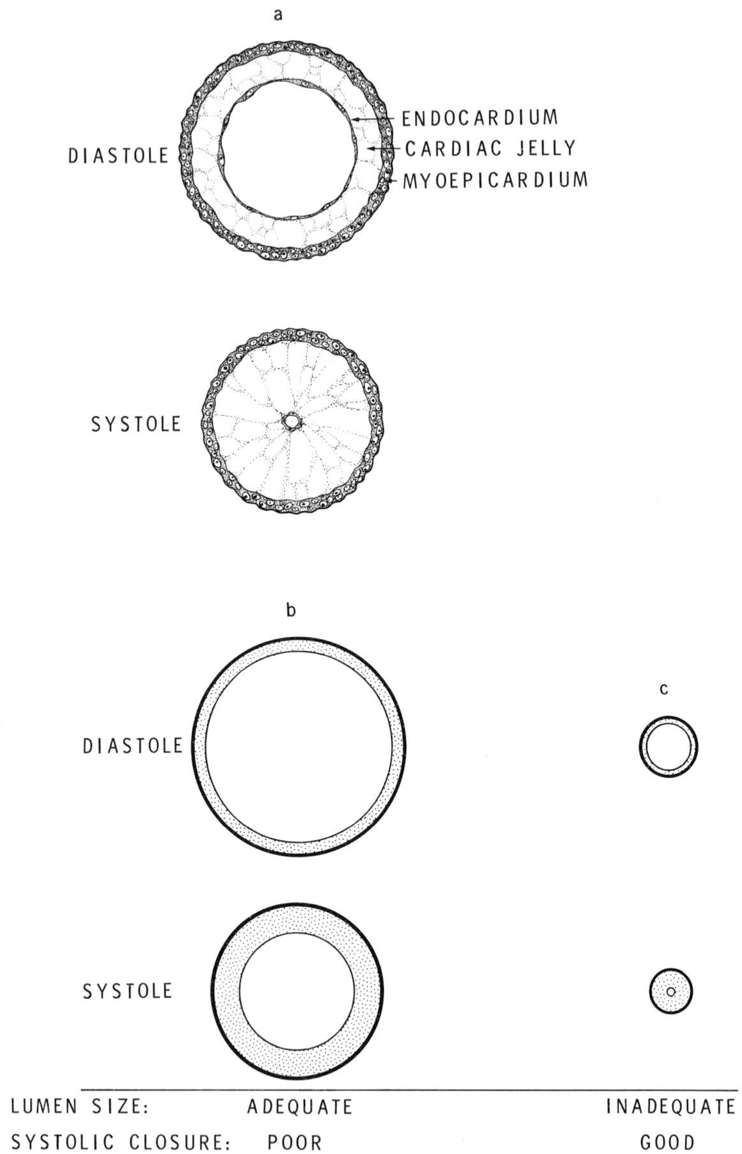

Figure 9. (a) One function of cardiac jelly is to increase wall thickness so that an adequate lumen size during diastole and an adequate closure during systole are obtained. (b) If the heart tube is thin walled and the lumen large enough to provide adequate flow, then adequate systolic closure cannot be obtained. (c) If the tube is thin walled but small enough to allow systolic closure, then the lumen volume is inadequate. (Adapted from Barry, A. 1948. The functional significance of the cardiac jelly in the tubular heart of the chick embryo. Anat. Rec. 102: 289.)

such as some cases of persistent patent ductus arteriosus and valvar pulmonic stenosis, the origin may be later in fetal life. Infants born with congenital heart anomalies most likely represent only a fraction of the total incidence of intrauterine cardiac anomalies, since the more severely affected embryos die early in embryonic life.

EARLY DEVELOPMENT OF THE HEART

At the end of the third week after fertilization, a horseshoe-shaped vascular plexus appears (Figure 7). Each limb of the horseshoe forms a single endothelial tube. Primarily because of growth of the embryo, which alters the embryo's form and spatial relationships, these bilateral endothelial tubes eventually meet in midline. At about the twenty-third day these tubes fuse to form a single, rhythmically beating heart tube.

The heart tube is composed of three layers (Figure 8): an inner layer of endocardium lines the lumen, the outer, or myoepicardial, layer eventually forms both the epicardium and myocardium, and between these two lies a thicker layer composed of an acellular, transparent material known as cardiac jelly. Cardiac jelly, a relatively noncompressible but malleable substance, has important physiologic implications. In order for a tubular heart to propel a sufficient quantity of blood in one direction only, the tube must have walls thick enough to provide both systolic closure (valve action) and an effective stroke volume (Figure 9a). A thin-walled tube could perform effectively only one of these functions; cardiac jelly provides the necessary thickness (Figure 9b,c). Apposition of mounds of cardiac jelly results in a primitive type of valve action to ensure unidirectional flow. Since cardiac jelly is plastic, flow of blood through the heart tube may mold the cardiac jelly and influence cardiac development. The biochemistry of cardiac jelly has been of interest recently. It contains a large amount of glycosaminoglycans (acid mucopolysaccharides) that are derived for the most part, if not entirely, from the endothelial lining.

FURTHER DEVELOPMENT OF THE HEART TUBE

The paired atria communicate with the caudal end of the heart tube through the atrioventricular orifice. Continuing in the direction of blood flow, the initial portion of the heart tube dilates and can be identified as the early embryonic ventricle. The middle portion will become the bulbus cordis, and the cranial, or arterial, portion forms the aortic sac, which gives rise to the aortic arches. The heart tube, lying within the confines of the pericardial cavity, is fixed only at its cranial and caudal ends. It grows more rapidly than the pericardial cavity and thus is forced to bend sharply. This results in a C-shaped loop with the convexity directed anteriorly and rightward. Further growth results in a more complex S-shaped curve (Figure 10). As a consequence of these changes, the atrioventricular junction and the early embryonic ventricle move to the left. The atria enlarge dorsocranially and thus soon come to lie cranial to the ventricular region, the orientation found in the completed heart. As the atrial and ventricular portions enlarge, their junction, which remains relatively narrow, becomes the atrioventricular canal. Similarly, the first and second portions of the heart tube (i.e., the embryonic ventricle and the bulbus cordis) dilate while their junction, which will become the interventricular foramen, remains relatively narrow. Approximately 25 days after fertilization, two areas break down on the ventral surface of the heart tube, on either side of the interventricular foramen. This process, called trabeculation, is the mechanism by which the definitive ventricles are formed.

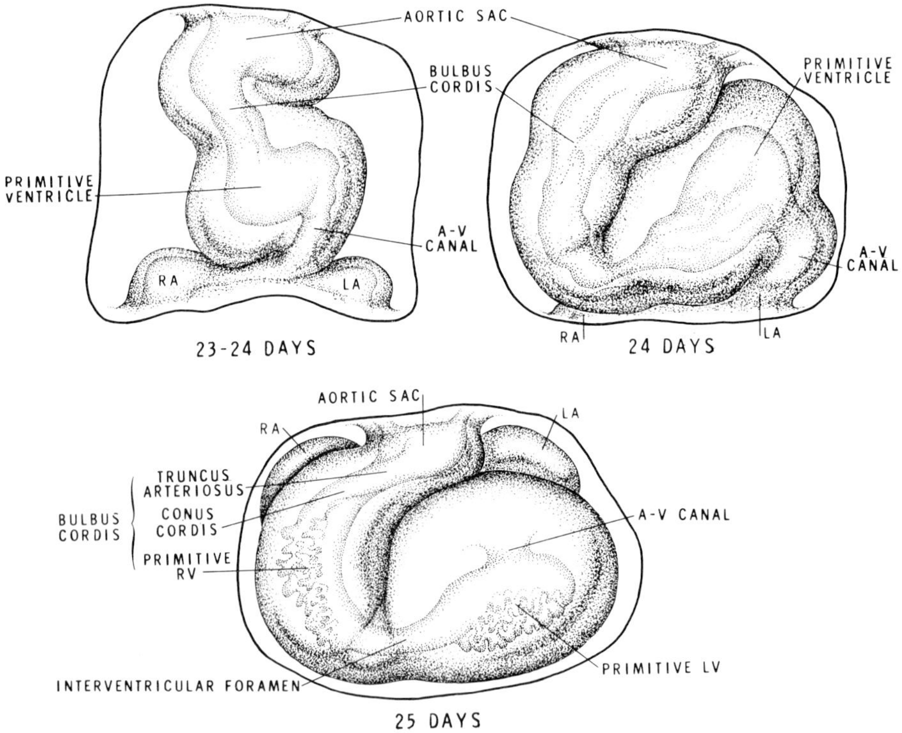

Figure 10. Evolution of the heart tube from simple to complex form. At 23 days of age, bending of the heart tube is just beginning; by 24 days, a C-shaped loop has formed. At 25 days, the atria have grown posterosuperiorly, reorienting the AV canal, trabeculation has begun, indicating the site of both ventricles, and the components of the bulbus cordis can be identified. (Adapted from Van Mierop, L. H. S. 1969. Sections on Anatomy of the Heart: Embryology of the Heart and Congenital Heart Disease. In the CIBA Collection of Medical Illustrations, Vol. 5, Circulatory System, Part 1.)

The trabeculated area distal, or downstream, to the interventricular foramen lies at the beginning of the bulbus cordis. As the early heart tube was divided into three components (primitive ventricle, bulbus cordis, and aortic sac), so the bulbus cordis can also be divided into three parts. The proximal portion becomes trabeculated and will form the right ventricle. The middle portion, which will form both the left and right ventricular outflow tracts, is called the conus cordis. The distal portion, which will form the proximal aorta and pulmonary trunk, is called the truncus arteriosus.

CONVERSION OF THE HEART TUBE TO FINAL FORM

Two basic architectural changes convert the heart tube from its original to its final form. The first, *rotation* of the bulbus cordis from right to left, brings the bulbus cordis into its adult relationship to the embryonic (left) ventricle. The growth force factors responsible for this have not been determined, although two can be suggested. Rapid growth of the atria might push the distal portion of the bulbus cordis toward the left, or, since the heart lies within a confined space, posterior growth of the right ventricle might push the right side toward the left.

The second basic change is *partitioning,* or *septation*. Formation of the various cardiac septa begins on approximately day 27 of gestation, and continues for 10 days. There are two quite different mechanisms for septal formation. A septum may be elaborated passively because of the increasing growth of the chambers it separates. In other words, the septum is left behind as the chambers enlarge. In man, the atrial septum secundum, the muscular ventricular septum, and the aorticopulmonary septum are formed passively. A septum may also form by active growth into a lumen of opposing tissue mounds, which then fuse. Such actively formed septa are the atrioventricular canal septum, the conus cordis septum, and the truncus arteriosus septum. The atrial septum primum is formed by both mechanisms.

Partitioning events are divided into five phases for purposes of this discussion. Keep in mind, however, that all of these events are occurring simultaneously:

1. Division of the atrioventricular canal into mitral and tricuspid orifices
2. Formation of the proximal ascending aorta and the pulmonary trunk from the truncus arteriosus
3. Formation of the right and left ventricular outflow tracts
4. Formation of the muscular portion of the ventricular septum
5. Formation of the atrial septa

At the end of the fourth embryonic week, two mounds of mesenchymal tissue—the superior and inferior endocardial cushions—appear on the superior and inferior walls of the atrioventricular canal (Figure 11). At this time,

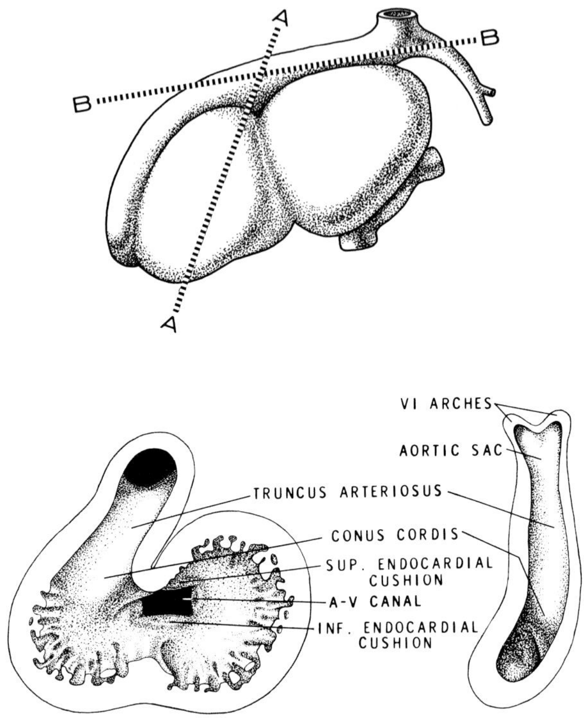

27 DAYS

Figure 11. The upper figure is to aid orientation to the remainder of Figure 11 and to Figure 12. Line A-A indicates the plane of the left-hand series of drawings, and line B-B indicates the plane of the right-hand series. At age 27 days, the initial stage of endocardial cushion formation, before truncoconal septation, has begun. (Adapted from Van Mierop, L. H. S. 1969. Sections on Anatomy of the Heart: Embryology of the Heart and Congenital Heart Disease. In the CIBA Collection of Medical Illustrations, Vol. 5, Circulatory System, Part I.)

the atrioventricular orifice has begun to shift medially, but is separated from the conus cordis by the bulboventricular flange. This flange is the internal expression of the infolding of the wall of the primitive heart tube, brought about by its bending to the right. The bulboventricular flange is created passively and has no inherent growth potential. Still, it must recede, which it does over the next several days (Figure 12a), allowing direct access of the right side of the atrioventricular canal to the right ventricle, as well as permitting access from the left ventricle directly into the posteromedial portion of the conus cordis and therefore into the aorta. As the superior and inferior cushions enlarge and approximate each other, two smaller lateral cushions appear at the right and left edges of the atrioventricular canal. Fusion of the major cushions divides the atrioventricular canal into two orifices. The fused cushions then arch posteriorly, presenting a convexity to the atria (Figure 12b).

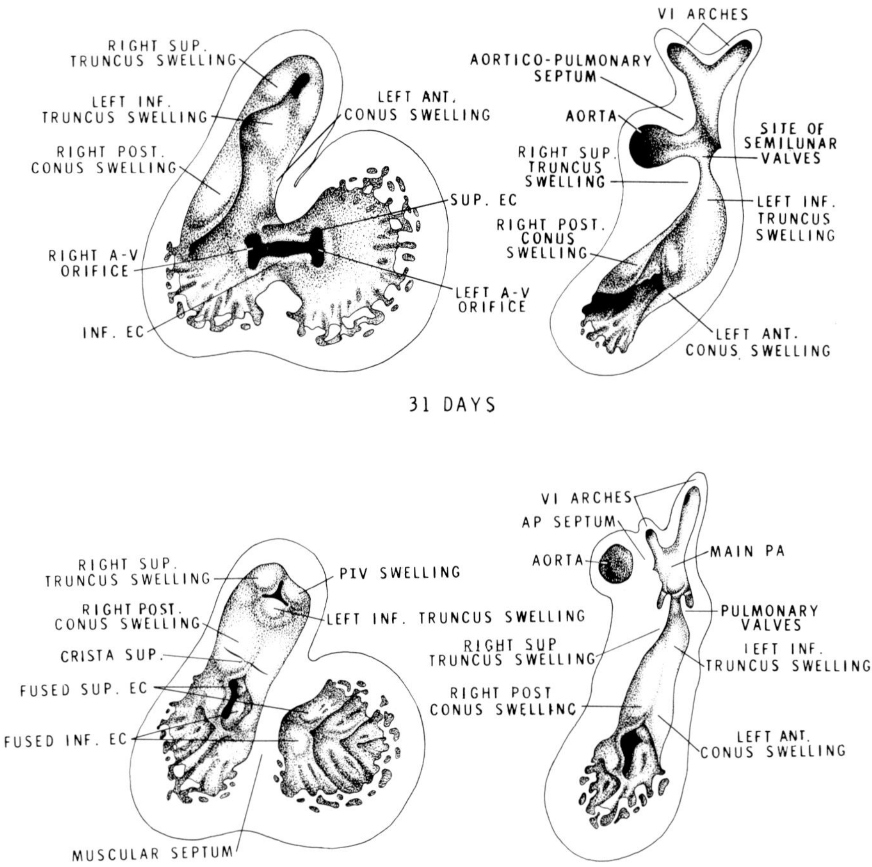

37 DAYS

Figure 12. (a) Age 31 days: on the left, endocardial cushion development has progressed and the process of division of the atrioventricular canal into two openings can be seen. The truncoconal septa are well formed. The right-hand drawing depicts division of the truncus arteriosus. The site of the semilunar valves can be identified. (b) Age 37 days: septation is almost complete, the right and left circulations are separate, and the pulmonic valve is nearing completion. (Adapted from Van Mierop, L. H. S. 1969. Sections on Anatomy of the Heart: Embryology of the Heart and Congenital Heart Disease. In the CIBA Collection of Medical Illustrations, Vol. 5, Circulatory System, Part I.)

This is met by the down-growing septum primum, which reaches and joins the posterior surface of the cushion (Figure 13). Once fusion of these structures occurs, there is little subsequent growth; therefore their close relationship is retained in the adult heart.

Similarly, two opposing mounds of endocardial cushion-like tissue appear on the right superior and the left inferior walls of the truncus arteriosus, along a spiral course of approximately 180° (see Figure 12). Fusion of these spiral truncal swellings divides the truncus arteriosus into the proximal ascending aorta and the pulmonary trunk, and accounts for their characteristic entwined structure. It should be emphasized that the truncus septum does not begin in one location and then grow along a spiral course, but rather the opposing spiral tissue masses arise simultaneously and grow inward until they meet. In the chick embryo, two streams of blood can be seen to spiral around each other in the truncus prior to the beginning of truncal septal development. This has led to the hypothesis that spiraling of blood determines the spiraling of the septum. Proximally, the truncus swellings meet with another pair of similar swellings that have developed in the conus cordis. Distally, the truncus swellings approach the aortic sac. Expansion of the aortic sac and shifting of the fourth and sixth arches result in an invagination between the origins of these two pairs of arches. This passively formed aorticopulmonary septum fuses with the truncus septa, completing formation of the aortic and pulmonary channels.

The two swellings that appear on the right posterior and the left anterior walls of the conus cordis fuse with each other and become continuous with the right superior and left inferior truncus swellings, respectively. Proximally, the right posterior conus swelling terminates at the tricuspid orifice, joining the superior endocardial cushion, and the left anterior conus swelling extends to

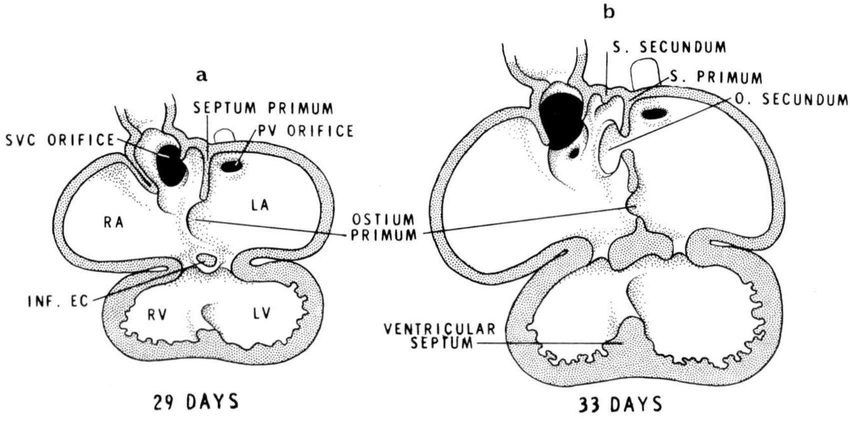

Figure 13. Stages in development of the atrial and ventricular septa. (a) At 29 days the septum primum is growing down toward the endocardial cushions, which are just appearing. (b) At 33 days, ostium secundum has appeared in septum primum and septum secundum has just begun to be elaborated. The interventricular septum is well defined. (c) At 37 days, ostium primum has closed. The endocardial cushions have curved with the convexity posterosuperiorly toward the atria. The atrioventricular valves are forming. (d) At 55 days, the ventricular septum is complete, as are the AV valves. Septum secundum now overlies the septum primum, forming the foramen ovale.

Key: S = septum, O = ostium, PV = pulmonary vein. (Adapted from Van Mierop, L. H. S. 1969. Sections on Anatomy of the Heart: Embryology of the Heart and Congenital Heart Disease. In the CIBA Collection of Medical Illustrations, Vol. 5, Circulatory System, Part 1.)

the anterior portion of the muscular ventricular septum. On the right side, the process results in the formation of the right ventricular infundibulum and accounts for the fact that the tricuspid and pulmonic valves are separated by muscular tissue, the crista supraventricularis. Since muscular tissue later grows more than connective tissue elements, the tricuspid and pulmonic valves become widely separated in the adult heart. In contrast, the aortic and

c

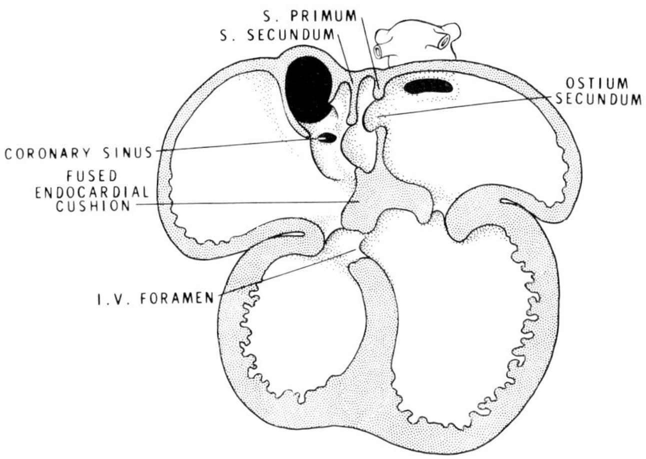

37 DAYS

d

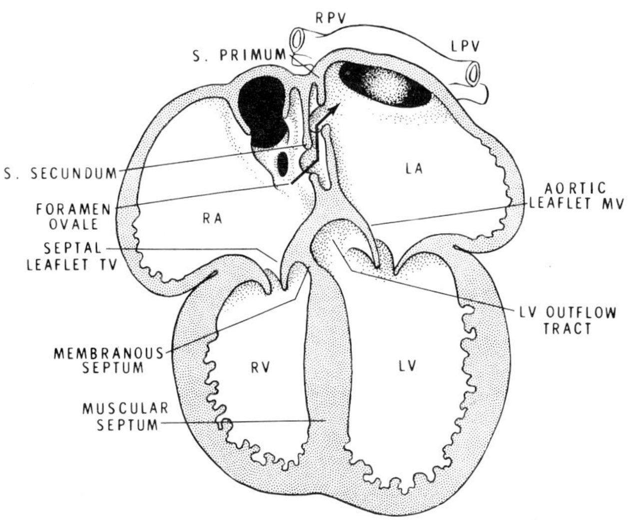

55 DAYS

Figure 13. *continued*

mitral valves, which are joined by connective tissue that grows little after fusion, remain intimately related.

The muscular portion of the ventricular septum is elaborated passively as the ventricles enlarge (Figure 14). The septum does not begin distally and grow up into the interventricular canal; rather, its completion is accomplished by growth of tissue originating from the inferior endocardial cushion and the conus septum.

As the endocardial cushions and conal swellings develop and join, the plane of the interventricular foramen changes so that it is bounded by the muscular ventricular septum anteroinferiorly and by the endocardial cushions and the conus septum posterosuperiorly. It is along this rightward-inclined plane that completion of the ventricular septum occurs. This reorientation of the interventricular foramen along an axis almost perpendicular to the long axis of the left ventricle accounts for the sharp bend in the left ventricular outflow tract of the adult heart, where it leads into the root of the aorta (see Figure 13d). This angulation of the aortic root also accounts for its relationship to the right ventricle. Thus, in any large membranous ventricular septal defect, the aorta seems to originate in part from the right ventricle, ''overriding'' the ventricular septum.

The truncus arteriosus, as it crosses the roof of the common atrium, results in a depression in the expanding atria, which internally creates septum primum (see Figure 13a). The superior and inferior limbs of this septum reach the endocardial cushions and thus encircle an opening known as ostium

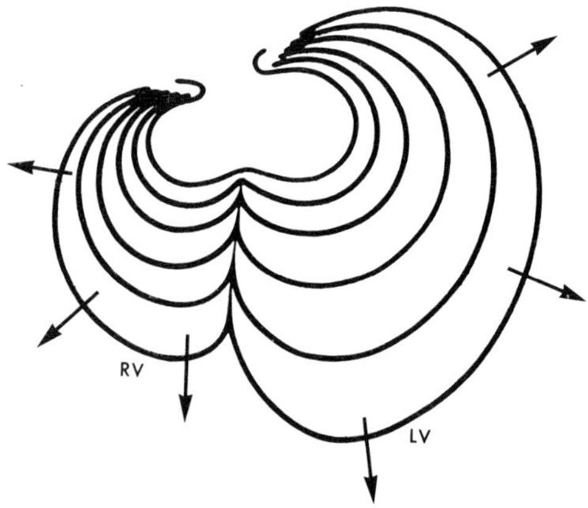

Figure 14. Schematic representation of the passive elaboration of the interventricular septum. Each concentric line represents a further stage in the development of the ventricles. As can be seen, enlargement of the ventricles results in a progressively larger wall (septum) between them. (From Van Mierop, L. H. S., Alley, R. D., Kausel, H. W., and Stranahan, A. 1963. Pathogenesis of transposition complexes. I. Embryology of the ventricles and great arteries. Am. J. Cardiol. 12:216.)

primum. Extensions of tissue from the superior and inferior endocardial cushions and actively growing tissue on the free edge of septum primum grow together and fuse, obliterating ostium primum. Before this closure occurs, a degeneration must take place in septum primum and a second opening (ostium secundum) must appear. This opening is essential for the continued passage of blood from the right atrium to the left atrium. Continued growth of the atria results in another passively formed septum, septum secundum, lying just to the right of septum primum. The leading edge of septum secundum soon comes to overlie ostium secundum, creating the foramen ovale (see Figure 13d). Prenatally, right atrial pressure is greater than left atrial pressure, and blood flows from the right atrium to the left atrium through the foramen ovale. Within minutes after birth, pulmonary blood flow increases and left atrial pressure exceeds right atrial pressure. Septum primum is forced against septum secundum, functionally obliterating the passage between the atria. Anatomic closure occurs within a few weeks in most individuals, although approximately 20% of the population maintains indefinitely some degree of anatomic patency of foramen ovale.

FORMATION OF THE VALVES

A significant portion of the atrioventricular valves is formed from the endocardial cushions. The superior and inferior portions of the aortic leaflet of the mitral valve are formed from the superior and inferior endocardial cushions, respectively. The inferior cushion also forms the major part of the septal leaflet of the tricuspid valve. The remaining AV valve cusps are formed by a process of excavation of the ventricular wall at the atrioventricular orifice (see Figures 12 and 13).

The semilunar valves are formed from the distal end of the truncus swellings and from a pair of smaller, intercalated valve swellings that are located on the walls of the truncus arteriosus in a line perpendicular to the line of fusion of the truncus swellings. Each of the two truncus swellings contributes one cusp to the aortic valve and one to the pulmonic valve. Together with a cusp derived from an intercalated valve swelling, this provides three cusps for each valve. The valve cusps themselves are formed by excavation of these swellings in a direction toward the ventricle (see Figure 12).

DEVELOPMENTAL HISTORY OF THE AORTIC ARCHES

A total of six aortic arches develop, although all are not present at any one time. Only three arch pairs persist: the third, fourth, and sixth (Figure 15). That portion of both dorsal aortae between the third and fourth arches disappears by the thirty-fifth day of gestation. With lengthening of the third arches

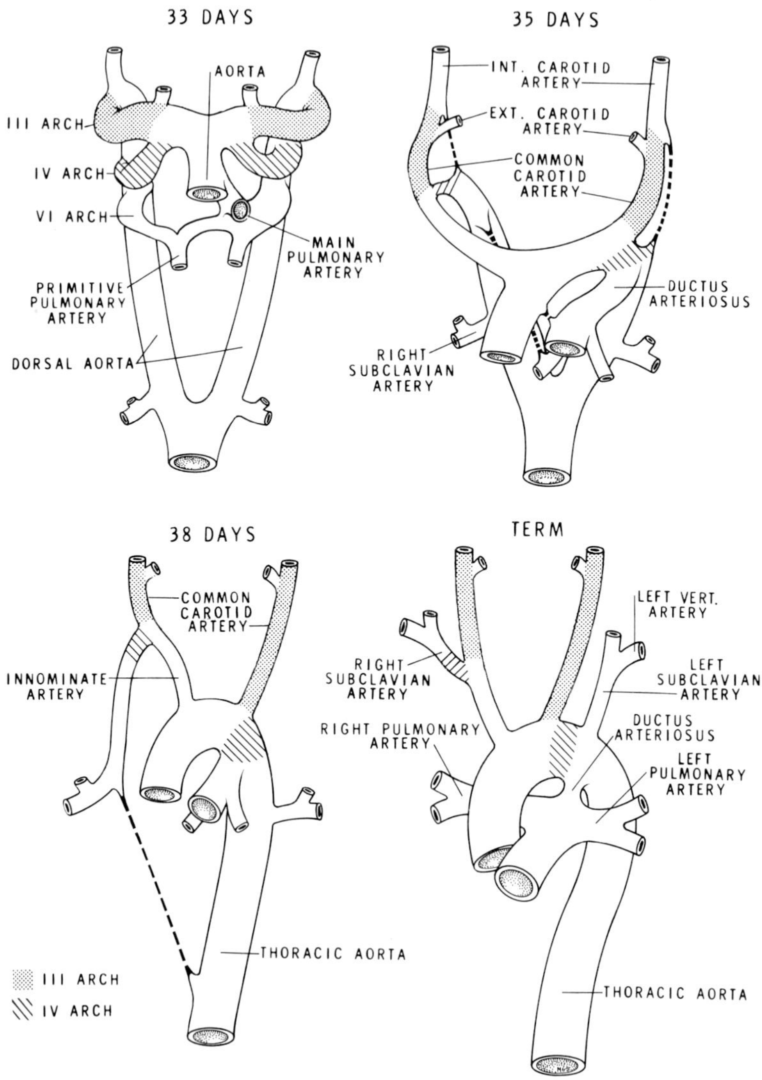

Figure 15. Stages in the development of the third, fourth, and sixth aortic arches. Note that the fourth arches form only a small part of the completed system. The right fourth arch forms the initial portion of the right subclavian artery. The left fourth arch forms only the portion of the aortic arch between the left common carotid and the left subclavian arteries. The innominate artery and the ascending aorta to the origin of the left common carotid artery are derived from the aortic sac and not from the arch system. (Adapted from Van Mierop, L. H. S. 1969. Sections on Anatomy of the Heart: Embryology of the Heart and Congenital Heart Disease. In the CIBA Collection of Medical Illustrations, Vol. 5, Circulatory System, Part 1.)

as the heart grows downward, the aortic sac lengthens to form the innominate artery on the right side and the aortic arch on the left side, up to the origin of the left common carotid artery.

The distal portion of the right dorsal aorta disappears by the thirty-eighth day of gestation, but the proximal portion remains as part of the right subclavian artery. Because of differences in growth rates along the aorta, the left subclavian artery appears to migrate toward the left common carotid artery.

The right fourth arch forms the initial portion of the right subclavian artery. The left fourth arch forms that portion of the definitive arch of the aorta between the left common carotid and the left subclavian arteries. The distal portion of the right sixth arch disappears by the thirty-fifth day of gestation, and the distal left sixth arch becomes the ductus arteriosus. The proximal portion of the sixth arch forms the initial segments of the pulmonary arteries.

The derivatives of the aortic arch system may be summarized as follows:

Truncus arteriosus	Proximal ascending aorta, main pulmonary artery
Aortic sac	Right segment: distal ascending aorta and innominate artery Left segment: arch of the aorta to origin of left common carotid artery
Third arches	Common carotid arteries and initial portion of the internal carotid arteries
Fourth arches	Right: Initial segment of right subclavian artery Left: Aortic arch between left common carotid and left subclavian arteries
Sixth arches	Right: Proximal portion forms initial segment of right pulmonary artery Left: Proximal portion forms initial segment of left pulmonary artery
Right dorsal aorta	Proximal portion becomes part of the right subclavian artery
Left dorsal aorta	Thoracic descending aorta

THE GREAT VEINS

The venous system, originally a bilaterally symmetric system, gradually becomes asymmetric as a result of obliteration of many of its channels. Initially, both the left and the right common cardinal veins, which drain the upper body, drain into the left and right horns of the sinus venosus. The right common cardinal vein develops preferentially and forms the superior vena cava. The left common cardinal vein usually loses its connection with the sinus venosus and disappears. The transverse portion of the sinus venosus persists as the coronary sinus. A number of venous systems that drain the lower body contribute to the formation of the inferior vena cava.

The common pulmonary vein originates as a single vessel growing out from the posterior wall of the left atrium, just to the left of septum primum (see Figure 13a). It connects with a plexus of veins in the area of the lung buds that is known as the splanchnic plexus. Initially, this plexus has connections with systemic venous plexuses both above and below the diaphragm (septum transversum), which gradually disappear. The common pulmonary vein and its first four branches enlarge and finally become incorporated into the left atrium (see Figure 13b).

BIBLIOGRAPHY

Barry, A. 1948. The functional significance of the cardiac jelly in the tubular heart of the chick embryo. Anat. Rec. 102:289–298.

Bremer, J. L. 1932. The presence and influence of two spiral streams in the heart of the chick embryo. Am. J. Anat. 49:409–440.

deVries, P. A., and Saunders, J. B. de C. M. 1962. Development of the ventricles and spiral outflow tract in the human heart. A contribution to the development of the human heart from age group IX to age group XV. Contrib. Embryol. 37:89–114.

Grant, R. P. 1962. The embryology of ventricular flow pathways in man. Circulation 25:756–779.

Patten, B. M. 1953. Human Embryology, 2nd ed. Blakiston, New York.

Patten, B. M., Kramer, T. C., and Barry, A. 1948. Valvular action in the embryonic chick heart by localized apposition of the endocardial masses. Anat. Rec. 102:299–308.

Rudolph, A. M. 1974. Congenital Diseases of the Heart. Year Book Medical Publishers, Inc., Chicago.

Van Mierop, L. H. S. 1969. Sections on anatomy of the heart; embryology of the heart and congenital heart disease. In the Ciba Collection of Medical Illustrations, Vol. 5, Circulatory System, Part 1. CIBA Pharmaceutical Co., Summit, N.J.

chapter 3

EXPERIMENTAL PRODUCTION OF CONGENITAL HEART DEFECTS

A variety of physical and chemical agents have been reported to cause congenital heart defects in experimental animals. In most instances, experimentally produced heart defects are only part of a general catastrophe in which many organ systems are affected. However, when the teratogen is applied directly to the heart, as in the case of x-irradiation or mechanical devices, heart defects alone can be produced. A mechanism of action has not been established for any of the cardiac teratogens.

Dr. James G. Wilson has proposed five general principles of experimental teratology (see bibliography):

1. Susceptibility of an embryo to a teratogen depends on the developmental stage at which an agent is applied.
2. Each teratogenic agent acts in a specific way on a particular aspect of cellular metabolism.
3. Genotype influences to a greater or lesser degree an animal's reaction to a teratogenic agent.
4. Any agent capable of causing malformation also causes an increase in embryonic mortality.
5. A teratogenic agent need not be deleterious to the maternal organism.

In recent years many agents capable of causing congenital heart defects in experimental animals have been described. These included drugs, chemicals, deficiency states, infectious agents, and mechanical devices. In addition, some investigators have operated on late gestational fetuses to cause specific defects for intrauterine hemodynamic investigations. A few examples are presented of experimental teratology of the cardiovascular system, as well as those human teratogens that have been established with reasonable certainty.

EXPERIMENTAL ANIMAL TERATOGENS

Application of a teratogen to pregnant experimental animals will result in varying ratios of affected offspring depending on the potency of the teratogen, the time of application, and the susceptibility of the species. Within an exposed litter, there will often be normal as well as affected embryos. This illustrates an important teratologic principle that is analogous to the finding in human twin studies—it is unusual for both twins to have congenital heart defects, even when the twins are identical (see further discussion in Chapter 4).

Maternal vitamin deficiency states (vitamin A, riboflavin, folic acid, pantothenic acid) in the rat have caused predominantly ventricular septal defects or aortic arch anomalies. Both vitamin A and vitamin D intoxication can also produce heart defects. Vitamin D intoxication in the rabbit can produce lesions analogous to those seen in humans with supravalvar aortic stenosis syndrome, thought to be related to hypercalcemia prior to birth.

Trypan blue (an azo dye) is a potent teratogen when injected into a pregnant rat. Heart defects produced include ventricular septal defects, aortic arch anomalies, transposition complexes, atrial septal defects, anomalies of the atrioventricular valves, and great vein anomalies, especially involving the left superior vena cava. The incidence of heart defects may be as high as 60%. Trypan blue is a potent inhibitor of synthesis of glycosaminoglycans, compounds that are abundant in cardiac jelly. Sibling variation may be very marked, and species variation is also great. In contrast to almost all other

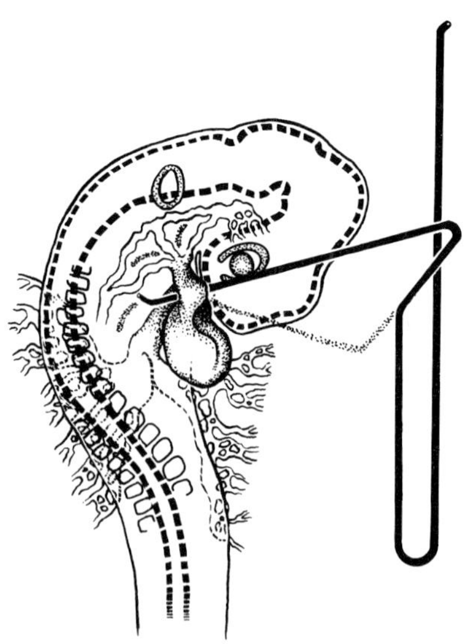

Figure 16. Diagram of a 3-day-old chick embryo with a fine wire in place. Note that, in reference to the embryo, the wire is lifting the truncoconal region of the heart tube rightward and anteriorly.

maternally administered teratogens, a cardiac defect may occur in the absence of any other demonstrable congenital abnormality.

Salicylates, also glycosaminoglycan synthesis inhibitors, have caused congenital heart defects in the chick. In the human fetus aspirin has been implicated in premature closure of the ductus arteriosus by means of the ability of aspirin to inhibit prostaglandin synthesis. Whether or not aspirin can cause structural heart defects in the human embryo is unknown.

X-irradiation of the chick embryo heart results in ventricular septal defects, aortic arch and truncoconal abnormalities, and semilunar valve anomalies. Endocardial cushion derivatives seem to be the most sensitive cardiac tissues, and the muscular septum the least sensitive. It is also possible to produce ventricular septal defects and aortic arch anomalies by irradiating neighboring tissues while the heart itself is shielded. Direct radiation of the

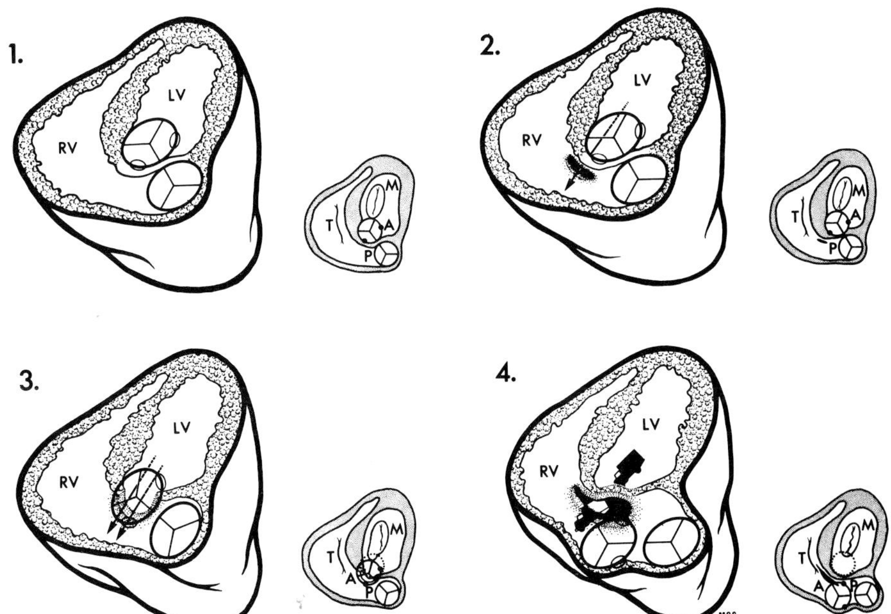

Figure 17. (1) Normal chick heart anatomy. The various defects found following the mechanical interference illustrated in Figure 16 are: (2) ventricular septal defect; (3) ventricular septal defect and movement of the aorta so as to override the ventricular septum; and (4) large ventricular septal defect and displacement of the aorta so that it now exits entirely from the right ventricle (origin of both great vessels from the right ventricle).

The smaller drawings schematically illustrate the "ventricular skeleton," emphasizing the anatomic relationship of the valves and the ventricular septum. The larger drawings give a three-dimensional representation emphasizing relationships of the semilunar valves and the ventricular septum. The coronary ostia, illustrated in all drawings, are always found in the two aortic sinuses on either side of the aorticopulmonary septum.

Key: RV = right ventricle, LV = left ventricle, M = mitral valve, AV = aortic valve, T = tricuspid orifice, and P = pulmonic valve.

Table 1. Spectrum of anomalies versus duration of injury

Type of anomaly	Hours of wire placement 24	48	60
Normal	12		
Widened left ventricular outflow tract	15		
Widened left ventricular outflow tract plus ventricular septal defect	20	32	15
Ventricular septal defect with overriding aorta		35	15
Double outlet right ventricle		30	35
Double inlet left ventricle (usually with double outlet right ventricle)		15	50

exposed rat fetus affects predominantly endocardial cushion tissue derivatives. Aortic arch and great vein anomalies may also be seen, as in trypan blue–induced defects. Cardiac anomalies may be produced in as many as 25% of the rats.

Manipulative procedures have also been developed for producing congenital heart defects in the chick embryo. *Surgical occlusion* of the developing aortic arches produces ventricular septal, aortic arch, and truncoconal defects. A ventricular septal defect is always present concurrent with certain aortic arch abnormalities; its incidence depends on which aortic arches are occluded. Occlusion of nonfunctioning arches (first, second, and fifth) may not result in defects, while occlusion of definitive arches will always result in anomalies.

Mechanical interference with the developing embryonic heart produces anomalies in approximately 90% of embryos. Temporary distortion of the truncoconal area of the chick embryo heart tube (Figure 16) results in ventricular septal defects, ventricular septal defects with overriding aorta, double outlet from the right ventricle, and double inlet to the left ventricle (Figure 17). The severity of the malformation depends on the duration of the interference (Table 1).

HUMAN CARDIAC TERATOGENS

Maternal rubella has been shown to produce ventricular septal defects, patent ductus arteriosus, valvar pulmonic stenosis, and multiple peripheral coarctations of the pulmonary arteries. The incidence of cardiac defects when maternal rubella occurs in early pregnancy is probably not less than 20% and possibly as high as 80%. Studies have shown that infection of the fetus with rubella virus can occur without clinical evidence of disease in the mother. In addition, the fetus may continue to harbor the virus even after it is no longer recoverable from the mother. Cultures of rubella virus have been grown from prenatally infected babies as long as 18 months after birth. Thus, these infants have the capacity to infect personnel involved in their care.

Thalidomide, when ingested by a pregnant woman, produces phocomelia, as well as many other severe congenital defects, among her offspring. The most frequent cause of death among affected children is congenital heart disease. The most common anomaly is truncus arteriosus, followed by tetralogy of Fallot. Ventricular septal defects, atrial septal defects, transposition complexes, and anomalous pulmonary venous connections have also been reported. The incidence of cardiac anomalies among live-born infants with the thalidomide syndrome is at least 40%.

The fetal alcohol syndrome, initially described in France in 1968, has been elucidated over the past 5 years in several publications from the University of Washington. Born to women with severe chronic alcoholism, these infants demonstrate numerous abnormalities, including a 50% incidence of cardiac defects, mainly of the cardiac septa.

Anticonvulsants, particularly diphenylhydantoin (Dilantin), have been strongly implicated in producing heart defects in infants of mothers on chronic therapy. Multiple defects of other organ systems are also present.

Sex hormones remain controversial as a human cardiac teratogen, but most of the evidence strongly implicates them. A retrospective study of infant deaths from congenital heart disease published in 1977 revealed a substantial incidence of exposure to sex hormones. Other studies have given similar results, including some that have suggested transposition of the great vessels as a particular risk.

Exposure to *lithium,* a psychiatric drug, can result in a variety of congenital heart defects, most notably Ebstein's anomaly.

Although *Coxsackie virus* has been implicated in production of congenital heart defects in both human and experimental animals, the data is not totally convincing. Most workers would agree, however, that it is unlikely that rubella would be the only virus capable of producing human heart defects.

Finally, it is well known that infants born to *diabetic mothers* have a substantially increased incidence of congenital heart disease. In one review of 470 such infants, 4% had heart defects, with transposition of the great vessels, ventricular septal defect, or coarctation of the aorta being the most common.

BIBLIOGRAPHY

Anderson, R. C. 1976. Cardiac defects in children of mothers receiving anticonvulsant therapy during pregnancy. J. Pediatr. 89:318–319.

Gessner, I. H. 1966. Spectrum of congenital cardiac anomalies produced in chick embryos by mechanical interference with cardiogenesis. Circ. Res. 18:625–633.

Gessner, I. H., and Van Mierop, L. H. S. 1970. Experimental production of cardiac defects: The spectrum of dextroposition of the aorta. Am. J. Cardiol. (DeHaan Symposium) 25:272–278.

Hanson, J. W., Jones, K. L., and Smith, D. W. 1976. Fetal Alcohol Syndrome. JAMA 235:1458–1460.

Hanson, J. W., Myrianthopoulos, N. C., Harvey, M. A. S., and Smith, D. W. 1976. Risks to the offspring of women treated with hydantoin anti-convulsants, with emphasis on the fetal hydantoin syndrome. J. Pediatr. 89:662–668.

Janerich, D. T., Dugan, J. M., Standfast, S. J., and Strite, L. 1977. Congenital heart disease and prenatal exposure to exogenous sex hormones. Br. Med. J. 1:1058–1060.

Krugman, S. (ed.) 1965. Rubella symposium. Am. J. Dis. Child. 110:345–476.

Nora, J. J., Nora, A. H., and Toews, W. H. 1974. Lithium, Ebstein's Anomaly, and other congenital heart defects. Lancet 2:594–595.

Overall, J. C., Jr. 1972. Intrauterine virus infections and congenital heart disease. Am. Heart J. 84:823–833.

Rowland, T. W., Hubbell, J. P., Jr., and Nadas, A. S. 1973. Congenital heart disease in infants of diabetic mothers. J. Pediatr. 83:815–820.

Wilson, J. G. 1960. Experimental production of congenital cardiac defects. In A. D. Bass and G. K. Moe (eds.), Congenital Heart Disease, pp. 65–82. American Association for the Advancement of Science, Washington, D. C.

chapter 4

GENETICS AND CARDIAC ANOMALIES

Congenital heart defects occur as part of several well-established syndromes, some involving chromosomal abnormalities. Cardiac anomalies also occur in familial patterns unassociated with any currently detectable chromosomal abnormality. Most congenital heart disease, however, occurs in the absence of any known genetic mechanism.

CHROMOSOMAL ABNORMALITIES

A normal idiogram has 22 pairs of autosomes, which can be classified into seven groups on the basis of their morphology, i.e., the relative length of the chromosome arms and the position of the junction or centromere (Figure 18). These groups are 1-3, 4-5, 6-12, 13-15, 16-18, 19-20, and 21-22 (Figure 19). They are also classified by the letters A through G, respectively. Autoradiographic techniques now allow precise identification of all chromosomes by

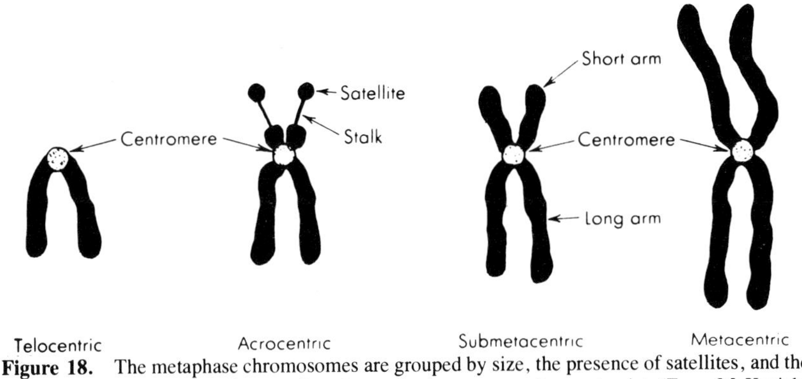

Figure 18. The metaphase chromosomes are grouped by size, the presence of satellites, and the location of the centromere. In man the telocentric chromosome does not exist. (From McKusick, V. A. 1964. Human Genetics. Prentice-Hall, Englewood Cliffs, N.J.)

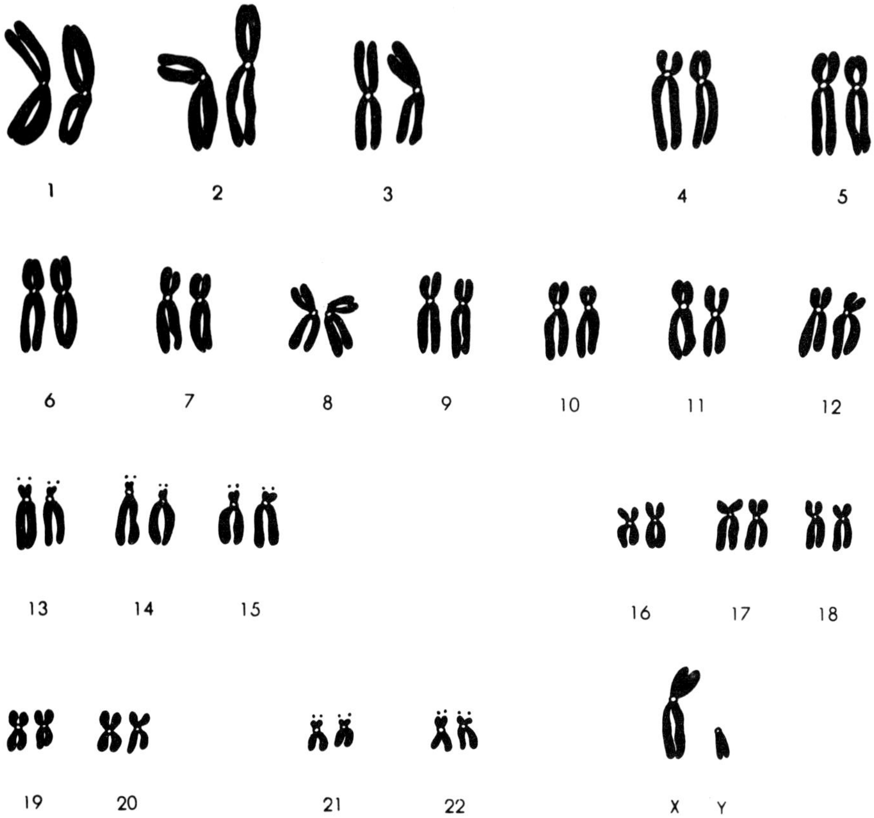

Figure 19. The mitotic metaphase chromosomes of a somatic cell of a normal male arranged in karyotype. (From McKusick, V. A. 1964. Human Genetics. Prentice-Hall, Englewood Cliffs, N.J.)

number. Normally there is one pair of sex chromosomes, either two X chromosomes (female) or one X and one Y (male).

Chromosomal abnormalities are characterized either by the presence of extra chromosomal material, by the absence of a sex chromosome, or by partial absence of an autosome (Table 2). Apparently, absence of an autosome is incompatible with life. In the typical trisomy syndromes, there is an additional chromosome converting the affected pair into a triplet (e.g., trisomy 21, the Down syndrome), and the individual has 47 chromosomes. In the Turner syndrome, a sex chromosome is missing, and the individual has only 45 chromosomes.

The occurrence of a trisomy may be due to nondisjunction. If, during formation of ovum or sperm, one of a pair of chromosomes divides but fails to separate, nondisjunction occurs. The resulting sex cell contains 22 single chromosomes and one chromosome pair rather than 23 single chromosomes.

Table 2. Summary of known chromosomal aberrations associated with congenital heart disease

Type	Frequency in live births	Common heart defects[a]
Trisomy 21 (Mongolism, Down syndrome)	1:600	AV canal, VSD, PDA
Turner syndome	1:3000 females	Coarctation, pulmonic stenosis
Trisomy 13	1:5000	VSD, PDA, ASD, dextroposition
Trisomy 18	1:3000	VSD, PDA
Cri-Du-Chat	< 100 cases reported	Variable

[a] VSD = ventricular septal defect, PDA = patent ductus arteriosus, and ASD = atrial septal defect.

Subsequent fertilization by a sperm or ovum with a normal number of chromosomes results in three of that particular chromosome (Figure 20). Theoretically, trisomy can occur after a normal fertilization. During the first cleavage division, faulty distribution of a chromosome may give rise to one trisomic cell and one monosomic cell. The latter is unlikely to survive, and the embryo will derive entirely from the trisomic cell. It is thus possible that in some cases trisomy may actually be an acquired disease. Another hypothesis for the cause of trisomy is based on an abnormality of a replicator gene, which controls chromosome division. Several autosomal trisomy syndromes have been identified.

Trisomy 13 syndrome has as its principal clinical features low-set, malformed ears and a sloping forehead, microphthalmus, colobomata, cleft lips, cleft palates, flexion deformity in the fingers, and polydactylism involving both the hands and the feet (Figure 21). Capillary hemangiomata, cryptorchidism, apneic spells, minor motor seizures, and apparent deafness are also found in a majority of affected infants. Cardiac defects, seen in 80% or more of the affected infants, include ventricular septal defect, patent ductus arteriosus, atrial septal defect, and dextroposition. Less commonly, anomalous pulmonary venous drainage, bicuspid aortic valve, and pulmonic stenosis have been reported.

Trisomy 18 commonly manifests itself in low-set, malformed ears, a prominent occiput, micrognathia, and a narrow palatal arch. Approximately 80% of affected infants are female. As in trisomy 13 syndrome, there is a flexion deformity in the fingers, but in trisomy 18 this involves primarily the index fingers, which overlap the third fingers. A dorsiflexed hallux is also characteristic. Polyhydramnios, a small placenta, low birth weight, and failure to thrive are also common features. Spasticity of the extremities occurs frequently. Cardiac anomalies are found in nearly every instance of trisomy 18.

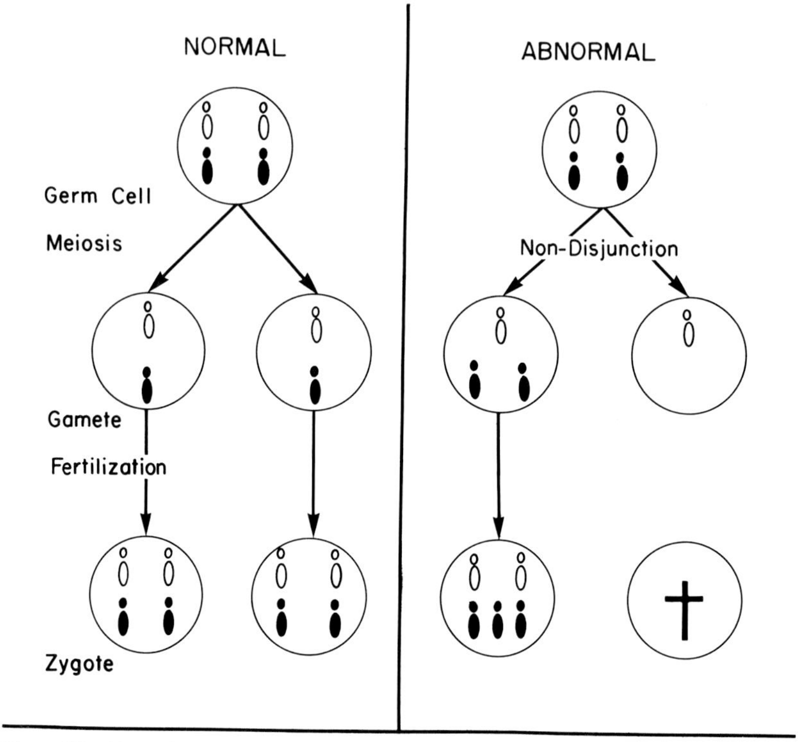

Figure 20. Formation of a trisomic cell due to nondisjunction. The monosomic cell apparently dies, since absence of an autosomal chromosome has not been reported.

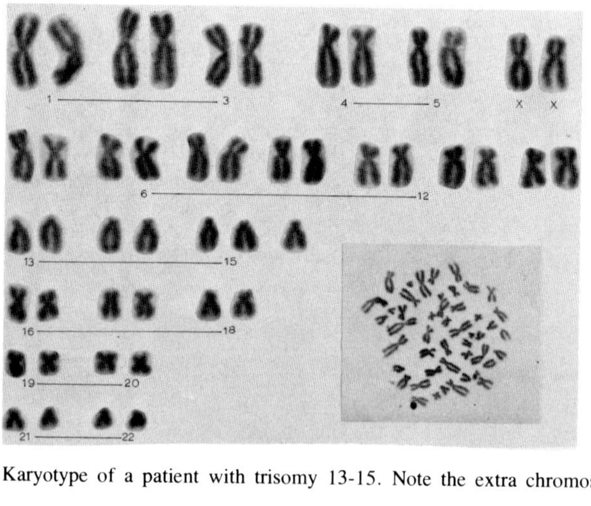

Figure 21. Karyotype of a patient with trisomy 13-15. Note the extra chromosome in this group.

Ventricular septal defect and patent ductus arteriosus, either isolated or in combination, account for more than half of these. Atrial septal defects, bicuspid semilunar valves, and pulmonic stenosis occur less commonly.

Trisomy 21, which results in mongolism (the Down syndrome), is usually sporadic in occurrence. Approximately 40% of all mongoloid children have heart defects. Rarely, the Down syndrome may be familial, in which cases the abnormality is due to the presence of additional 21-chromosomal material on another chromosome (translocation). The heart defect most commonly seen in trisomy 21 is some form of endocardial cushion defect, usually a complete AV canal; but ventricular and secundum atrial septal defects are also common. These three lesions account for 75% of all the congenital heart anomalies seen (Table 3). Individuals with the Down syndrome and cardiac disease apparently develop pulmonary vascular disease more frequently than do other individuals with similar anomalies. The reason for this apparent increased susceptibility is undetermined. About one-third of our patients with the Eisenmenger syndrome also have trisomy 21. Tetralogy of Fallot is the only other significant cause of cyanotic heart disease in patients with Down syndrome—complex types of cyanotic cardiac anomalies are rarely seen.

Turner syndrome is caused by absence of a sex chromosome; thus the karyotype is designated XO. Heart defects occur in 20% of affected individuals, with coarctation of the aorta being the most common, accounting for 70% of the heart defects seen.

Noonan syndrome has been identified in individuals of either sex with similar physical features and normal chromosomes (Table 4). This has also been called the "male Turner syndrome," but this designation is inappropriate since the Noonan syndrome occurs in both sexes. Furthermore, the resemblance to the Turner syndrome is at best superficial. Pertinent differences are the presence in Noonan syndrome of mental retardation, significant pectus

Table 3. Nature and frequency of cardiac defects in the Down syndrome

Defect	Berg (1960)	Rowe (1961)	Krovetz (1978)	Total	Percentage
Atrioventricular canal				87	40
Complete	16	23	31	(70)	
Incomplete	6	3	8	(17)	
Ventricular septal defect	20	23	20	63	29
Atrial septal defect	22	6	3	31	14
Patent ductus arteriosus	0	7	2	9	4
Tetralogy of Fallot	4	1	1	6	3
Miscellaneous	11	8	2	21	10
Totals	79	71	67	217	100

Table 4. Distinguishing features of the Turner and Noonan syndromes

Feature	Turner	Noonan
Sex	Females	Either
Karyotype	XO	Normal
Mental retardation	Rare	Common
Pectus excavatum	Rare	Common
Most common heart anomaly	Coarctation	Pulmonary valve dysplasia

excavatum, and a 50% incidence of heart disease, most commonly pulmonic stenosis. A cardiomyopathy similar to idiopathic hypertrophic subaortic stenosis also occurs (see Chapter 26).

FAMILIAR PATTERNS WITHOUT DEMONSTRABLE CHROMOSOMAL ABNORMALITY

Occasionally, families will be seen with multiple occurrences of the same or similar congenital heart defects. No chromosomal abnormalities can be detected, and it is assumed that these events represent single-gene mutations. There have been a number of reports of a specific heart defect in several generations of a family tree without other evidence of congenital malformations (Figure 22). These have been mainly atrial septal defects, patent ductus arteriosus, and pulmonic valve stenosis.

In addition, a number of familial syndromes are known in which congenital heart defects occur as part of the disease. Again, chromosomal abnormalities cannot be detected and it is thought that single-gene mutations are responsible.

Atriodigital dysplasia (Holt-Oram syndrome) is a complex including atrial septal defects of the ostium secundum type and skeletal malformations, particularly of the thumb and forearm. Cardiac dysrhythmias, especially sinus bradycardia with prolonged AV conduction time (first degree AV block), and inhibition of normal atrial activation because of sinus arrest or SA block are frequent. Occurrence of this syndrome in multiple generations of a family suggests an autosomal dominant mode of transmission.

Hereditary familial cardiomyopathy is the general name of an ill-defined group that is probably composed of several entities with the single common denominator of cardiomegaly. It is characterized by a high incidence in affected families, probably inherited as a Mendelian dominant. In one type, hypertrophy of the ventricular septum obstructs the left ventricular outflow

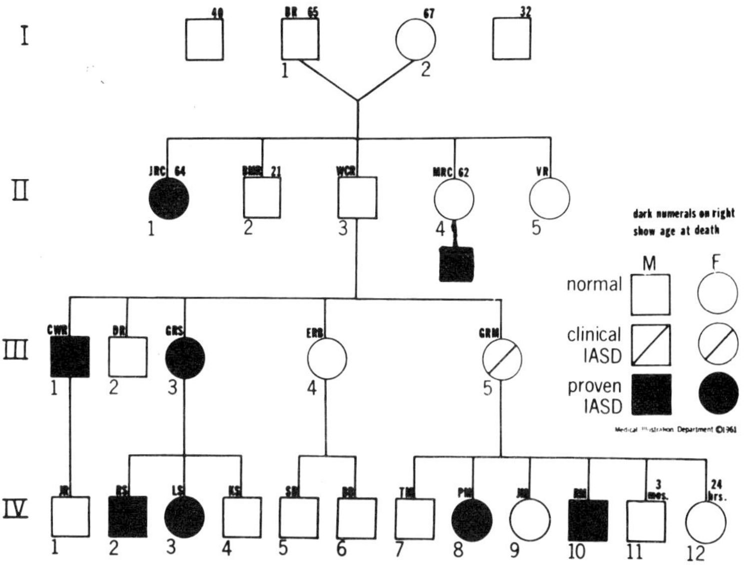

Figure 22. A family tree showing the occurrence of atrial septal defects in three generations. (From Zuckerman, H. S., Zuckerman, G. H., Mammen, R. E., and Wassermil, M. 1962. Atrial septal defect. Familial occurrence in four generations of one family. Am. J. Cardiol. 9:515.

tract, resulting in idiopathic hypertrophic subaortic stenosis (see Chapter 26). Arrhythmias may occur, as well as sudden death due to Stokes-Adams attacks.

Supravalvar aortic stenosis occurs in two groupings. The first is thought to be inherited as a Mendelian dominant with incomplete penetrance, and the intelligence of these children is normal. Supravalvar aortic stenosis also occurs sporadically as part of a syndrome involving mental retardation and an abnormal appearance characterized by a round elfin face with pouting lips and hypertelorism (see Figure 182). These cases are nonfamilial. Some patients with this type of supravalvar aortic stenosis are thought to have had severe infantile hypercalcemia. Peripheral pulmonary artery stenosis may be part of the syndrome.

Glycogen storage disease of the heart is characterized by large amounts of glycogen in all tissues, especially the myocardium. It is transmitted as an autosomal recessive trait and affects either sex. Most affected children die during the first year of life, only rarely surviving early infancy. Symptoms are mainly cardiac failure, muscular weakness, macroglossia, and growth retardation. Enormous hypertrophy of the ventricles, especially the left, is seen. In some cases, hemodynamic studies have indicated left ventricular outflow obstruction, probably secondary to massive septal hypertrophy.

Carpenter syndrome (Figure 23) is characterized by mental retardation, obesity, acrocephaly, polydactyly, syndactyly, and cryptorchidism. It may be confused with Laurence-Moon-Biedl-Bardet syndrome and includes a variety of congenital defects generally occurring in afflicted males. Left ventricular hypertrophy, usually associated with renal disease and frequently with systemic hypertension, is also common.

Ellis–van Creveld syndrome (chondroectodermal dysplasia) is an autosomal recessive abnormality characterized by small stature, short extremities, polydactyly of the fingers and occasionally of the toes, small thorax, hypoplastic nails, and hypoplasia of the alveolar ridge with abnormal teeth. Approximately one-half of these patients have a cardiac defect, most frequently common atrium.

Congenital heart defects occur in other dysmorphic syndromes; thus, the above should be considered as examples.

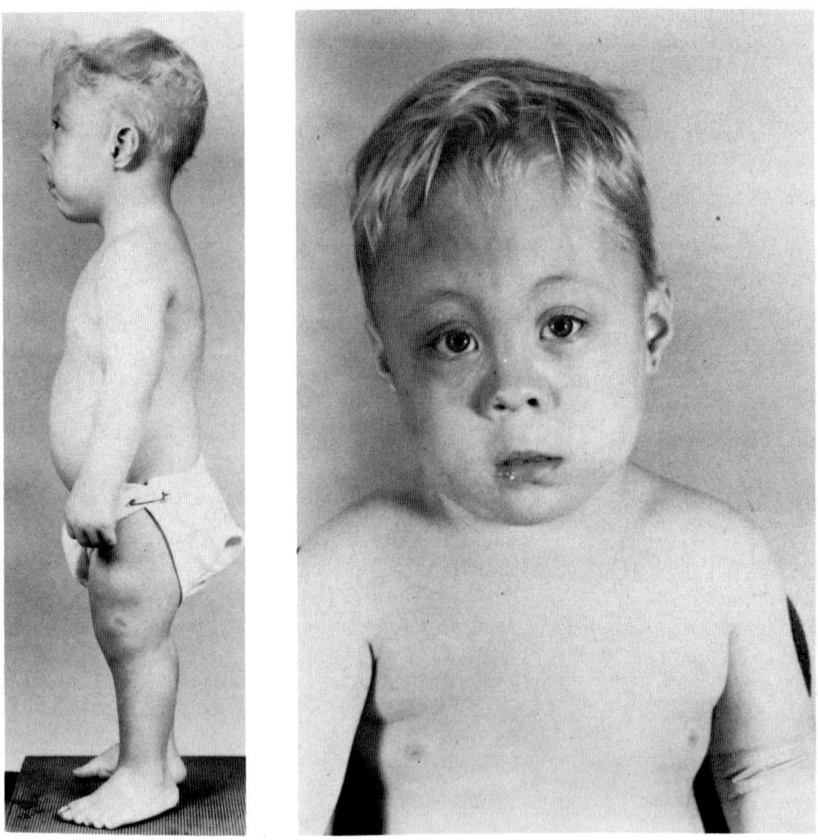

Figure 23. One of three siblings with the Carpenter syndrome. Note the six toes on the left foot, the brachiocephalic skull, and the dull facies.

ROLE OF GENETICS IN CONGENITAL HEART DISEASE

It is helpful to consider the etiology of congenital heart disease as a spectrum ranging from pure genetic to pure environmental factors (Figure 24). For example, the occurrence of congenital heart disease secondary to a teratogenic agent is clearly at the environmental end of the spectrum. In contrast, some cardiomyopathies are genetic in etiology and familial patterns are readily discernible. The vast majority of heart disease in children falls between these two extremes. For example, patent ductus arteriosus is sometimes related to neonatal distress, at other times clearly familial, and in still other cases secondary to maternal rubella. In most cases, however, abnormal patency of the ductus is of sporadic occurrence and unknown etiology.

Clear-cut genetic factors are known to operate in domestic animals. Certain inbred strains of chickens and rats have a high incidence of ventricular septal defects. The higher prevalence of spontaneously occurring congenital heart disease in purebred (up to 3.2%) than in mixed dogs (0.44%) and the apparent predisposition of certain breeds to specific malformations suggest the operation of genetic factors. Additionally, several strains of dogs have been developed in which specific defects occur with high frequency.

Studies of heart defects in human twins offer some interesting data that provide insight into the interaction of genetic events and the environment. When one of a set of fraternal twins has a heart defect, the probability of the second twin having that (or a similar) defect is equivalent to that for all siblings—2% to 5%. For identical twins, if the defect was inherited according to Mendelian laws, then the concordance rate would be 100%; that is, the twins, being identical, should have the same defect. If no genetic forces were

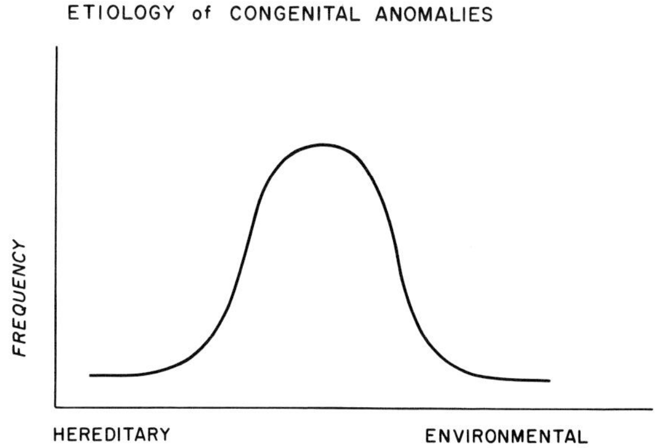

Figure 24. Schematic representation of the etiology of congenital heart disease. At one end are cases caused entirely by genetic factors, and at the opposite end are those caused entirely by environmental factors. The vast majority of congenital anomalies are found between these two extremes and are caused by complex and as yet largely unknown interrelationships of both genetic predisposition and environmental enhancement.

operative, then the incidence of concordance would be the same as it is for fraternal twins (or any siblings). The actual concordance rate falls in between these figures. The best information in the literature indicates a concordance rate for heart defects in human identical twins of 10%–25%. (One study, giving a rate of 46%, the highest ever reported, is not supported by other investigations.) These twin data are taken as strong evidence for the concept of polygenic inheritance as the mode of determination in these individuals. According to Smith, a polygenetically determined abnormality is one that is the consequence of minor differences at many gene loci, no one of which may be held fully responsible for the abnormality. Present evidence in the human supports the conclusion that polygenic inheritance is the primary mechanism in the etiology of many single localized morphogenic defects. Thus it is likely that much congenital heart disease is acquired in utero, perhaps from complicated interactions between genetic susceptibility and subtle factors in the intrauterine environment.

GENETIC COUNSELING

Although the majority of cases of congenital heart diseases occur as isolates with no familial pattern, the question of the risk of repeated occurrence in the family is frequently asked. In families having one child with a congenital heart defect, the incidence of congenital heart defects in the affected child's siblings varies from 2% to 5%. Congenital heart anomalies in siblings tend to be the same or similar, especially in the acyanotic types. If two pregnancies result in cardiac defects, the same parents may have a risk of 25% to 50% in subsequent offspring, particularly if the defects that occurred are developmentally similar.

BIBLIOGRAPHY

Berg, J. M., Crome, L., and France, N. E. 1960. Congenital cardiac malformation in mongolism. Br. Heart J. 22:331–346.

Chi, T. P. L., and Krovetz, L. J. 1975. The pulmonary vascular bed in children with Down Syndrome. J. Pediatr. 86:533–538.

Lamy, M., de Grouchy, J., and Schweisguth, O. 1957. Genetic and non-genetic factors in the etiology of congenital heart disease: A study of 1188 cases. Am. J. Human Genet. 9:17–41.

McKusick, V. A. 1964. A genetical view of cardiovascular disease. Circulation 30:326–357.

Ross, L. J. 1969. Congenital cardiovascular anomalies in twins. Circulation 20:327–342.

Rowe, R. D., and Uchida, I. A. 1961. Cardiac malformation in mongolism. A prospective study in 184 mongoloid children. Am. J. Med. 31:726–735.

Smith, D. W. 1964. Autosomal abnormalities. Am. J. Obstet. Gynecol. 90:1055–1077.

Smith, D. W. 1970. Recognizable Patterns of Human Malformation. W.B. Saunders Co., Philadelphia.

Van Praagh, R. 1973. Genetic implications of successful treatment of congenital heart disease. In B. G. Barratt-Boyes, J. M. Neutze, and E. A. Harris (eds.), Heart Disease in Infancy, pp. 331–339. Williams & Wilkins, Baltimore.

chapter 5

HEMODYNAMICS OF HEART DISEASE

For the beginner, there seems to be a hopeless variety of congenital and acquired malformations and combinations of these defects. From a pathophysiologic standpoint, however, there are five basic types of cardiovascular problems, whether of congenital or acquired origin. These are:

1. Volume overloading, in which an excess amount of blood is pumped by either or both ventricles
2. Obstruction of flow entering the ventricle
3. Obstruction of flow leaving the ventricle (pressure overloading)
4. Disorders of contraction or relaxation of the ventricles
5. Cardiac disorders secondary to systemic disease

We prefer to classify cardiac lesions on this basis rather than on the more traditional one of cyanotic versus acyanotic. Moderate degrees of arterial desaturation and cyanosis are difficult to detect clinically, particularly in the neonate. Furthermore, cyanosis may be due to pulmonary factors, such as pneumonia, or to a slow peripheral circulation secondary to the vasoconstriction associated with congestive heart failure. However, when evident, the degree and time of development of cyanosis may suggest certain entities.

Another proposed classification scheme is based on roentgenographic assessment of pulmonary vascular markings. Unfortunately, the assessment of cyanosis and pulmonary vascular markings is most difficult during infancy.

VOLUME OVERLOADING

Since the affected ventricle is filled with an excess of blood during each diastolic period, the term *diastolic overloading* has also been applied.

Left-to-Right Shunts

A left-to-right shunt may cause a volume overload of either one or both ventricles. In the case of left-to-right shunts at the atrial level, volume overloading occurs in the right ventricle. With shunts at the ventricular level, usually both ventricles are overloaded. Shunts above the semilunar valves (e.g., patent ductus arteriosus) cause left ventricular volume overloading (Table 5).

The increased pulmonary blood flow always present with left-to-right shunts (and some other entities; see "Obligatory Admixture Lesions," below) commonly overloads the carrying capacity of the mitral valve and produces a "relative" mitral stenosis. This overload will increase left atrial pressure, and so pulmonary arterial and right ventricular pressures must increase to keep blood flowing.

Left-to-right shunts at any level of the cardiovascular system require that excess blood flow through the pulmonary circuit. The cardiac chambers and vessels affected by the volume overloading differ depending on the location of the defect. Table 5 illustrates this point further. Note, for example, that with an atrial septal defect there is excessive blood flow through the right atrium, the right ventricle, the pulmonary artery, the pulmonary vascular bed, and the pulmonary veins. On returning to the left atrium, however, the excess flow is immediately shunted to the right atrium so that there is little stimulus for an increase in left atrial pressure or for left atrial enlargement. Further downstream, the left ventricle and aorta receive a normal amount of blood and are normal in size and activity.

Blood, like water, can only flow downhill. The direction of flow through a ventricular septal defect, for example, will be determined by the pressures in the right and left ventricles. If the ventricular septal defect is larger than 80% of the aortic root diameter, the pressures in the ventricles will be equal. The direction and magnitude of flow will then depend on the ratio of the resistances in the systemic and pulmonary circulation. Increased pulmonary artery blood flow (and usually increased pressure) eventually results in narrowing of the pulmonary arterioles and increasing resistance to pulmonary blood flow. If the resistance of the pulmonary arterioles bed exceeds that of the systemic

Table 5. Sites of volume overloading in left-to-right shunts

	Site of shunt		
	Atrial	Ventricular	Great vessels
Right atrium	+	0	0
Right ventricle	+	+	0
Pulmonary artery	+	+	+
Pulmonary vasculature	+	+	+
Pulmonary veins	+	+	+
Left atrium	0	+	+
Left ventricle	0	+	+
Aorta	0	0	+

circulation, then the dominant shunt will be from the venous to the arterial direction (i.e., right-to-left) and cyanosis will result. This situation is referred to as the Eisenmenger complex when the underlying anomaly is a ventricular septal defect and as the Eisenmenger syndrome or reaction when it occurs with other cardiac anomalies. Examples of left-to-right shunts are:

- Atrial level
  - Sinus venosus defect, commonly associated with anomalous pulmonary venous connection from the right lung
  - Ostium secundum defect (foramen ovale)
  - Ostium primum defect, associated with a cleft mitral valve
- Ventricular level
  - Ventricular septal defect
- Great vessel level
  - Patent ductus arteriosus
  - Truncus arteriosus
  - Aortic-pulmonic window
- Peripheral vessels
  - Arteriovenous fistulae

Obligatory Admixture Lesions

These are lesions in which both pulmonary venous and systemic venous blood must pass through a common chamber. This term is not totally satisfactory, since there may be a surprising amount of separation of blood streams even where there is no anatomical separation. In all of these anomalies there will be increased pulmonary flow unless there is either accompanying pulmonic stenosis or marked pulmonary arteriolar narrowing (Eisenmenger reaction).

These entities commonly present with a clinical triad of *cyanosis, congestive heart failure,* and *increased pulmonary arterial markings* on x-ray. The types of anomalies included in this classification are:

- Transposition of the great vessels
- Total anomalous pulmonary venous connection
- Truncus arteriosus
- Three-chambered hearts
  - Single atrium
  - Single ventricle (one pumping ventricle and one small, nonfunctioning ventricle located beneath either great vessel—double inlet left ventricle is one example)
- Complete atrioventricular canals

Valvar Regurgitation

The hemodynamics of these lesions are relatively simple. In order to maintain a normal cardiac output, the ventricle involved must eject an excessive amount of blood during each systole, since some of the blood ejected from the ventricle returns to it during the next diastole. The connecting great vessel or atrium must therefore carry an excess amount of blood flow and becomes enlarged. For example, in mitral insufficiency the left atrium enlarges. Since one consequence of valvar incompetence is to cause an augmentation of diastolic volume in the affected ventricle, these are also examples of volume overloading.

OBSTRUCTIVE LESIONS

Most obstructive lesions are well tolerated for long periods of time. Anomalies such as aortic stenosis, pulmonic stenosis, and coarctation of the aorta are quite compatible with athletic supremacy. When deterioration does set in, however, it may result in rapid decline, or, rarely, sudden death.

The pressure drop across the obstruction depends on both the severity of obstruction and the flow rate (Figure 25). The uncomplicated valve or vessel

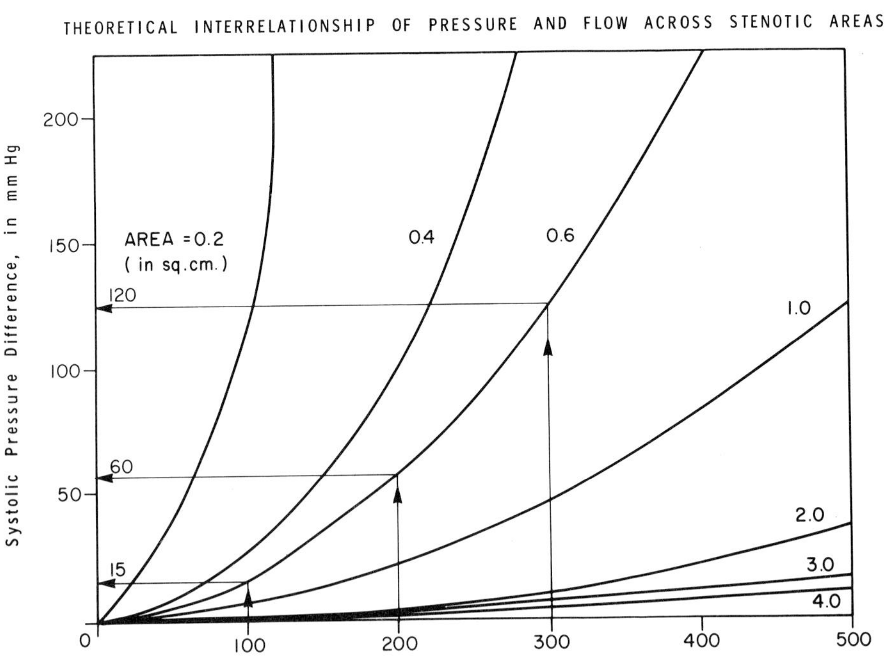

Figure 25. Theoretical interrelationships of pressure drop and flow across a stenotic valve. When the area of the valve has been reduced to about one-fourth of normal size, or about 0.6 cm^2 in the adult, and the flow is about normal, or 200 ml per systolic sec, the pressure drop is 60 mm Hg. With apprehension or exercise, flow might increase to 300 ml/sec and pressure difference to 120 mm Hg. Conversely, with cardiac decompensation, flow might decrease to 100 ml/sec and pressure difference to 15 mm Hg. Thus, cardiac output must be known in order to interpret pressure data.

stenosis must have the same amount of blood flowing on either side of the obstruction. This is not the case if there is a communication between the right and left sides of the heart, or, in the case of a vessel, if there is collateral circulation around the obstruction.

If there is a septal defect and obstruction, blood will flow across the defect in the direction of the pressure gradient. For example, in a case of pulmonic stenosis and a ventricular septal defect, if the pressure in the right ventricle exceeds that in the left, there will be a right-to-left shunt. This means that some of the blood bypasses the pulmonary bed, and the pulmonary blood flow will be less than the systemic blood flow. We then have two types of obstructive lesions: those with no communication between the right and left sides of the heart and those with such a communication.

Examples of *ventricular inflow obstructions* are:

LEFT HEART	RIGHT HEART
Mitral stenosis	Tricuspid stenosis
Cor triatriatum	Ebstein's anomaly

These entities result in increased venous pressure. In left-sided lesions, there will be increased pulmonary venous pressure and eventually pulmonary edema, whereas in right-sided lesions there will be increased systemic venous pressure with resultant peripheral edema and hepatosplenomegaly.

Examples of *ventricular outflow obstructions* are:

LEFT HEART	RIGHT HEART
Aortic stenosis	Pulmonic stenosis
Coarctation of the aorta	Pulmonary artery coarctation
Systemic hypertension	Pulmonary hypertension

Isolated outflow obstructions are, in general, well tolerated. The ventricles can maintain a normal cardiac output by increasing systolic pressure and by hypertrophy of their musculature. The chest x-ray and ECG are often completely normal. Unless a critical degree of narrowing is reached there is little or no cardiomegaly and few or no symptoms. This is not to say that ventricular outflow obstruction cannot be important during early infancy. When accompanied by a septal defect or if the orifice is so small that the ventricle cannot adapt effectively, severe decompensation may result.

DISORDERS OF CONTRACTION AND/OR RELAXATION

In these lesions the abnormality lies in the inability of the myocardium to contract or to relax sufficiently well to maintain an adequate cardiac output. The clinical pictures of these lesions differ in details such as age incidence, but the pathophysiologies present a number of similarities. In all of these diseases, filling or emptying of one or both ventricles is less efficient than usual. As one would expect, digitalis often is not very effective. Even nearly toxic levels of digitalis may fail to achieve any clinical response. When the inefficient myocardium is already producing nearly maximal amounts of effort, adding digitalis cannot cause a significant increase in efficiency.

In our experience, nonobstructive cardiomyopathy is the most common lesion in this category. Endocardial fibroelastosis is a classic example of this group, but for undetermined reasons has become less common in recent years.

EXTRINSIC DISORDERS

Under this heading we include those disorders in which the heart and cardiovascular system are adequate for ordinary needs but not for the special circumstances encountered. Included are the so-called high output failure syndromes of hyperthyroidism and anemia. Peripheral arteriovenous anastomoses in the cerebral, coronary, or hepatic circulations all cause rapid diastolic emptying of the systemic circulation, producing a widened pulse pressure. The heart compensates by increasing the left ventricular stroke volume.

Similarly, there are low output syndromes that are secondary to hypothyroidism or cardiac tamponade. One common feature of this group is that measures directed exclusively at the cardiovascular system are usually ineffective. *Successful therapy depends on treatment of the underlying disease.*

BIBLIOGRAPHY

Fishman, A. P. 1963. Dynamics of the pulmonary circulation. In W. F. Hamilton and P. Dow (eds.), Handbook on Physiology, Circulation, Vol. II, pp. 1667–1743. American Physiological Society, Washington, D.C.

Marshall, H. W., Helmholz, H. F., Jr., and Wood, E. H. 1962. Physiological consequences of congenital heart disease. In W. F. Hamilton and P. Dow (eds.), Handbook of Physiology, Circulation, Vol. I, pp. 417–487. American Physiological Society, Washington, D.C.

chapter 6

PHYSICAL EXAMINATION

Much can be gained by inspecting the patient prior to applying a stethoscope to the chest. One look may suggest that the child has a specific syndrome and thus suggest a specific cardiac defect. For example, the diagnosis of mongolism makes an endocardial cushion defect or a ventricular septal defect the most probable cardiac anomaly. (See Chapter 4 for further discussion of syndromes and heart disease.)

GROWTH PATTERNS

When the cardiac malformation has only minor hemodynamic significance, such as a small ventricular septal defect, there should be a normal growth pattern both for height and weight. If such a child is small for age, the growth problem should not be ascribed to the heart defect.

With obstructive anomalies, such as coarctation of the aorta, aortic stenosis, or pulmonic stenosis, growth is also usually normal. Even severe obstruction is compatible with superior physical development and normal exercise tolerance.

With large left-to-right shunts, growth may be markedly reduced, in weight usually more than in height. In an acyanotic child with congenital heart disease and marked growth retardation, a large left-to-right shunt is the most likely diagnosis.

EXTRACARDIAC ANOMALIES

Extracardiac anomalies may be a valuable clue to the type of cardiac defect, since they are more common with some cardiac anomalies than others. An extracardiac anomaly is quite uncommon in uncomplicated complete transposition of the great vessels, whereas such anomalies are frequent in tetralogy of Fallot. Conversely, children with multiple congenital anomalies frequently have an additional heart defect.

HEAD

The child who has been cyanotic since birth often has *a head that appears large* in relation to the rest of his body. There is marked frontal bossing and the anterior fontanel may remain open up to the age of 3 years.

The combination of *a small head and a heart defect* should suggest post-rubella syndrome. The complete syndrome is easy to recognize—the infant presents in congestive heart failure with microcephaly, eye anomalies (particularly cataracts and glaucoma; Figure 26), and deafness. Jaundice and thrombocytopenia may be seen in the newborn. The most common cardiac anomalies are patent ductus arteriosus, multiple coarctations of the pulmonary arteries, and valvar pulmonic stenosis. At times the post-rubella syndrome is difficult to detect. Deafness may cause the child to be a slow learner, and the

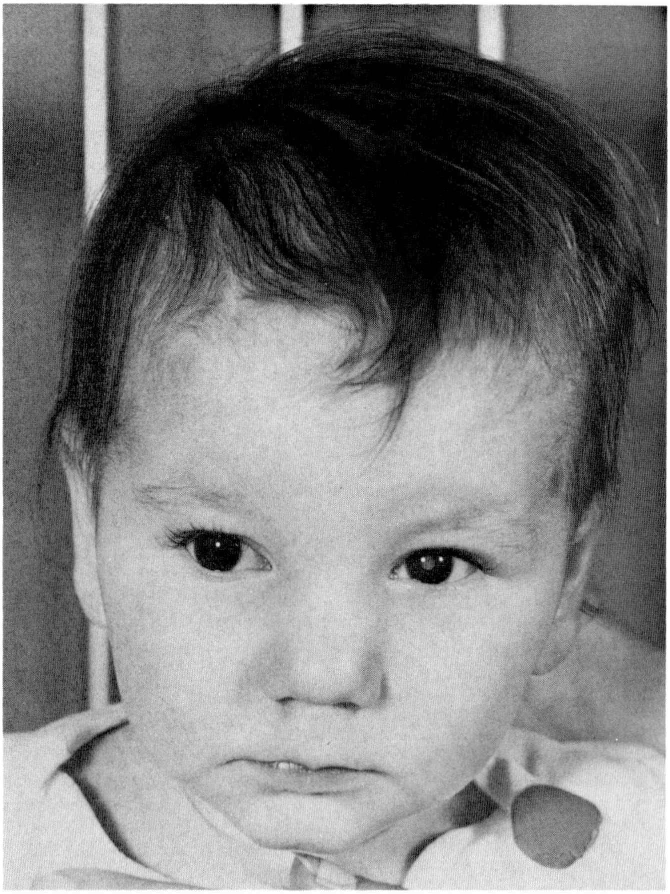

Figure 26. One-year-old girl with a unilateral cataract in the left eye and other features of the post-rubella syndrome. She had a patent ductus arteriosus transected, and pulmonic valvar stenosis and multiple coarctations of the pulmonary artery were present.

reduced head circumference may be subtle. Systolic murmurs, secondary to multiple coarctations of the pulmonary arteries, are loudest in either or both axillae, but may not be readily appreciated if only the precordium is auscultated.

With *hydrocephalus and a surgically inserted valve mechanism,* the drainage end of which lies in the superior vena cava, recurrent emboli from the catheter tip into the pulmonary bed will cause pulmonary hypertension in over 10% of cases. If the foramen ovale is not anatomically sealed, a right-to-left shunt at the atrial level may result. Such patients may also develop congestive heart failure.

FACE

The face of a child with supravalvar aortic stenosis is distinctive (see Figure 182). *Wide-set eyes in a full face* with a broad forehead and a small, pouting chin are characteristic. Hypertelorism alone with a full, round ("moon") face is seen with isolated pulmonic valve stenosis.

Edema of the eyelids, particularly noted on awakening, is a valuable clue to the presence of congestive heart failure. Edema of the eyelids, systemic hypertension, and often pulmonary edema suggest renal disease, especially acute glomerulonephritis.

Multiple small telangiectasias of the tongue and mucous membranes in a cyanotic individual should suggest hereditary telangiectasis (Weber-Osler-Rendu syndrome) with multiple pulmonary arteriovenous fistulae.

NECK

Examination of the neck may reveal *a large thyroid,* suggesting that the patient's tachycardia, cardiomegaly, and flow murmurs may be secondary to hyperthyroidism.

Thrills in the neck over the great vessels or in the suprasternal notch are most often associated with aortic or pulmonic stenosis. They may also be felt with coarctation of the aorta, patent ductus arteriosus, or truncus arteriosus.

Neck veins and jugular pulses are difficult to evaluate in an infant. In the older child and adolescent, more precise analysis of the venous wave is possible. *Engorged neck veins,* particularly with a prominent "a" wave, suggest right heart failure. *Prominent pulsations of arterial vessels* suggest a run-off lesion from the aorta, either into the left ventricle (as in aortic valve incompetence) or into the pulmonary artery (as in patent ductus arteriosus).

PERIPHERAL PULSES

Bounding arterial pulses caused by a wide pulse pressure may occur in any aortic run-off lesion. The combination of congestive heart failure and wide pulse pressures in an infant strongly suggests a patent ductus arteriosus, since failure from other causes usually decreases pulse pressure. Wide pulse pressures may also be seen with slow ventricular rates and a large stroke volume. The large left ventricular stroke volume in an infant with a large ventricular septal defect also increases pulse pressure.

The murmur of aortic stenosis and a wide pulse pressure suggest idiopathic hypertrophic subaortic stenosis. In other forms of aortic stenosis, the pulse pressure is either normal or narrowed.

Narrow pulse pressure occurs with low cardiac output, such as in shock or congestive heart failure. In the newborn, weak pulses are characteristic of hypoplastic left heart lesions, such as aortic atresia. Pulses may also be diminished in neonates with critically severe aortic stenosis.

Observation of the *difference between upper and lower extremity pulses* in coarctation of the aorta is decades old, but it is surprising how frequently it is missed. Palpation for the posterior tibial or dorsalis pedis pulses may be less disturbing to the infant or young child, and therefore more helpful than pressing the groin in search of the femoral pulse. If such foot pulses are readily palpable, coarctation is unlikely, but *not* definitely ruled out. Accurate measurement of at least systolic blood pressures in the arm and leg is mandatory as part of a complete cardiovascular examination.

Absence of individual arterial pulsations may be secondary to a vascular anomaly, previous use of an artery in palliative surgery (such as subclavian artery to pulmonary artery anastomosis), arteriotomy at cardiac catheterization, or thrombosis. *Decreased blood pressure in one arm* suggests an anomalous subclavian artery with a contralateral aortic arch; i.e., an anomalous right subclavian with a left aortic arch or an anomalous left subclavian with a right aortic arch.

DIGITS

An abnormal number of digits may be associated with a defect of the atrial septum. The Ellis–van Creveld syndrome exhibits polydactylism, usually with a single atrium. When *the thumb is missing or misplaced* in conjunction with other bony abnormalities of the forearm, an atrial septal defect should be suspected. This combination, known as the Holt-Oram syndrome, has a familial occurrence.

ARTERIAL DESATURATION AND CYANOSIS

Cyanosis is a colorometric determination in which the observer's eyes act as a spectrophotometer for the color of the blood. Approximately 3 g/dl of reduced or unoxygenated hemoglobin must be present in order to detect cyanosis. This amount is a minimum and is independent of the total hemoglobin. The actual oxygen saturation of a cyanotic individual may be quite variable depending on how much hemoglobin is available. For example, a patient with a total of 20 g/dl of available hemoglobin will appear cyanotic with 3 g/dl of reduced hemoglobin, leaving 17 g (or 85%) oxygenated hemoglobin. A patient with 10 g/dl of available hemoglobin still requires 3 g/dl of reduced hemoglobin to appear cyanotic, leaving 7 g/dl (or 70%) saturated. The point is that cyanosis in an anemic child implies a substantially lower oxygen saturation than in the usual cyanotic patient whose hemoglobin level is high.

When *overt cyanosis* is present, the arterial saturation is usually below 85%. Lesser degrees of arterial desaturation are difficult to detect. Reddening of the lips, cheeks, and fingertips may suggest desaturation when overt cyanosis is not present. An elevated hematocrit is of considerable value in confirming a clinical impression of cyanosis. Cyanosis of some duration precedes clubbing of the digits, which is most obvious in the great toes and the thumbs. The nail bed angle is lost and the nails themselves are softer and more curved than normal. The color of the nail bed is not uniform, the proximal portion being bluer.

Differential cyanosis has been described in the presence of a "reversing" patent ductus arteriosus. In an infant with severe coarctation of the aorta, particularly with a hypoplastic or atretic long segment of the aortic arch, desaturated blood may be carried from the pulmonary artery through the ductus to the descending aorta, while the ascending aorta receives normally saturated pulmonary venous blood. Such patients will have a pink upper body and a cyanotic abdomen and lower extremities. If the left subclavian artery arises distal to the aortic obstruction, then only the right upper chest, head, and right arm will be pink. On the other hand, most infants with an interrupted arch have a ventricular septal defect, in which case mixing occurs at the ventricular level, reducing the difference between aortic and pulmonary artery oxygen levels and thereby preventing observation of differential cyanosis.

Cyanotic children, particularly those with decreased pulmonary flow, may assume a *knee-chest squatting position*. Squatting, by occluding venous return from the legs, increases the arterial saturation of the reduced amount of blood returning to the heart, thus allowing greater oxygenation of blood flowing to the brain. The heart is also brought closer to the feet, thereby reducing gravity work.

The physician faced with a cyanotic newborn must differentiate between cyanosis secondary to a right-to-left shunt caused by a congenital heart lesion and *noncardiac causes of cyanosis*. The latter include: primary lung disease; accentuation of normal acrocyanosis; intrauterine maternal-to-fetal transfusion syndrome (producing a high hematocrit), cyanosis, and even heart failure; cerebral damage with depressed respiration; intrinsic or extrinsic airway anomalies; and congenital and acquired hemoglobinopathies.

CHEST AND RESPIRATION

The character of the respirations should be analyzed carefully. *Tachypnea* is often an early manifestation of congestive heart failure, usually because of increased pulmonary blood flow. Some cyanotic patients, such as those with complete transposition of the great vessels, have constant tachypnea, since arterial pO_2 and pCO_2 remain relatively steady. *Hyperpnea (deep respirations)* usually indicates hypoxemia secondary to decreased pulmonary blood flow. In tetralogy of Fallot, arterial saturation varies enormously depending on activity and peripheral oxygen demand. Thus, while sleeping, the patient's respirations may be normal, since pulmonary flow may be adequate for the resting metabolic needs. With increased activity systemic blood flow increases, but because pulmonary flow cannot increase proportionately cyanosis and hyperpnea result.

Examination of the lungs for pulmonary pathology, particularly pneumonia or congestive heart failure, is an important adjunct to the cardiac examination. In infants, the thoracic roentgenogram yields significantly more information than does the physical examination. Although we rely heavily on the former, examination of the lungs should not be slighted.

Chest deformities, especially left chest prominence, may occur with cardiac enlargement. Marked scalloping or scooping out of the lower chest bilaterally (Harrison's grooves) is commonly associated with a large left-to-right shunt. The chest is increased in anterior-posterior diameter because of stiffening of the lungs, chronic hyperinflation, and increased respiratory effort, causing the diaphragm to tug at a malleable chest cage.

Severe kyphoscoliosis may lead to cor pulmonale. A patient with kyphoscoliosis and heart disease should bring to mind the Marfan syndrome or Friedreich's ataxia. Atrial septal defects in adolescent females are associated with a significant incidence of chest cage and spinal anomalies. Mitral valve prolapse is also associated with skeletal anomalies, particularly thoracic scoliosis.

When *the spine is very straight* (the "straight back syndrome"), the position of the heart may be distorted. The pulmonary artery is prominent on chest x-ray and functional murmurs may be more prominent than usual.

Similarly, *pectus excavatum* causes distortion of the cardiac position, pushing the heart into the left chest. In this circumstance the electrocardiogram often has an rSr′ in the right precordial leads. Absence of a pathological murmur confirms that these children have no heart disease, even though the chest x-ray and electrocardiogram may suggest an abnormality.

DEXTROCARDIA

When the cardiac impulse is on the right side, the physician must determine whether *mirror-image dextrocardia* (situs inversus), *dextroversion* (a rotational anomaly), or *dextroposition* (cardiac shift secondary to chest cage or lung pathology) exists. Mirror-image dextrocardia (situs inversus) is associated with congenital heart disease less than 5% of the time. When the heart is rotated to the right (situs solitus with dextroversion) there is nearly always associated congenital heart disease. The P wave in lead I separates the first category from the other two. In mirror-image situs inversus, the atria are inverted; thus, the P wave is opposite from normal, i.e., negative in lead I. In dextroversion and dextroposition, the atria are in normal position and the P wave in lead I is upright.

ABDOMEN

Palpation of the liver and spleen are important in the cardiac evaluation. Enlargement of the liver is expected in right heart failure. Furthermore, following the distance of the liver edge below the right costal margin is an excellent way of judging response to digitalis therapy.

Palpation of equal amounts of liver on each side of the abdomen suggests the absent spleen syndrome (Ivemark syndrome, asplenia). In this condition the viscera have a similar structure on both sides, as if two right sides were pasted together rather than a right and a left side. Since one side is the mirror image of the other, the term *organ isomerism* is applied. Complex congenital heart anomalies are the rule. Most common are single ventricle with pulmonary outflow tract obstruction, anomalous pulmonary venous return, transposition of the great arteries, endocardial cushion defects, rotational anomalies of the heart, and systemic venous anomalies. The chest x-ray often shows the cardiac apex and stomach bubble on opposite sides. If the tracheobronchial tree can be identified on the chest x-ray, both main stem bronchi have the appearance of a right bronchus.

Ascites secondary to congestive heart failure occurs only in long-term severe congestive heart failure. When it is present in a relatively asymptomatic child, consider constructive pericarditis.

LEGS

In an infant, dependent *edema* secondary to congestive heart failure usually is found in the sacral area or in the face rather than in the legs. After the child starts walking, dependent edema is present in the lower extremities. Such edema is most severe in patients with endocardial fibroelastosis or renal disease. Infants with Turner syndrome often have lymphedema, particularly of the feet.

PALPATION

Palpation of the precordium localizes the position and activity of the heart and the apical impulse. In infants with complex cardiac malformations, it is sometimes difficult to decode left ventricular activity from right ventricular activity, especially since there is no guarantee that two separate ventricles are present.

The entire precordium may be hyperactive, particularly when there is increased volume work of the heart, such as in large left-to-right shunts or valve incompetence. Diminished precordial pulsations occur in pericardial disease, Ebstein's anomaly of the tricuspid valve, and some cardiomyopathies.

In the older child, particularly one with an isolated lesion, analysis of ventricular activity is more feasible. With the heel of the hand over the sternum and the fingers pointing toward the cardiac apex, a prominent left parasternal systolic impulse secondary to right ventricular hyperactivity lifts the heel of the hand; a prominent apical impulse secondary to left ventricular hyperactivity will elevate the fingers. Both ventricles may show increased activity, such as in a large ventricular septal defect. A sharp, quick impulse suggests volume overload of the ventricle, whereas a more prolonged, sustained impulse suggests pressure overload.

If a murmur is of sufficient intensity, its vibrations may be felt on the chest wall as a thrill. Diastolic thrills are far less common than systolic thrills. Although some observers prefer using the fingertips to sense thrills, for many the palm at the base of the fingers is more sensitive. With some practice, one can place the hand on the chest even on a 1-kg premature infant and accurately assess these tactile sensations.

AUSCULTATION

Analysis of the second heart sound and its components is one of the most rewarding phases of cardiac auscultation. This requires identification of the presence of both aortic and pulmonic closure sounds, and evaluation of their intensity, the time between them, and their movement with respiration. A single second heart sound (S_2) means that the aortic and pulmonic valves are closing simultaneously, one valve is absent, or one valve is closing inaudibly. When the pulmonic component of the second sound is accentuated, pulmonary hypertension is present.

The third heart sound (S_3) may be normally very prominent in older children and adolescents (Figure 27). The fourth heart sound (S_4) is more difficult to hear because it immediately precedes the first sound (S_1) and is quite low in frequency. When S_3 and S_4 are both prominent, suspect myocardial disease.

It has been estimated that three out of every four normal children have heart murmurs at one time or another. Physicians dealing with children are frequently called on to decide whether a murmur is of no consequence or deserves further investigation. There is no sure way of differentiating innocent murmurs from organic (pathologic) murmurs in all instances by auscultation alone. Occasionally, even experienced cardiologists have difficulty making

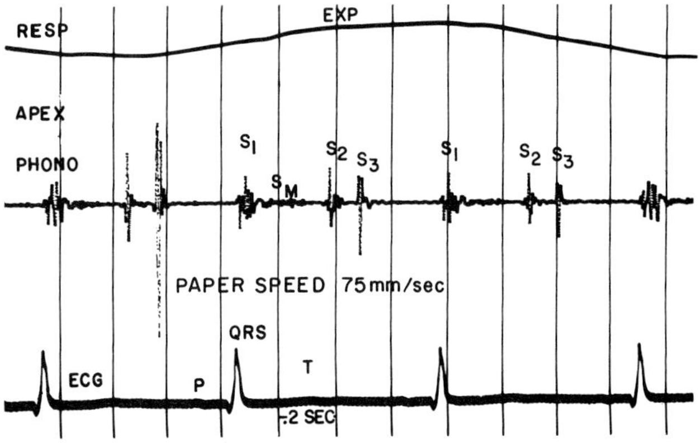

Figure 27. Phonocardiogram shows an early systolic murmur and a prominent third sound (S_3) in an 11-year-old girl with a normal heart. This is a common innnocent murmur, usually grade 3/6 or less, that is heard best over the mid-precordium and the second LICS at the sternal border. Note that the murmur is of low intensity, a characteristic of many innocent murmurs.

this decision when using only auscultatory findings. The following are a few guidelines to assist the physician:

1. Auscultation and its interpretation in the first few weeks of life are difficult. Having identified a murmur, do not commit yourself to a diagnosis too early, particularly in an acyanotic newborn who is doing well. Murmurs heard in the first few days of life may disappear completely, and other murmurs may appear. If the newborn's condition does not dictate urgency, another examination after a few weeks may be more revealing.
2. A loud murmur, not heard during the first week, but noted at the four-to-six–weeks examination, is most likely due to a left-to-right shunt, especially a ventricular septal defect. (See Table 6 for grading of murmurs.)
3. A murmur that is loud enough to produce a thrill should be considered abnormal.
4. Children often have murmurs with a fever, since fever increases cardiac output, thus increasing the intensity of a functional murmur. It is important to reevaluate the child after recovery before making a decision as to the significance of the murmur. Similar murmurs secondary to increased cardiac output are caused by anemia, thyrotoxicosis, a large AV fistula, exercise, or excitement.
5. Athletic children may have slow heart rate and a high stroke volume, again increasing the intensity of an innocent murmur.
6. An asymptomatic child with a grade 1 or 2 systolic murmur seldom has significant heart disease. Minor degrees of x-ray and electrocardiogram variations are found in many normal individuals. When in doubt, the physical examination, particularly auscultation, is often the best guide.
7. Do not become obsessed with making an anatomic diagnosis from physi-

Table 6. Grading of murmurs

Grade	Description
1	Faint murmur; audible on careful auscultation, but generally not heard during the first few seconds
2	Somewhat louder murmur; can be heard immediately
3	Moderately loud murmur; not accompanied by a thrill
4	Loud murmur with thrill
5	Very loud murmur; audible if one edge of the stethoscope is in contact with the chest
6	Loudest possible murmur; can be heard with the stethoscope 1 cm from the chest wall

cal examination alone. Simply identifying a murmur as possibly pathologic, particularly in an infant, is sufficient reason to seek further evaluation by a pediatric cardiologist.

Common Types of Innocent Murmurs

Vibratory Murmur ("Twanging String" Murmur; "Groaning" Murmur) This is an early to midsystolic musical murmur of low to medium intensity (grade 3 or less) with a "groaning" quality. The murmur is heard best over the mid-precordial area, but may be referred to the second left intercostal space, left sternal border, or apex (Figure 28). The intensity increases with exercise and varies with respiration.

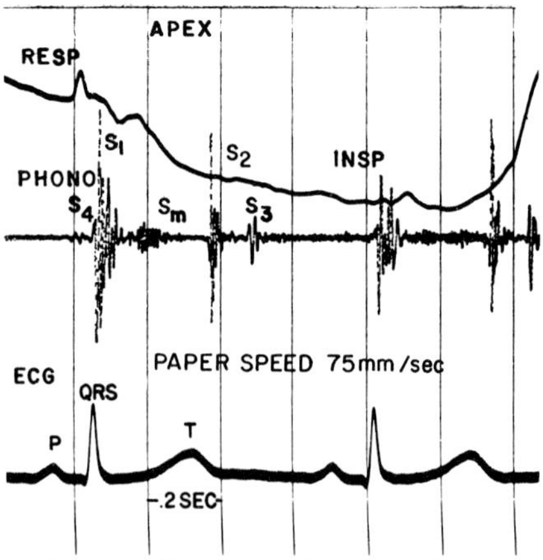

Figure 28. A "twanging string" or harmonic midsystolic murmur (SM), one of the most common and impressive of the innocent murmurs, in a 5-year-old boy with a normal heart. Such a murmur is usually maximal over the midprecordium, but is also well heard at the apex and second LICS. It usually has an intensity of grade 2 or 3. Note that the first sound complex (S_1) is not obscured. The murmur occupies primarily midsystole, has a "picket fence" configuration, and ends before the second sound (S_2).

Pulmonary Ejection Murmur This is an early to midstystolic murmur, grade 3 or less, loudest in the second and third left intercostal spaces parasternally, with radiation to the apex and lower left sternal border. It originates in the pulmonary artery and is generated by rapid ejection of blood into this vessel. Any condition that increases cardiac output increases the intensity of this murmur. It is particularly common in preadolescent youngsters. An uncommon variant sounds like the crunching of cellophane near the ears and is therefore called a "pulmonary artery crunch" (Figure 29).

Venous Hum This is a continuous, low-to-medium–pitched humming noise, best heard in the neck and second right intercostal space parasternally, with the patient sitting. Rarely it is loud enough to produce a thrill (Figure 30). In contrast to the murmur of a patent ductus arteriosus, maximal intensity occurs during diastole. The diastolic phase can usually be obliterated by compressing the neck veins, by turning the head, or lying the patient down. The systolic phase is also reduced by these same maneuvers, although less strikingly so.

Some Rarer Innocent Functional Murmurs

Cardiorespiratory Murmurs These are sharply localized, usually midsystolic murmurs that vary markedly with respiration. Murmurs that begin in midsystole, vary with respiration, and are maximal in the second left intercostal space are probably benign. Those that are maximal at the apex and often initiated by a midsystolic click are usually due to congenital mitral valve prolapse.

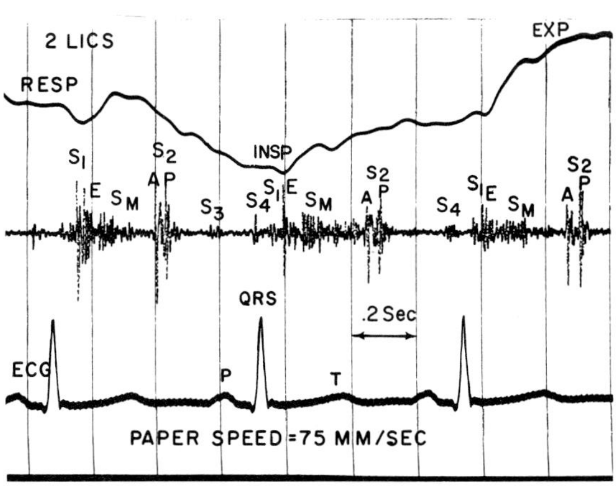

Figure 29. A dramatic, but innocent, systolic murmur recorded in a 13-year-old girl. This pulmonary artery "crunch" is an unusual variant of the common pulmonary ejection murmur. On expiration, it achieves its maximal intensity and sounds like the crunching of cellophane held close to the ear. Note the third and fourth heart sounds, S_3 and S_4, heard well in many normal adolescents, as is the ejection sound (E).

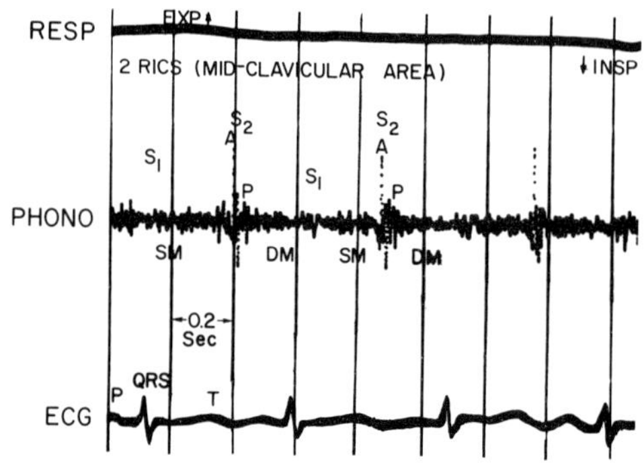

Figure 30. A venous hum, another common innocent murmur, recorded in a 2-year-old boy in the sitting position. This prominent continuous murmur is noted best in the right midclavicular area, and usually disappears or diminishes in intensity when the patient lies down.

Carotid Bruits These murmurs are thought to originate in the right carotid artery at its site of origin from the innominate artery. This murmur occurs at the time of rapid ejection of blood into this vessel; hence, it is a brief early to midsystolic murmur. Maximal intensity is over the right side of the neck, rather than in the second right intercostal space, differentiating it from valvar aortic stenosis.

Ejection Clicks

Ejection sounds usually occur in the latter part of the first heart sound. Because they sound similar to the striking of a pair of coins, they have been labeled ejection clicks. They have been attributed to the opening of the aortic or pulmonic valves or to sounds generated in the great vessels when blood suddenly fills them.

Pulmonary ejection sounds are heard maximally in the second left intercostal space and are not transmitted to the apex. As is usual with sounds emanating from the pulmonary artery, their intensity increases during expiration and diminishes markedly with inspiration. Aortic ejection sounds are maximal at the apex or second right intercostal space, vary little with respiration, and are more widely transmitted.

Pulmonary ejection clicks may occur in normal children, often associated with transiently increased blood flow. They also may be heard in association with an enlarged pulmonary artery caused by valvar pulmonic stenosis, pulmonic insufficiency, or large left-to-right shunts. *Aortic ejection clicks,* on the other hand, are usually pathologic, occurring most often in conditions resulting from a large ascending aorta, e.g., valvar aortic stenosis, aortic insufficiency, and tetralogy of Fallot.

FUNCTIONAL CLASSIFICATION

It is helpful to grade the functional and therapeutic status of the patient. The classification given in Table 7 is widely used.

Table 7. Classification of cardiac patients

Functional capacity	Therapeutic
Class I No limitation of physical activity No symptoms with ordinary physical activity	Class A Physical activity not restricted
Class II Slight limitation of physical activity Symptoms occur with ordinary physical activity	Class B Ordinary physical activity not restricted Severe or competitive physical activity not advised
Class III Marked limitation of physical activity; comfortable at rest Symptoms occur with less than ordinary physical activity	Class C Ordinary physical activity moderately restricted Strenuous activity discontinued
Class IV Symptoms with any physical activity and may occur at rest Symptoms increase in severity with any physical activity	Class D Ordinary physical activity markedly restricted
	Class E Complete rest advised Confined to bed or chair

BIBLIOGRAPHY

Castle, R. F., and Craige, E. 1961. Auscultation of the heart in infants and children. Pediatrics 26 (Suppl.):511–561.

Curtiss, E. I., Matthew, R. G., and Shaver, J. A. 1975. Mechanism of normal splitting of the second heart sounds. Circulation 51:157–164.

Kusukawa, R., Bruce, D. W., Sakamoto, T., MacCanon, D. M., and Luisada, A. A. 1966. Hemodynamic determinants of the amplitude of the second sound. J. Appl. Physiol. 21:938–946.

Ongley, P. A., Sprague, H. B., Rappaport, M. B., and Nadas, A. S. Heart Sounds and Murmurs. A Clinical Phonocardiographic Study. Grune & Stratton, New York.

chapter 7

ELECTROCARDIOGRAPHY

Many physicians suffer from electrocardiographobia. To help alleviate this dire syndrome (characterized by blurred vision, dry mouth, and trembling hands), the following guide is offered to supply a few fundamentals of ECG interpretation.

The distribution of electrical charges in a resting cell and the movement of a wave of depolarization from negative to positive areas are shown in Figure 31. The myocardium is composed of many cells producing a composite depolarization sequence (Figure 32). In most instances, electrical information produced by the heart is sampled at a distance (on the surface of the chest). Both logical deduction and empirical induction are needed to project such information into a picture of the electrical activity of the heart itself.

TERMINOLOGY OF ELECTROCARDIOGRAPHIC WAVE FORMS (Figure 33)

The *P wave* is the result of atrial depolarization. The *QRS complex* is the result of ventricular depolarization. Within the QRS complex, the *Q wave* is

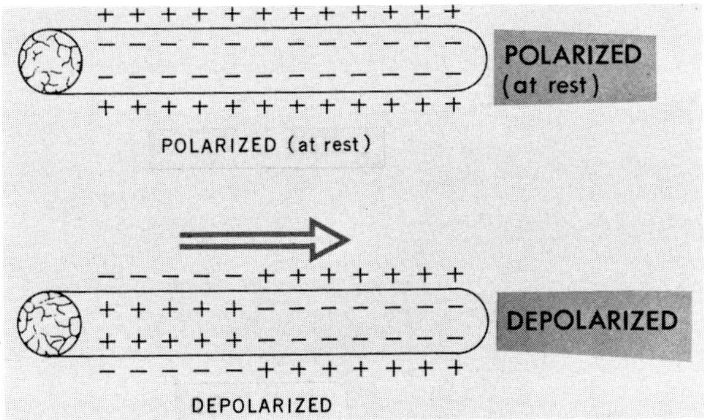

Figure 31. (Top) Illustrates the distribution of electrical charges in a resting cell, with the inside being negative as compared with the outside. (Bottom) Shows a wave of depolarization (a wave of negativity) sweeping down the cell. By convention, positive vectors point from a negative area to the positive area.

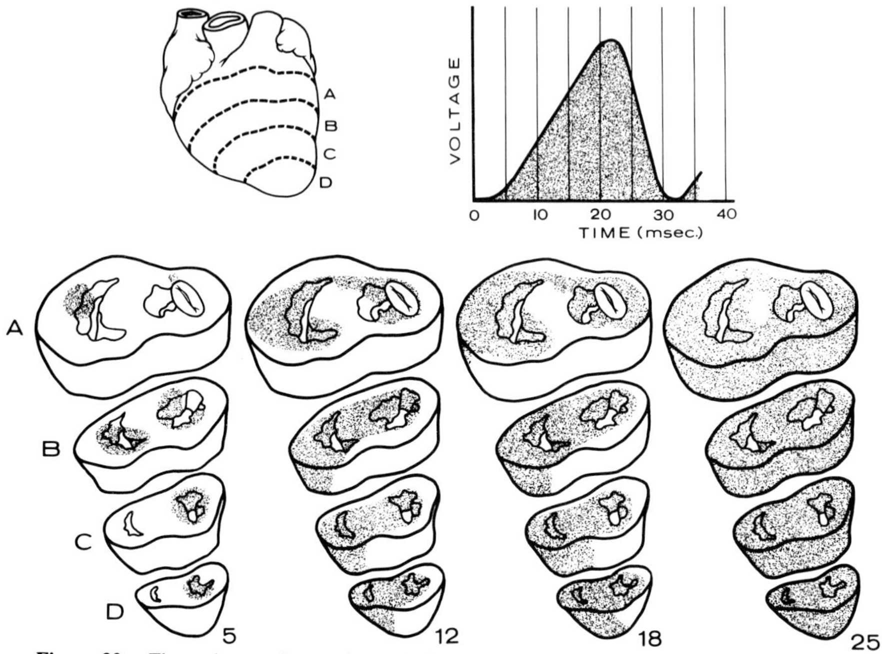

Figure 32. The pathway of normal ventricular excitation in the dog. Note the extent of depolarization at 5, 12, 18, and 25 msec after the initiation of the QRS complex. The small drawing of the heart (upper left) indicates the positions of planes labeled A, B, C, and D. The insert (upper right) indicates the total duration of ventricular depolarization. (From Scher, A. M. 1965. Electrical correlates of the cardiac cycle. In T. C. Ruch and H. D. Patton (eds.), Medical Physiology and Biophysics, 19th ed. W. B. Saunders Company, Philadelphia.)

the initial negative wave, the *R wave* the first positive wave, and the *S wave* a negative wave following the R wave. When there is only a negative component to the QRS complex, it is called a *QS wave*. *R′ and S′ waves* refer to second positive and negative waves following R and S waves, respectively, in the same QRS complex. The *ST segment* lies between the end of the QRS complex and the beginning of the T wave. The *T wave* arises from ventricular

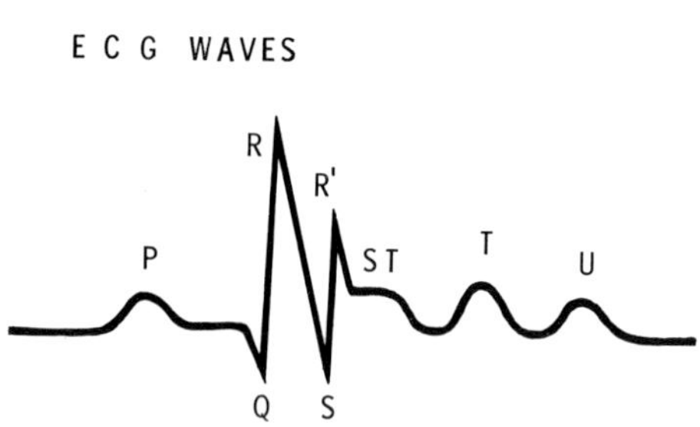

Figure 33. Diagram showing the components of the cardiac cycle as depicted by ECG wave forms. See text for complete description.

repolarization, which creates a wave usually of lower amplitude and longer duration than the preceding QRS complex. The *U wave* is a small wave occasionally seen following the T wave. U waves may be noted in electrocardiograms of normal adolescents or in individuals with hypokalemia.

COMMON TECHNICAL ERRORS

1. Negative P and T waves in lead I suggest either that there is a reversed position of the atria, as in mirror-image dextrocardia, or that the technician has inadvertently reversed the arm leads (Figure 34).
2. If all precordial chest leads look exactly alike, the technician has probably forgotten to change the switch on the panel of the ECG machine from aVF to the precordial position (V leads); or the technician has smeared electrode paste across the chest to "save time," and has formed a single precordial electrode in doing so (Figure 35).
3. Improper placement of V_1 electrode too high on the chest or too far to the right may cause an rSR′ pattern rather than the expected normal rS pattern.

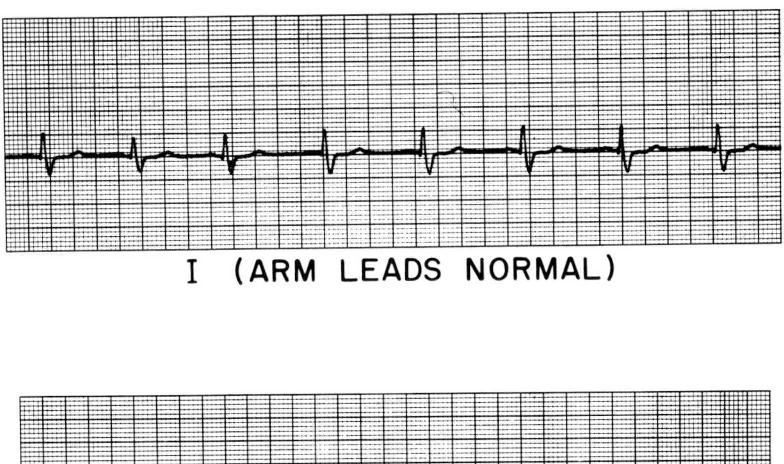

I (ARM LEADS NORMAL)

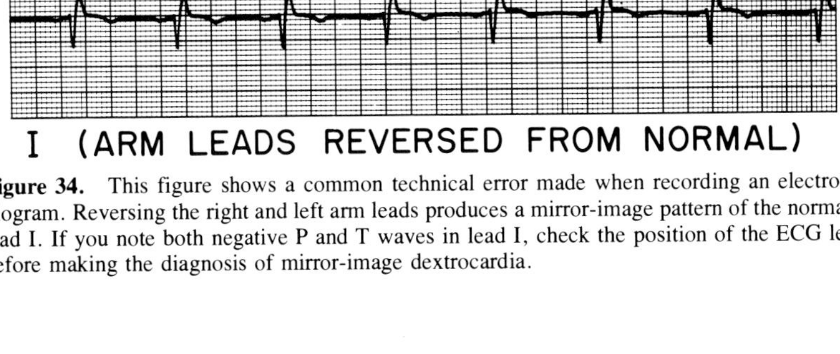

I (ARM LEADS REVERSED FROM NORMAL)

Figure 34. This figure shows a common technical error made when recording an electrocardiogram. Reversing the right and left arm leads produces a mirror-image pattern of the normal in lead I. If you note both negative P and T waves in lead I, check the position of the ECG leads before making the diagnosis of mirror-image dextrocardia.

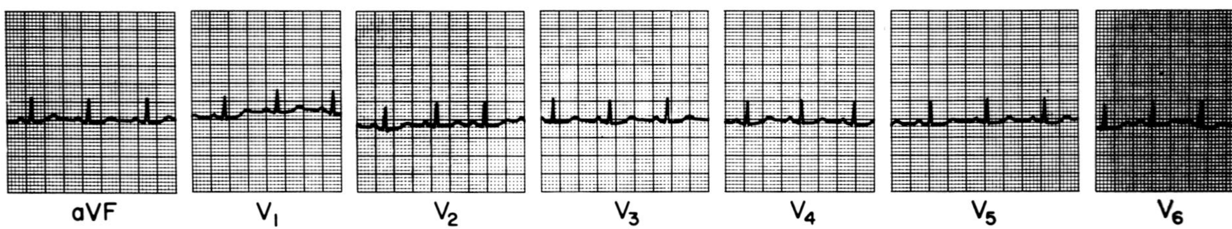

Figure 35. Another common technical error made while recording an electrocardiogram is to forget to switch the dial on the ECG panel from the aVF to the V (precordial) lead position. When the precordial leads are identical, look immediately at lead aVF. If lead aVF has the same configuration as the precordial leads, you have made this particular technical error.

ELECTROCARDIOGRAPHIC INTERPRETATION

As with most laboratory tests, the electrocardiogram needs statistical analysis for proper interpretation. When dealing with groups of patients, we can usually sort out certain features that distinguish the majority of those with an abnormality from the normal group. However, biologic populations can rarely be clearly separated by a single test; frequently there is a great deal of overlap. It is a further statistical truism that the more criteria that are used intelligently to differentiate normal from abnormal, the better the separation. Thus, when interpreting electrocardiograms, the more criteria of abnormality that are satisfied, the more likely the electrocardiogram is to be abnormal.

A sound policy is to insist on *not* interpreting an electrocardiogram—or any other laboratory data, for that matter—as an isolated item. Relatively few electrocardiograms are diagnostic by themselves, but they can be powerful adjuncts when viewed as part of a clinical picture. For example, there is a great deal of overlap between infants with normal electrocardiograms and those with right ventricular hypertrophy. Similarly, electrocardiograms of normal young boys and of those with left ventricular hypertrophy also overlap. If the total clinical picture suggests a cardiac lesion, then this information should be applied in interpreting the electrocardiogram.

ELECTROCARDIOGRAPHIC COMPONENTS

The *P-R interval,* the time from the beginning of the P wave to the beginning of the QRS complex (Figure 36), increases with age (see Table 8). *A shortened P-R interval* may be seen occasionally in otherwise normal children, with an ectopic atrial pacemaker closer to the AV node, in glycogen storage disease of the heart, or when conduction is partially through an aberrant shorter pathway (Wolff-Parkinson-White syndrome, Figure 37). *A prolonged P-R interval* may be seen in 1%–2% of normal persons, or in patients with

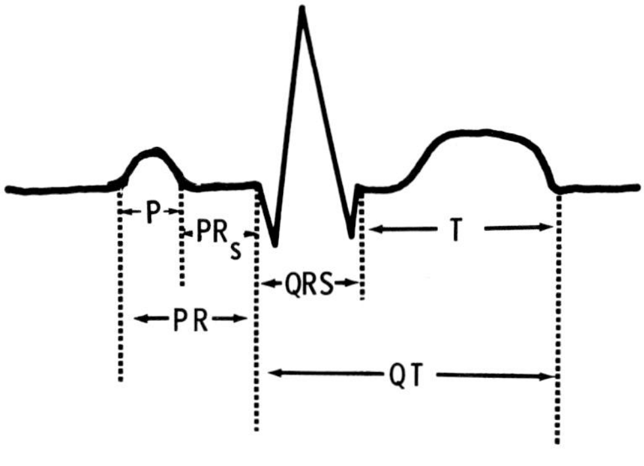

Figure 36. Diagram showing the various time intervals measured on an electrocardiogram. See text for details.

Table 8. Duration of electrocardiographic intervals (values are given in seconds)[a]

Age	P-R intervals		QRS duration		QT_c	
	Lower limit	Upper limit	Lower limit	Upper limit	Lower limit	Upper limit
Birth–1 day	0.08	0.12	0.04	0.10	0.34	0.54
1 day–1 week	0.08	0.12	0.04	0.08	0.34	0.54
1 week–1 month	0.08	0.12	0.04	0.07	0.30	0.50
1–3 months	0.08	0.16	0.05	0.08	0.32	0.47
3–6 months	0.08	0.12	0.05	0.08	0.35	0.46
6 months–1 year	0.08	0.14	0.04	0.08	0.31	0.49
1–3 years	0.08	0.16	0.04	0.08	0.34	0.43
3–5 years	0.10	0.16	0.04	0.09	0.34	0.46
5–8 years	0.10	0.18	0.04	0.09	0.33	0.51
8–12 years	0.10	0.20	0.05	0.10	0.35	0.44
12–16 years	0.10	0.20	0.04	0.10	0.30	0.46
Adult males	0.11	0.21	0.05	0.10	0.30	0.45
Adult females	0.11	0.21	0.05	0.10	0.30	0.45

[a] Adapted from Dittmer, D. S., and Grebe, R. M. (eds.) 1959. Handbook of Circulation, p. 141. W. B. Saunders Company, Philadelphia.

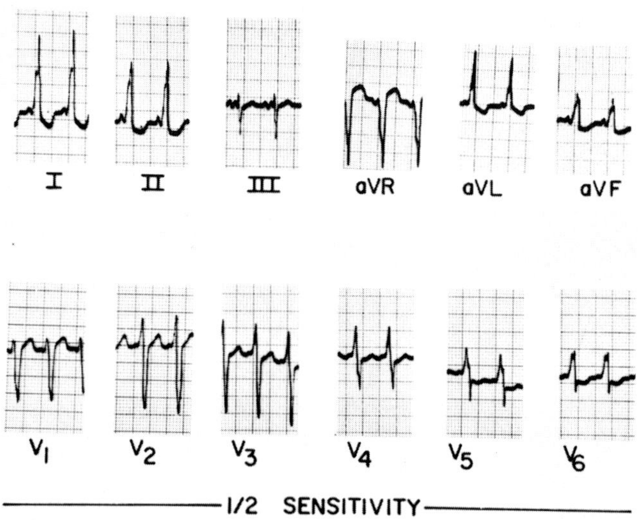

Figure 37. Wolff-Parkinson-White (WPW) syndrome consists of a short P-R interval, and a slow slurred onset of the QRS complex (delta wave), resulting in a prolonged QRS duration. Note the marked ST segment and T wave changes. This electrocardiogram was recorded in a 6-month-old male child with recurrent bouts of supraventricular tachycardia and congestive heart failure. This particular WPW pattern mimics left bundle branch block. (Adapted from Schiebler, G. L., Wood, R. S., and Johnson, W. S. 1963. Paroxysmal pseudoventricular tachycardia in an infant with the Wolff-Parkinson-White syndrome. J. Florida Med. Assn. 49:804–807.)

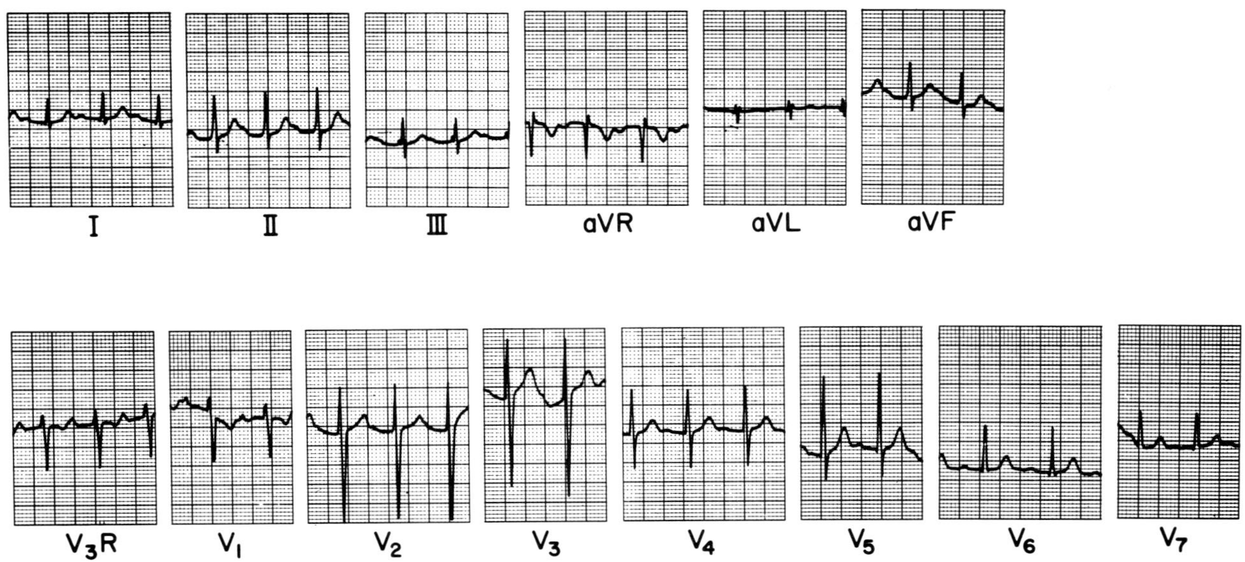

Figure 38. With a delay in atrioventricular conduction, the P-R interval increases. When this time interval exceeds the normal maximum value for age, first degree AV block is present. In the above electrocardiogram, the P-R interval is 0.22 sec.

acute rheumatic fever, following administration of digitalis, or in hyperthyroidism (Figure 38). First degree atrioventricular block is not infrequently seen in patients with thyrotoxicosis. Thus fever, tachycardia, first degree atrioventricular block, and the murmur of mitral insufficiency occur as part of the clinical picture of thyrotoxicosis, and should not be construed as evidence of rheumatic fever. *No regular P-R interval* is seen in complete AV block. There is no regular relationship between P waves and QRS complexes.

The *P wave* has a normal maximum amplitude in any lead of 0.3 mV (3 mm).* The P wave should always be positive in leads I and II. It is negative in lead III in 10% of otherwise normal children.

The *QRS duration,* measured from the beginning to the end of the QRS wave (see Figure 36), indicates prolonged ventricular excitation if longer than 0.08 sec in infants or 0.10 sec in older children (see Table 8).

The *R wave* should be more than 5 mm in at least one lead (see Table 10). An rSr′ pattern in the right precordial leads or in lead aVR occurs in about 5% of normal children.

ST segment duration is the time interval between the end of the QRS complex and the beginning of the T wave (see Figure 36). A depression or elevation of this segment of more than 2 mm in any lead is abnormal.

T waves are normally positive in leads I and II and negative in aVR. A positive T wave in leads V_3R or V_1 is normal at birth, but after 3 days of age it indicates right ventricular hypertrophy. In some normal children, it may become upright again after 8 years. Negative T waves in leads II, V_5, and V_6 are evidence of myocardial damage. Negative T waves in leads III and aVL are usually abnormal (see Figures 33 and 36).

QRS-T angle is the angle between the mean QRS vector (axis) and the mean T vector (axis) in any plane, but usually refers to the frontal plane. In normal newborns, it may be as great as 160°, but in older infants and children a QRS-T angle of more than 45° is usually abnormal.

The *Q-T interval,* measured from the beginning of the QRS complex to the end of the T wave (see Figure 36), is inversely proportional to heart rate. Correction for rate may be made by dividing the measured Q-T interval by the square root of the R-R interval. This corrected measurement is referred to as the Q-T_c interval (see Table 8). A prolonged Q-T_c interval may be seen in active carditis, in calcium depletion, or after quinidine administration. A shortened Q-T_c interval occurs with digitalis administration and hypercalcemia.

CRITERIA FOR DIAGNOSIS OF CHAMBER ENLARGEMENT

Before discussing the criteria for diagnosis of chamber enlargement, a few cautions should be noted.

*Throughout the book, when speaking of ECGs, it will be assumed that 1 mV = 10 mm.

Caution No. 1: The criteria that follow assume a normal position of the heart in the chest and a normal depolarization sequence. Interpretation of the ECG when either of these conditions is not present may be difficult.

Caution No. 2: Interpretation of the ECG is strongly influenced by the frequency response of the machine. A quick test of this may be done by using

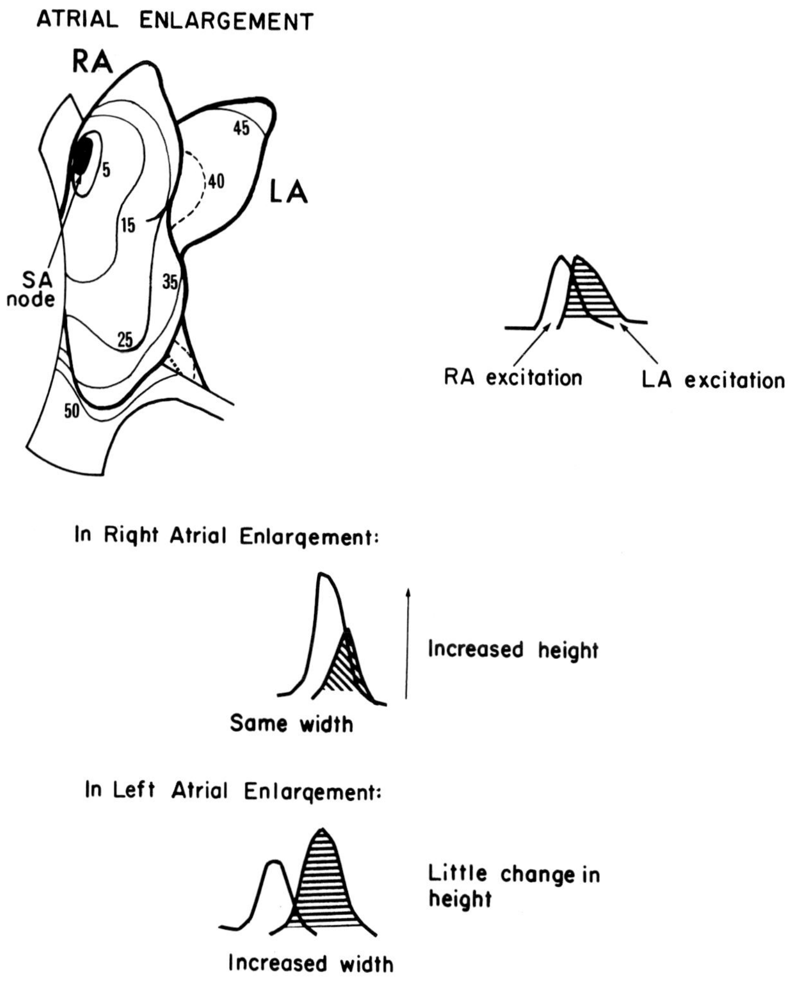

Figure 39. Schematic concept of electrical excitation of the atria. Note that the right atrium is depolarized before the left atrium. Summation of these two potentials results in a smooth-contoured P wave. When the right atrium is enlarged, its potential is increased, but it still occurs during the early portion of P wave inscription. Thus, an increase in P wave height results, but the total wave time remains the same duration. When the left atrium is enlarged, depolarization begins at the usual time, but now takes longer. As a result, there is little increase in P wave height, but the total duration of the wave form is longer. The effect is a broad, notched P wave.

the calibration button. First, with the sensitivity switch set at ×2 (i.e., 20 mm/mV) and the paper running, depress and release the button several times. The result should be a series of vertical lines with a sharp corner or a 1–2-mm overshoot.

Next, using the same settings and with the paper running, keep the calibration button depressed until the tracing returns almost to the baseline. The time required for the stylus to move from 20 mm above the baseline to a point 7 mm above the baseline should be at least 3.0 sec.

Caution No. 3: Many ECG machines are equipped with frequency cutoff switches, usually labeled Hi and Low. The low setting reduces 60-Hz noise but also affects the amplitudes of the QRS complexes. Always record with the switch in the high setting and reduce 60-Hz interference by other means (e.g., better electrical grounding or better cleaning of the skin beneath the electrodes).

Caution No. 4: The hotter the stylus in thermal recording ECG machines, the lower the frequency response. Always use the lowest setting that produces a clear tracing.

Left Atrial Enlargement (Figure 39)

1. Broad, notched P waves (P mitrale). These are best seen in leads I, II, V_5, and V_6 (see Figure 190).
2. Negative P waves in lead V_3R or V_1.
3. Diphasic P waves in lead V_3R or V_1 when the negative part is of greater duration than the preceding positive portion (see Figure 214).
4. A useful rule for deciding if the P wave is broad is to compare the duration of the P wave (P) to the duration of the PR segment (PR_S). The latter is the time from the end of the P wave to the beginning of the next QRS complex (see Figure 36). A ratio greater than 1.6 suggests left atrial enlargement.

Right Atrial Enlargement (Figure 39)

1. Peaked P waves taller than 3 mm. This is best appreciated in leads II, III, aVF, V_3R, V_1, and V_2 (see Figure 136).
2. A P:PR_S ratio of less than 1.0.

Right Ventricular Hypertrophy (RVH)

Major Criteria

1. Taller than normal R waves in right precordial leads V_3R and V_1, with deeper than normal S waves in V_6 (see Table 10).
2. A pure R wave in lead V_1 before 1 week of age or after 3 months of age.
3. R:RS ratio in lead V_1 greater than normal for age (see Table 9).
4. Positive T wave in lead V_1 or V_3R after first 3 or 4 days of life. **Impor-**

Table 9. R wave expressed as percentage of RS deflection (values in parentheses are upper and lower extremes of normal)[a]

	Lead	
Age	V_1	V_6
Birth–1 day	62 (26–96)	50 (0–100)
1 day–1 week	58 (35–81)	65 (25–100)
1 week–1 month	66 (34–94)	76 (30–100)
1–3 months	63 (27–100)	78 (60–100)
3–6 months	60 (33–86)	86 (60–100)
6 months–1 year	56 (28–84)	88 (70–100)
1–3 years	45 (32–67)	94 (75–100)
3–5 years	42 (21–67)	95 (68–100)
5–8 years	35 (10–55)	94 (69–100)
8–12 years	34 (16–50)	95 (80–100)
12–16 years	27 (10–55)	90 (70–100)

[a] Adapted from Dittmer, D. S., and Grebe, R. M. (eds.) 1959. Handbook of Circulation, p. 145. W. B. Saunders Company, Philadelphia.

tant exception: when T waves are negative in lead V_6 because of left ventricular pressure overloading.

5. A Q wave in lead V_1 is abnormal after 3 or 4 days of age. It represents either right ventricular hypertrophy or an altered conduction pattern, such as occurs in single ventricle or ventricular inversion.
6. An rsR′ pattern in right chest leads with the R′ greater than 1.0 mV without prolongation of the QRS duration.

Minor Criteria

1. Right axis deviation beyond +135°.
2. R or R′ in lead aVR greater than 0.5 mV, or more than half of the total QRS amplitude.
3. Intrinsicoid deflection (beginning of QRS to maximum amplitude) in lead V_1 greater than 0.035 sec in absence of right bundle branch block.

Left Ventricular Hypertrophy

Major Criteria

1. No Q wave in lead V_5 or V_6 with either depressed ST segments or flat or inverted T waves. The R wave voltage may be normal or increased (Figure 40) (left ventricular pressure overloading).
2. Q wave deeper than 4 mm with tall, peaked symmetrical T waves in lead V_5 or V_6 (Figure 40) (left ventricular volume overloading).

Minor Criteria

1. R wave in lead V_5 or V_6 greater than normal for age.
2. S wave in lead V_1 greater than normal for age.

Table 10. Amplitudes of electrocardiographic waves at various ages [values are in millimeters (1 mV = 10 mm); values in parentheses are ranges][a]

Age	Wave				
	P	Q	R	S	T
LEAD I					
Birth–1 day	0.8(0–1.8)	0.3(0–0.5)	1.5(0–5.5)	6.4(0–12.5)	2.0(0–3.0)
1 day–1 week	0.8(0–1.8)	0.8(0–1.0)	2.0(0–6.0)	5.0(0–10.0)	1.0(0.6–3.0)
1 week–1 month	0.9(0–1.8)	1.0(0–3.0)	3.5(1.0–8.5)	4.6(0–9.3)	2.1(1.0–4.0)
1–3 months	0.4(0–2.0)	1.1(0–2.5)	6.0(2.0–14.0)	3.6(0–9.0)	2.2(0.2–4.3)
3–6 months	1.0(0–2.0)	1.2(0–2.0)	7.8(2.0–13.0)	3.3(0–7.0)	2.6(0.2–5.2)
6 months–1 year	1.0(0.5–2.5)	1.6(0–4.5)	8.0(3.0–17.0)	3.7(0–10.0)	2.4(1.0–6.0)
1–3 years	1.1(0.5–2.5)	1.5(0–3.0)	8.0(3.0–17.0)	3.1(0–8.0)	2.9(1.0–6.6)
3–5 years	1.1(0.5–2.0)	1.2(0–2.0)	6.5(3.0–16.0)	2.1(0–6.0)	2.5(1.0–6.0)
5–8 years	1.0(0.5–2.0)	1.1(0–2.5)	6.2(1.0–15.5)	2.0(0–7.0)	2.6(1.0–5.5)
8–12 years	1.0(0–2.0)	1.3(0–3.0)	6.5(1.0–16.0)	1.5(0–8.0)	2.9(1.0–6.0)
12–16 years	0.9(0–2.0)	1.0(0–3.0)	5.9(0–12.0)	1.3(0–10.0)	2.5(1.0–6.0)
LEAD II					
Birth–1 day	1.4(0–2.5)	1.5(0–5.0)	5.5(0–23.0)	2.0(0–7.0)	1.0(−1.0 to 3.0)
1 day–1 week	1.8(0–2.8)	1.8(0–4.0)	5.0(2.0–12.0)	2.3(0–8.0)	1.6(0–4.0)
1 week–1 month	1.5(0.5–2.0)	1.6(0–4.0)	7.5(2.0–14.0)	1.4(0–6.5)	2.7(0–5.6)
1–3 months	1.5(0.5–2.0)	1.8(0–5.0)	11.5(5.0–19.0)	1.9(0–6.0)	3.1(0.5–5.6)
3–6 months	1.6(0.5–2.5)	2.3(0–5.5)	13.5(3.0–23.0)	1.7(0–6.0)	3.4(0.2–6.7)
6 months–1 year	1.7(0–2.5)	2.4(0–5.0)	13.0(2.5–25.0)	2.2(0–6.0)	3.2(0.3–5.8)
1–3 years	1.6(0.5–3.0)	2.1(0–4.5)	12.5(1.5–23.0)	1.6(0–6.0)	3.0(0.2–5.7)
3–5 years	1.7(0.5–3.0)	1.6(0–4.5)	12.5(3.0–21.0)	1.3(0–5.0)	3.1(0.1–5.9)
5–8 years	1.7(0.5–3.0)	1.4(0–5.0)	12.5(3.5–21.5)	1.7(0–6.0)	3.3(0.6–5.9)
8–12 years	1.5(1.5–3.0)	1.4(0–3.0)	13.5(4.0–23.5)	1.5(0–6.0)	3.6(−0.5 to 8.2)
12–16 years	1.6(1.0–3.0)	1.2(0–2.5)	13.5(3.5–24.5)	1.4(0–7.0)	3.3(−0.2 to 6.7)

LEAD III					
Birth–1 day	0.6(−1.0 to 2.0)	2.5(0–9.0)	9.0(2.0–23.0)	0.2(0–3.0)	1.0(−1.2 to 3.0)
1 day–1 week	0.8(0–2.0)	2.5(0–5.0)	7.5(3.0–15.0)	0.3(0–4.0)	0.5(−2.3 to 3.1)
1 week–1 month	0.8(−0.5 to 2.0)	2.4(0–5.0)	7.9(2.0–17.0)	0.2(0–2.0)	0.6(−2.2 to 3.5)
1–3 months	0.6(−1.0 to 2.0)	3.3(0–7.0)	8.5(4.0–15.0)	0.6(0–5.0)	0.9(−1.7 to 3.7)
3–6 months	0.8(0–2.0)	4.5(0–9.0)	10.2(3.0–22.0)	0.6(0–6.0)	1.2(−2.1 to 4.6)
6 months–1 year	0.8(0–2.0)	4.1(0–8.0)	9.8(2.0–22.0)	0.8(0–6.0)	0.7(−2.7 to 4.0)
1–3 years	0.7(−1.5 to 2.0)	3.5(0–8.0)	7.5(1.0–19.0)	0.8(0–8.0)	0.2(−3.2 to 3.6)
3–5 years	0.6(−1.0 to 2.0)	2.5(0–6.0)	8.5(1.0–18.0)	0.8(0–7.0)	0.3(−2.2 to 3.4)
5–8 years	0.6(−1.0 to 2.0)	2.2(0–5.5)	8.5(1.0–20.0)	0.8(0–8.0)	1.6(−2.2 to 4.4)
8–12 years	0.6(−1.5 to 2.0)	1.9(0–5.0)	9.2(1.0–24.0)	1.0(0–5.0)	0.7(−1.8 to 3.5)
12–16 years	(−0.5 to 2.0)	1.6(0–5.0)	9.0(1.0–26.0)	1.0(0–9.0)	0.8(−1.6 to 3.5)
LEAD aVR					
Birth–1 day	−0.9(−2.0 to 1.5)	2.4(0–4.0)	3.9(0–9.0)	0.3(0–9.5)	−0.5(−3.2 to 2.4)
1 day–1 week	−1.2(−2.0 to 0)	2.7(0–4.0)	2.7(0–7.0)	1.9(0–7.0)	−1.6(−3.2 to 0)
1 week–1 month	−1.0(−2.0 to 1.0)	4.0(0–9.0)	2.2(0–6.0)	2.0(0–8.0)	−2.3(−3.9 to −0.6)
1–3 months	−1.1(−2.0 to 0)	7.1(0–12.0)	2.1(0–4.0)	4.3(0–14.5)	−2.3(−4.7 to −0.2)
3–6 months	−1.1(−2.0 to 0)	8.0(0–12.0)	1.8(0–5.0)	6.0(0–15.0)	−2.9(−4.5 to −0.3)
6 months–1 year	−1.2(−2.5 to 0)	8.1(0–13.0)	2.3(0–5.0)	5.0(0–18.0)	−2.8(−5.1 to −0.4)
1–3 years	−1.3(−2.0 to 0)	7.3(0–14.0)	2.2(0–6.0)	5.0(0–15.0)	−2.9(−5.2 to −0.6)
3–5 years	−1.2(−2.0 to 1.0)	7.4(0–13.5)	1.7(0–5.0)	5.0(0–14.0)	−2.6(−5.6 to −0.5)
5–8 years	−2.0(−2.1 to 0)	8.2(0–13.0)	1.6(0–5.0)	5.2(0–15.0)	−2.6(−4.9 to −0.6)
8–12 years	−1.2(−2.5 to −0.5)	8.2(0–12.5)	1.3(0–4.0)	1.0(0–16.0)	−3.2(−5.3 to −0.7)
12–16 years	−1.1(−2.0 to −0.5)	7.9(0–14.0)	1.2(0–3.0)	0.8(0–14.0)	−2.9(−5.2 to −0.5)

continued

Table 10. *continued*

	Wave				
Age	P	Q	R	S	T
LEAD aVL					
Birth–1 day	0.1(−1.5 to 1.5)	1.3(0–2.0)	2.0(1.0–6.0)	6.5(0–16.0)	0(−2.4 to 2.6)
1 day–1 week	0.1(−1.5 to 1.0)	0.7(0–1.0)	1.6(0–3.0)	5.5(0–13.0)	0.9(−0.8 to 2.7)
1 week–1 month	0.3(−1.0 to 1.5)	1.3(0–1.5)	2.3(0–7.0)	6.0(0–11.0)	1.0(−1.2 to 3.1)
1–3 months	0.2(−1.0 to 1.0)	1.7(0–2.0)	3.6(1.0–9.0)	4.8(0–9.5)	0.7(−1.5 to 3.1)
3–6 months	0.4(−0.5 to 1.0)	1.1(0–1.5)	3.9(0–8.0)	4.0(0–7.0)	0.8(−0.6 to 2.4)
6 months–1 year	0.3(−1.5 to 1.0)	1.8(0–5.5)	4.6(1.0–10.0)	4.2(0–11.0)	1.2(−1.0 to 3.6)
1–3 years	0.4(−1.0 to 1.0)	1.3(0–4.0)	4.3(1.0–10.0)	3.8(0–9.0)	1.4(−0.5 to 3.4)
3–5 years	0.4(−1.0 to 1.0)	1.3(0–3.0)	3.3(0–7.0)	3.3(0–10.0)	1.2(−1.0 to 3.6)
5–8 years	0.3(−1.0 to 1.5)	1.2(0–4.0)	2.6(0–7.0)	3.2(0–10.0)	1.0(−1.2 to 3.3)
8–12 years	0.5(−1.0 to 1.0)	1.2(0–6.0)	2.7(0–8.0)	3.0(0–14.0)	1.3(−0.7 to 3.6)
12–16 years	0.3(−1.0 to 1.0)	1.3(0–6.0)	2.4(0–12.0)	3.0(0–20.0)	1.1(−1.1 to 3.6)
LEAD aVF					
Birth–1 day	1.1(−1.0 to 2.0)	1.9(0–6.0)	6.5(2.0–20.0)	0.8(0–7.0)	0.9(−1.2 to 3.0)
1 day–1 week	1.2(0–2.0)	2.0(0–4.0)	5.8(2.0–13.0)	0.7(0–3.0)	0.2(−1.6 to 3.8)
1 week–1 month	1.2(−1.0 to 3.0)	1.9(0–4.0)	6.8(2.0–15.0)	0.5(0–5.0)	0.5(−0.5 to 3.7)
1–3 months	1.2(0–2.0)	2.5(0–5.0)	8.8(0.5–17.8)	0.8(0–4.0)	2.0(−0.1 to 3.9)
3–6 months	1.1(0.5–2.0)	2.7(0–6.0)	10.1(0.5–20.2)	0.9(0–6.0)	2.2(0–4.2)
6 months–1 year	1.2(0–2.0)	2.9(0–6.0)	9.4(0–17.2)	1.1(0–4.0)	1.9(−0.1 to 3.7)
1–3 years	1.2(0–2.0)	2.2(0–5.0)	8.2(1.0–20.0)	0.8(0–5.0)	1.7(−0.6 to 4.1)
3–5 years	1.2(0–2.0)	1.7(0–5.0)	9.8(0.5–18.8)	0.7(0–3.5)	2.1(−0.7 to 4.9)
5–8 years	1.2(0–2.0)	1.5(0–5.0)	9.7(0.5–18.7)	0.9(0–7.0)	2.0(−0.6 to 4.5)
8–12 years	1.1(0–2.0)	1.5(0–3.0)	10.2(0.7–20.0)	1.0(0–5.0)	2.3(−0.5 to 4.7)
12–16 years	1.2(0–2.0)	1.3(0–3.0)	10.5(0.1–21.8)	1.0(0–5.0)	2.4(−0.7 to 5.4)

LEAD V_1					
Birth–1 day	1.0	0	16.0(6.0–27.0)	10.0(0–28.0)	0.6(−4.0 to 5.0)
1 day–1 week	1.1	0	17.0(4.0–30.0)	11.0(4.0–25.0)	−3.6(−6.0 to −2.0)
1 week–1 month	0.6(−1.0 to 2.0)	0	13.5(2.6–24.0)	7.0(0–17.0)	−2.8(−8.0 to −0.8)
1–3 months	0.4(−1.0 to 1.5)	0	10.0(1.5–19.0)	6.5(0–20.0)	−2.7(−7.0 to 2.0)
3–6 months	0.4	0	12.0(5.0–19.0)	7.0(3.0–12.0)	−4.2(−7.5 to −0.4)
6 months–1 year	0.7(−1.0 to 1.0)	0	12.8(1.5–20.0)	8.0(3.0–18.0)	−3.9(−7.4 to 0)
1–3 years	0.8(−1.0 to 2.0)	0	9.0(3.9–18.0)	7.0(0–28.0)	−3.7(−6.0 to −2.0)
3–5 years	1.0	0	7.0(2.0–16.0)	13.0(6.0–33.0)	−3.8(−6.2 to −1.0)
5–8 years	0.9	0	7.0(1.2–20.0)	14.0(4.0–26.0)	−3.5(−6.0 to −0.8)
8–12 years	0.7	0	6.0(1.8–16.0)	13.0(5.0–26.0)	−2.9(−5.6 to −0.5)
12–16 years	0.7	0	5.5(0–16.0)	14.5(5.0–26.0)	−1.5(−4.0 to 7.0)
LEAD V_2					
Birth–1 day	1.0	0	21.0(12.0–30.0)	22.0(7.0–37.0)	1.2(−7.5 to 10.0)
1 day–1 week	1.2	0	21.0(12.0–34.0)	21.5(3.0–40.0)	−4.2(−7.9 to −1.0)
1 week–1 month	1.3(0.5–2.0)	0	20.5(5.5–34.0)	17.0(4.0–29.0)	−4.5(−5.5 to 4.0)
1–3 months	0.8	0	15.5(3.5–28.0)	13.0(3.0–24.0)	−3.0(−7.0 to 2.0)
3–6 months	1.4(0.5–2.0)	0	24.0(13.0–35.0)	16.0(4.0–30.0)	−5.0(−9.0 to 6.0)
6 months–1 year	1.0	0	19.0(6.3–32.0)	17.0(2.0–34.0)	−4.5(−8.0 to 0)
1–3 years	1.4	0	16.0(5.5–25.0)	21.0(7.0–35.0)	−3.8(−8.8 to 1.0)
3–5 years	1.0	0	13.5(1.0–25.0)	22.0(16.0–34.0)	−4.1(−7.0 to −1.0)
5–8 years	1.0	0	12.0(1.0–26.0)	23.0(11.0–40.0)	−1.2(−6.0 to 6.0)
8–12 years	0.9	0	10.0(1.0–20.0)	23.0(12.0–40.0)	1.0(−7.5 to 10.0)
12–16 years	1.0	0	8.5(2.0–20.5)	23.0(8.0–51.0)	6.0(0.8–13.0)

continued

Table 10. *continued*

Age	Wave				
	P	Q	R	S	T
LEAD V_3					
Birth–1 day	1.7(1.0–3.0)	0(0–0)	20.0(11.0–29.0)	26.0(12.0–36.0)	−4.0(−7.0 to 4.0)
1 day–1 week	1.9(1.0–3.0)	0.1(0–3.0)	20.0(5.0–35.0)	19.0(0–36.0)	−1.5(−5.0 to 4.0)
1 week–1 month	1.4	0.1(0–1.0)	20.2(3.0–37.0)	14.0(2.0–26.0)	−0.5(−4.0 to 6.0)
1–3 months	0.9	0.2(0–1.0)	22.5(12.0–33.0)	15.0(5.0–25.0)	−0.2(−7.0 to 3.0)
3–6 months	1.5(0.5–2.5)	0.1(0–1.0)	21.0(12.0–31.0)	16.0(0–32.0)	−0.3(−5.0 to 4.0)
6 months–1 year	1.3(1.0–2.0)	0(0–3.0)	19.0(9.0–29.0)	13.5(2.0–26.0)	−2.5(−5.0 to 2.0)
1–3 years	1.2	0.2(0–1.0)	17.0(10.0–33.0)	14.5(6.0–25.0)	−1.5(−7.0 to 7.0)
3–5 years	1.0	0(0–0)	16.0(6.0–27.0)	13.0(4.0–24.0)	0.5(−4.0 to 4.0)
5–8 years	0.9(0–1.5)	0.1(0–1.0)	14.5(4.0–30.0)	16.0(2.0–31.0)	1.8(−6.0 to 11.0)
8–12 years	0.9(0–1.5)	0.05(0–0.5)	11.5(2.0–30.0)	15.5(1.0–30.5)	2.4(−8.0 to 6.0)
12–16 years	1.0(0–1.5)	0(0–0)	11.2(2.0–26.0)	13.0(3.0–34.0)	5.5(−1.5–13.0)
LEAD V_4					
Birth–1 day	1.1(0.5–2.0)	0.3(0–2.5)	19.0(6.0–32.0)	23.0(2.0–44.0)	−0.6(−7.0 to 3.0)
1 day–1 week	1.0(0.5–1.5)	1.0(0–5.0)	20.0(7.0–35.0)	13.0(1.0–30.0)	2.5(−2.0 to 6.5)
1 week–1 month	1.2(0.5–1.5)	1.0(0–4.0)	19.0(6.0–37.0)	9.0(2.0–18.0)	3.2(0.5–6.5)
1–3 months	0.9(0.5–1.5)	1.4(0–3.0)	21.0(9.0–33.0)	11.5(0–22.0)	3.0(−1.5 to 7.2)
3–6 months	1.0(0.5–1.5)	1.8(0–2.5)	21.5(8.0–36.0)	8.0(0–22.0)	3.2(0.4–6.8)
6 months–1 year	1.2(0–2.0)	1.6(0–3.0)	25.0(14.0–35.0)	11.0(0–27.0)	3.0(−2.0 to 8.0)
1–3 years	1.1(0.5–1.5)	2.5(0–5.0)	22.0(10.0–40.0)	7.5(0–19.0)	4.5(−1.6 to 11.0)
3–5 years	0.9(0.5–1.5)	1.7(0–5.0)	24.0(12.0–42.0)	6.5(1.0–18.0)	4.8(−1.2 to 10.5)
5–8 years	0.8(0–1.5)	1.6(0–5.0)	25.5(15.0–50.0)	8.0(1.0–20.0)	5.8(−0.8 to 11.5)
8–12 years	0.8(0–1.5)	1.8(0–4.5)	25.0(2.5–50.0)	7.0(1.5–20.0)	5.6(−0.2 to 11.2)
12–16 years	0.8(0–1.5)	0.5(0–3.0)	30.0(6.0–51.0)	6.5(1.0–17.0)	7.2(0–15.0)

LEAD V_5					
Birth–1 day	1.3(1.0–2.0)	2.2(0–5.5)	12.0(0–24.0)	11.0(0–30.0)	1.5(−3.8 to 6.3)
1 day–1 week	1.0(0.8–2.0)	2.0(0–5.0)	12.0(2.0–28.0)	8.0(0–18.0)	2.9(0.5–5.6)
1 week–1 month	1.1(1.0–2.0)	2.0(0–4.5)	13.5(4.0–34.0)	6.0(0–14.0)	3.4(0.5–5.7)
1–3 months	0.8(0.5–1.0)	2.0(0–3.0)	14.5(6.0–24.0)	5.5(0–14.0)	3.6(1.0–6.3)
3–6 months	1.1(1.0–1.5)	2.1(0–3.5)	19.0(11.0–39.0)	5.0(0–15.0)	3.7(0.2–7.6)
6 months–1 year	0.9(0–1.5)	2.3(0–5.0)	18.5(9.0–30.0)	3.0(0–9.0)	3.6(0.8–6.2)
1–3 years	1.0(0.5–1.5)	2.3(0–4.0)	19.0(11.)–39.0)	3.0(0–9.0)	4.3(0.2–8.3)
3–5 years	0.8(0.5–1.0)	2.1(0–5.0)	20.0(10.0–34.0)	2.5(0–8.5)	4.5(0.6–8.5)
5–8 years	0.8(0–1.5)	1.9(0–7.0)	22.0(13.0–39.0)	3.0(0–9.0)	5.7(0–11.0)
8–12 years	0.7(0–1.5)	1.9(0–4.5)	22.5(10.0–36.0)	3.0(0–11.5)	5.8(0.5–11.0)
12–16 years	0.8(0–1.0)	1.3(0–4.0)	18.0(5.0–31.0)	3.0(0–7.5)	5.9(0.5–11.5)
LEAD V_6					
Birth–1 day	0.9(0–2.0)	1.3(0–2.0)	4.5(0–8.0)	3.5(0–13.0)	1.3(0.8–3.4)
1 day–1 week	0.8(0.5–1.5)	1.3(0–2.0)	6.5(1.0–16.0)	3.2(0–13.0)	1.9(0.3–3.6)
1 week–1 month	0.9(0.5–1.0)	1.4(0–2.0)	8.5(1.0–24.0)	2.6(0–10.0)	2.7(0.1–5.6)
1–3 months	0.8(0.5–1.0)	1.4(0–3.5)	9.5(3.0–16.0)	2.0(0–6.0)	2.7(0.6–4.8)
3–6 months	0.8(0–1.5)	1.8(0–4.0)	10.0(0.5–17.0)	1.7(0–5.0)	2.7(−0.5 to 6.0)
6 months–1 year	0.8(0–1.5)	2.4(0–5.0)	13.0(4.5–21.0)	2.0(0–3.0)	2.9(0.7–5.0)
1–3 years	0.8(0.5–1.5)	1.7(0–4.5)	12.0(2.5–21.5)	1.2(0–4.0)	3.3(0.6–5.6)
3–5 years	0.8(0.5–1.0)	1.8(0–4.0)	13.0(3.5–22.0)	0.7(0–3.0)	3.6(0.8–6.4)
5–8 years	0.7(0–1.5)	1.7(0–5.0)	14.0(6.5–21.5)	0.9(0–5.0)	4.0(0.3–7.7)
8–12 years	0.7(0–1.5)	1.7(0–4.0)	13.5(10.0–22.0)	1.1(0–3.0)	4.4(0.5–8.4)
12–16 years	0.7(0–1.5)	1.3(0–2.5)	13.5(7.0–21.0)	1.2(0.2–5.0)	4.0(0.8–7.2)

[a] Adapted from Dittmer, D.S., and Grebe, R. M. (eds.) 1959. Handbook of Circulation, p. 141. W. B. Saunders Company, Philadelphia.

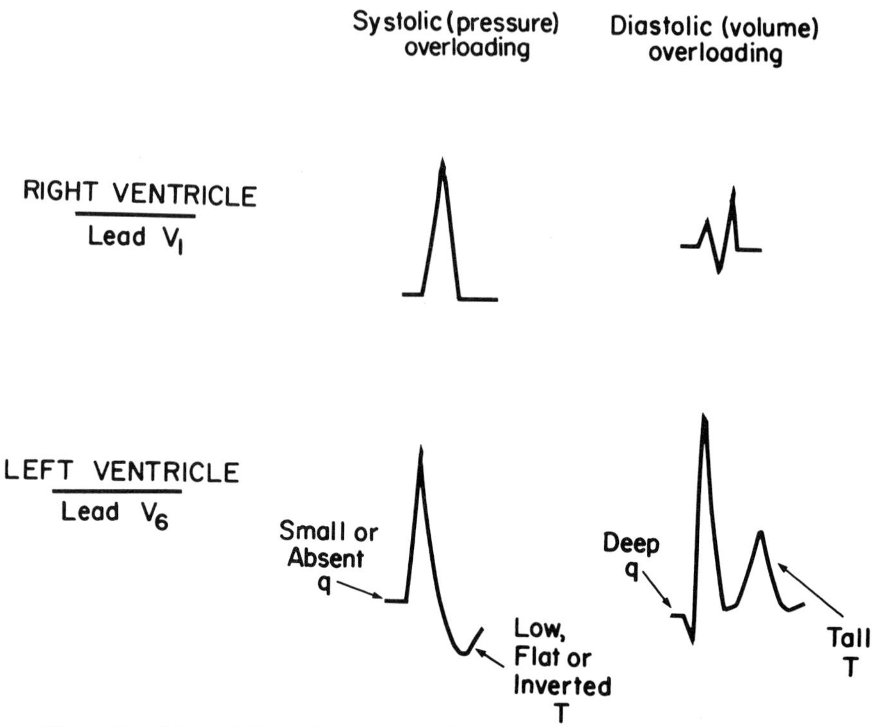

Figure 40. Schematic illustration of right and left ventricular pressure and volume overloading electrocardiographic patterns.

A dominant or monophasic R wave in V_1 (upper left) is usually present with an increase in pressure in the right ventricle. A low voltage rSR′ complex (upper right) is frequently noted with increased right ventricular volume.

A diminished or absent q wave, normal or increased R wave, and low, flat, or inverted T waves are noted with increased pressure in the left ventricle (lower left). A deep q wave, a tall R wave, and tall, symmetrical, narrow peaked T waves are noted with an increased volume in the left ventricle (lower right).

Combined Ventricular Hypertrophy

Combined ventricular hypertrophy (CVH or BVH) is suggested by evidence of overloading of both ventricles. Evidence of right ventricular hypertrophy plus any of the following suggests combined ventricular hypertrophy:

1. Dominant R waves (voltage not necessarily abnormal) with tall, positive T waves in lead V_5 or V_6.
2. Q wave in lead V_5 or V_6 greater than 3 mm.
3. Left axis deviation.

Evidence of left ventricular hypertrophy plus any of the following suggests combined ventricular hypertrophy:

1. Dominant R or R′ in right chest leads (voltage not necessarily abnormal).
2. R wave greater than Q wave in lead aVR.
3. S wave greater than R wave in lead V_6.

Large, biphasic QRS complexes (greater than 60 mm) in mid-precordial leads suggest biventricular hypertrophy, although isolated right or left ventricular hypertrophy also can cause such a pattern.

ELECTROLYTE IMBALANCE

Rarely, if ever, does a particular electrolyte abnormality occur as an isolated event. Invariably, concomitant changes in other electrolytes and in acid-base balance are present. The following paragraphs must be interpreted in that light.

Hyperkalemia results in tall, symmetrical, narrow T waves, and wide, flat P waves. The decreased amplitudes of such P waves may reach the point where they fuse with the baseline. Lengthening of the P-R interval and QRS duration, as well as various conduction disturbances, are also seen.

Hypokalemia is suggested by low-amplitude T waves. Prominent U waves or U waves blended with T waves may be found, as well as depressed ST segments, increased duration of QRS complexes, and increased amplitude of P waves.

Hypercalcemia causes a shortened Q-T interval due to a shortened ST segment. The T wave may be normal or narrow and peaked.

Hypocalcemia may be diagnosed by a prolonged Q-T interval that results from prolonged isoelectric ST segment.

DIGITALIS EFFECT

Digitalis causes prolonged AV conduction and hence a prolonged P-R interval. A shortened Q-T interval and ST segment changes, opposite in direction to the QRS complex, are found with therapeutic doses. Digitalis may decrease the amplitude of the T wave, but the direction of the T wave is usually unchanged.

Arrhythmias such as paroxysmal atrial tachycardia with block, various degrees of AV block, and frequent premature ventricular contractions are often associated with digitalis intoxication.

BIBLIOGRAPHY

Burch, G. E., and DePasquale, N. P. 1964. A History of Electrocardiography. Year Book Medical Publishers, Inc., Chicago.

Cabrera, E., and Monroy, J. R. 1952. Systolic and diastolic loading of the heart.

I. Physiologic and clinical data. II. Electrocardiographic data. Am. Heart J. 43: 661–686.
Masica, D. J., Maron, B. J., and Krovetz, L. J. 1972. Racial variations in the childhood electrocardiogram. Am. Heart J. 84:153–160.
Moss, A. J., and Emmanouilides, G. C. 1973. Practical Pediatric Electrocardiography. J. B. Lippincott, Philadelphia.
Traywick, J. P., Maron, B. J., Schuberth, K., and Krovetz, L. J. 1973. The electrocardiographic diagnosis of left ventricular hypertrophy in apparently normal children. J. Pediatr. 83:201–205.
Walsh, S. Z. 1963. Evolution of the electrocardiogram of healthy premature infants during the first year of life. Acta Paediatr. (Suppl.) 145.
Ziegler, R. F. 1954. Some aspects of electrocardiography in infants and children with congenital heart disease. Dis. Chest 25:490–497.

chapter 8

VECTORCARDIOGRAPHY

DEFINITIONS

Having now passed safely through the perils of electrocardiography, we would like to introduce some elementary concepts of vectorcardiography. At first glance, this three-dimensional version of electrocardiography seems three times as complicated. Actually, the vectorcardiogram (VCG) is far simpler to comprehend and interpret. It has been our finding with many groups of students that understanding the fundamentals of vectorcardiography greatly simplifies electrocardiographic interpretation.

The ECG and VCG are merely two different ways of looking at the same electrical forces. It may be that in a particular case one will be easier to interpret or more diagnostic than the other. Nonetheless, they offer the same

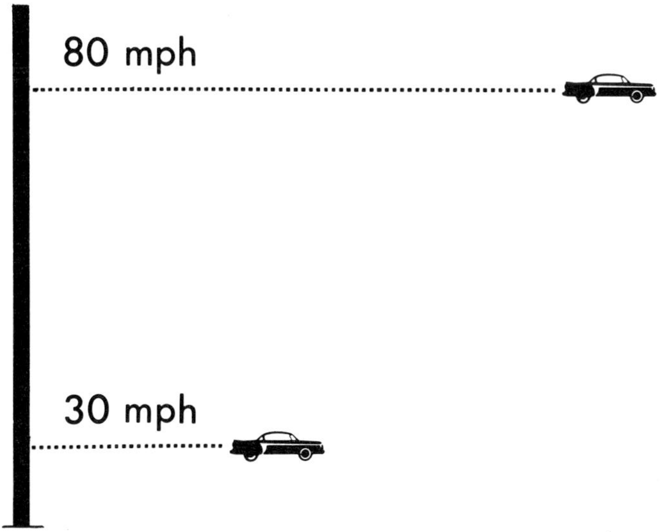

Figure 41. A scalar is a quantity that has only magnitude. It can be fully described by a number. This is illustrated in the figure by use of a bar graph and a number to describe the automobile's speed.

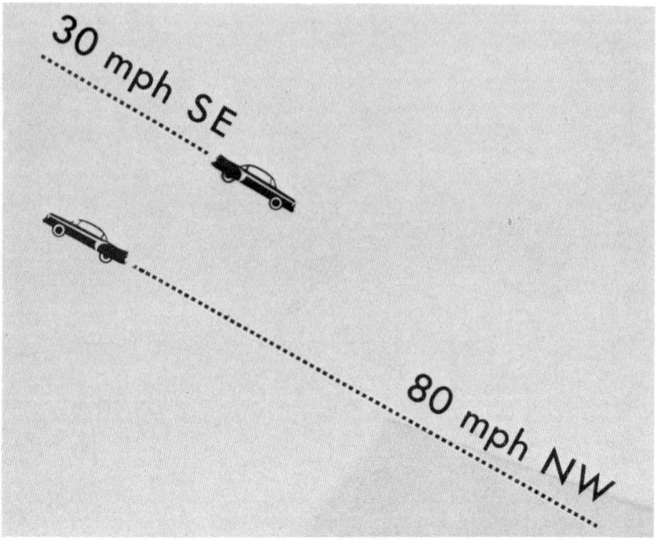

Figure 42. A vector is a quantity that has both magnitude and direction. In this case, each automobile is described both as to speed and direction. This combination is properly referred to as velocity.

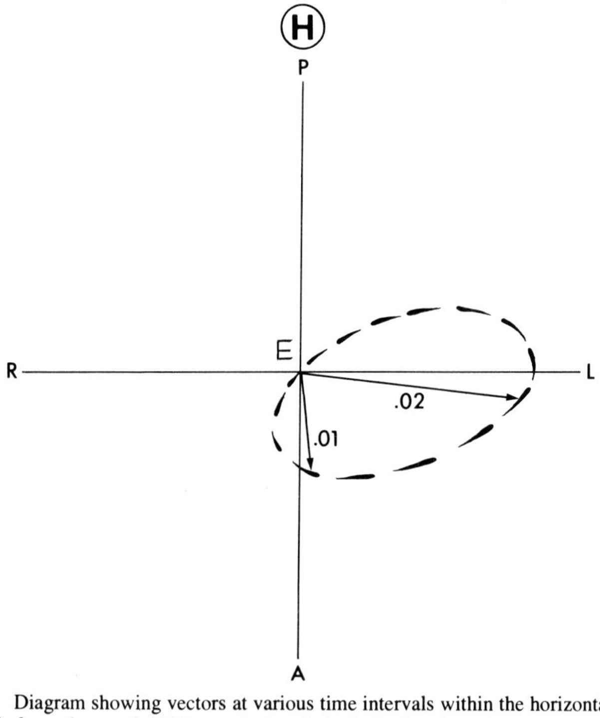

Figure 43. Diagram showing vectors at various time intervals within the horizontal QRS loop. Since a dot is formed every 0.0025 sec, the fourth dot is the location of the QRS loop at 0.01 sec. A line drawn between this position and the E point establishes the 0.01-sec vector. In a similar manner, the 0.02-sec, 0.03-sec, etc., vectors can be formulated. Each such vector has its own magnitude and direction.

information. Obviously then, a diagnosis of right ventricular hypertrophy on the ECG and one of left ventricular hypertrophy on the VCG of the same patient are irreconcilable; understanding their basic natures should prevent such an error.

The differences between electrocardiography and vectorcardiography may be described in the following manner. The ordinary ECG is recorded in a single plane, with a scalar quantity (voltage) on the vertical axis plotted against time on the horizontal axis. This is similar to a bar graph (Figure 41), which shows magnitude alone.

A vector adds a sense of direction, thus denoting both magnitude and direction (Figure 42). The VCG plots the movement of the electrical forces of the heart by indicating both the direction and the magnitude of these forces at any given instant. Whereas the ECG records time on the horizontal axis by using the smallest division (0.04 sec, at the usual paper speed of 25 mm per sec), the VCG indicates time by interrupting the tracing, usually every 2.5

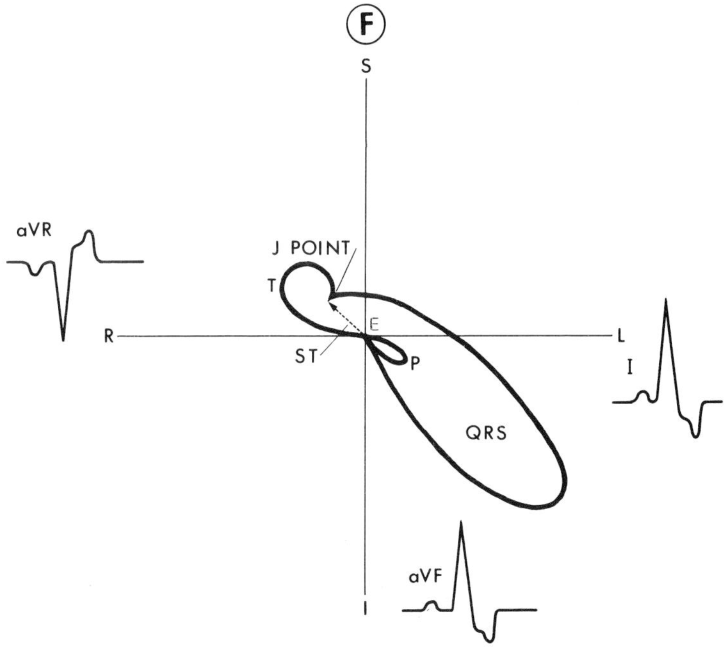

Figure 44. Under certain conditions, the QRS loop does not "close," i.e., it does not return to the E point. The diagram illustrates the formation of an ST vector by an imaginary line running from the E point to the junction of the QRS loop and T loops (the J point). Leads I, aVR, and aVF are depicted to show that the ST segment is positive or negative depending on the position of the ECG electrodes in relation to the ST vector.

msec, to form a series of dots. Thus, time, direction, and magnitude are recorded simultaneously. When the dots are far apart, the electrical wave is traveling very rapidly through the heart. When the dots are closer together, the wave is traveling more slowly. There is usually some initial and terminal slowing of all normal QRS loops.

In the vectorcardiogram, the zero voltage baseline is represented by the point of initial excitation (E point). The various waveforms—P, QRS, and T—normally inscribe loops that begin and terminate at the E point. The duration of each loop can be ascertained by counting the dots in each loop and multiplying by 0.0025 sec. Furthermore, the time and position of the fourth dot (0.01 sec) establish the apex of a vector running between that 0.01-sec dot and the E point. In the same way, the eighth dot defines the position of the 0.02-sec vector, etc. (Figure 43).

In pathologic circumstances, the QRS loop may fail to end at the E point. Then a vector can be drawn from the E point to the junction of the QRS and T loops, called the J point. This vector is the ST vector (Figure 44).

Ideally, vectors are plotted in three mutually perpendicular planes, in an orthogonal system (Figure 45). Many different lead systems have been de-

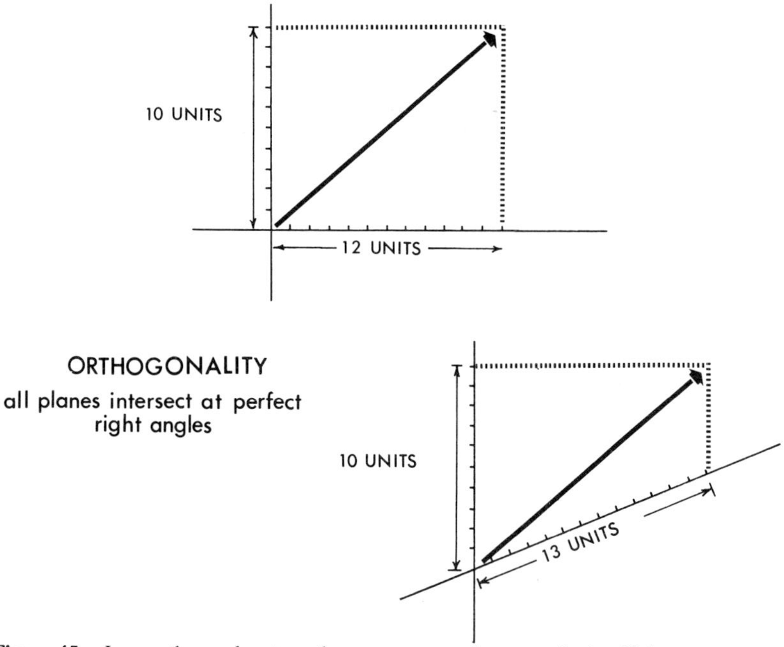

Figure 45. In an orthogonal system, the axes are mutually perpendicular. If the axes are not at 90° angles from each other, then the projection of a vector on the tilted axis will give a false reading, as in the illustration. A great deal has been written about orthogonal lead systems, but we believe that a perfectly orthogonal lead system will require a far more sophisticated and complex lead system than any now available. Obviously, it will be extremely difficult to design a lead system that will be orthogonal both for a small premature infant and for an obese adult.

signed, each claiming to be the best in achieving orthogonality. The clearest vectorcardiographic lead system to visualize is the Grishman cube method, which utilizes only four electrodes (Figure 46). When attached to the thorax, these four electrodes and their interconnections transform the chest into a "cube." The purpose of this cube is to record the electrical activity of the heart in three different planes—frontal, sagittal, and horizontal (or transverse). Each plane records the electrical activity of the heart in the form of various wave loops. With a knowledge of the forms of the loops in two planes, one can deduce those appearing in the third. The most commonly employed clinical lead system (Frank) uses seven leads (plus the right leg as ground) and weights the inputs for further correction. However, the end result is the projection of electrical activity onto the same three planes.

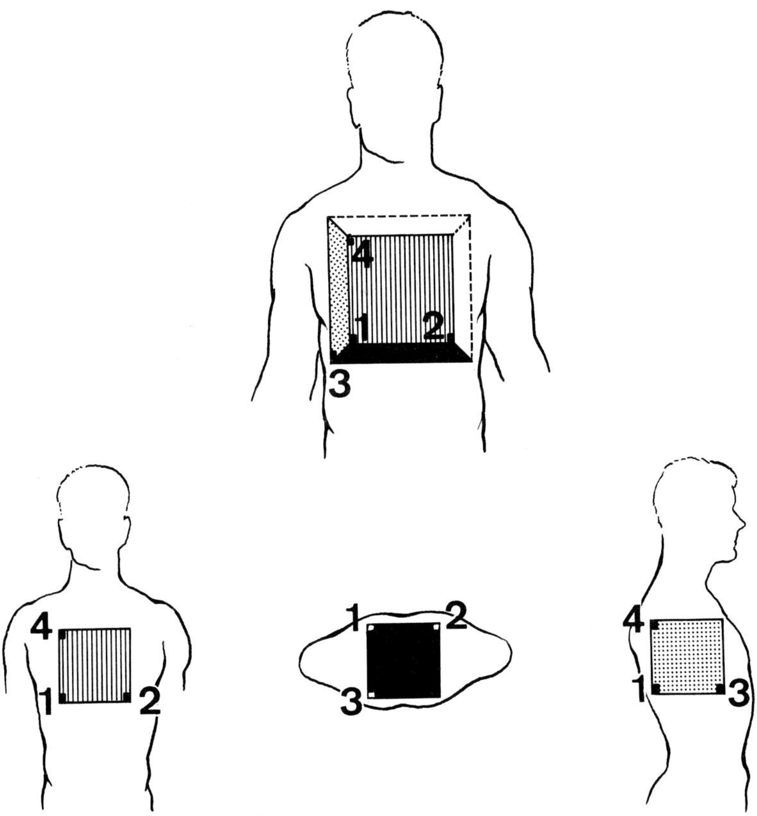

Figure 46. This illustrates the Grishman cube system in relation to the human thorax. Note that only four electrodes are attached to the chest. Using these in groups of three yields the various projections. Leads 1, 2, and 4, when connected, form the frontal plane (lower left); leads 1, 2, and 3 together form the horizontal plane (lower middle), and leads 1, 3, and 4 together form the right sagittal plane (lower right). Other lead systems use more electrodes and weight the information to yield systems that are orthogonal for more body configurations than the cube system.

The frontal plane is divided into superior and inferior portions and right and left sides, producing four quadrants—right superior, right inferior, left superior, and left inferior. Six leads of the ECG are related to the frontal plane—leads I, II, III, aVR, aVL, and aVF. These six ECG leads are located 60° apart at points on the body (Figure 47). In a sense, the vectorcardiogram provides a picture of the object from the front, whereas the ECG is more like six men each looking through a small porthole, describing the object as he sees it from his position. These six individual sources of information can be assembled to reproduce the frontal plane vectorcardiogram or they can be derived from the VCG (Figure 48). Similarly, the precordial leads relate to the vectorcardiogram as recorded in the horizontal plane (Figures 49–51). The horizontal plane is divided into anterior and posterior halves and right and left sides, again forming four quadrants. The multiple precordial leads are again utilized in an attempt to visualize a moving object, while the horizontal VCG

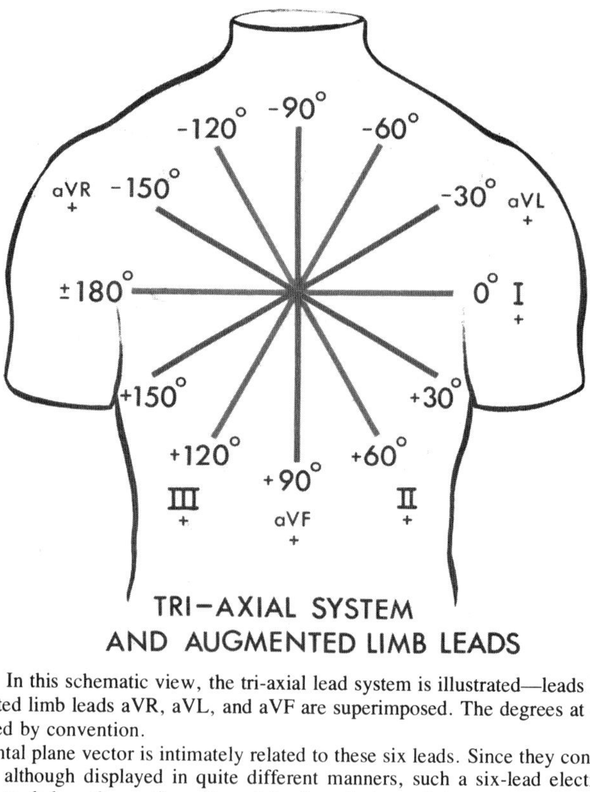

Figure 47. In this schematic view, the tri-axial lead system is illustrated—leads I, II, and III. The augmented limb leads aVR, aVL, and aVF are superimposed. The degrees at each lead are those assigned by convention.

The frontal plane vector is intimately related to these six leads. Since they contain the same information, although displayed in quite different manners, such a six-lead electrocardiogram may be used to deduce the configuration of the frontal plane of the vectorcardiogram, and vice versa.

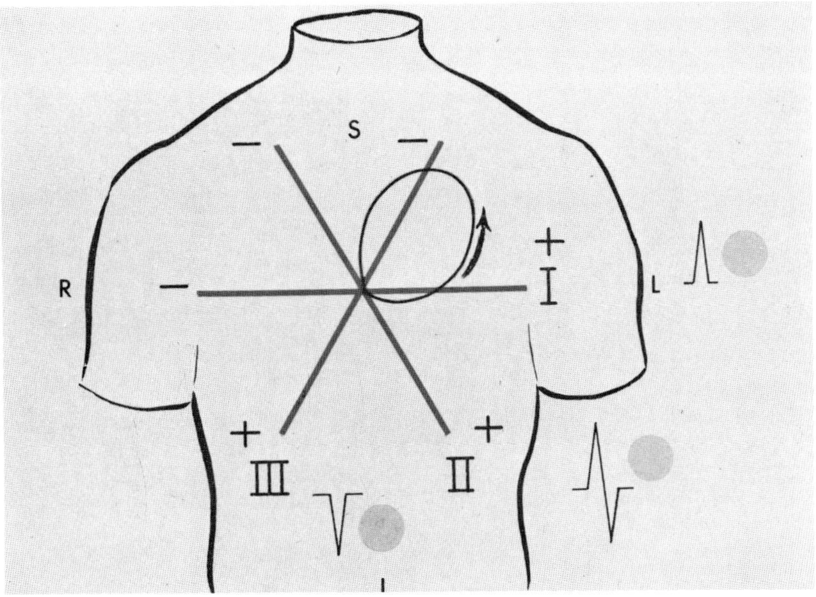

Figure 48. To convert from a vectorcardiogram recorded in the frontal plane to the standard and augmented electrocardiographic leads, draw a line from the location of the particular electrocardiographic lead in which you are interested through the E point (the imaginary starting point for all the electrical forces represented in the figure as the point of interaction of leads I, II, and III). Then through this E point draw a perpendicular to the initial line. Now all forces between the E point and the exploring electrode of the particular ECG lead are positive; and all forces away from the electrode are negative. In the illustration above, the electrical forces are entirely on the distant side of the lead III electrode; hence, one sees only a QS (negative) complex in lead III. As lead I ''sees'' the QRS loop, the electrical forces are all positive. From its vantage point, lead II visualizes the QRS vector loop as initially positive and then negative. Hence, lead II has an RS complex.

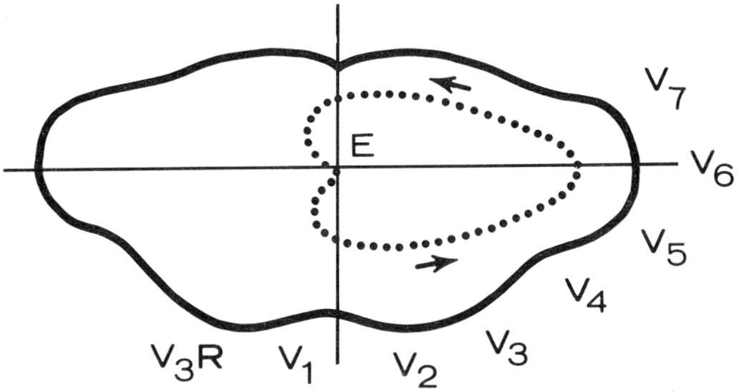

Figure 49. This illustration is the counterpart of Figure 48, in that it shows relationships between the precordial electrocardiographic leads (V_3R-V_7) and the horizontal plane of the vectorcardiogram. The precordial leads are not, however, attached in the same plane, but vary from the second to the fourth intercostal spaces. Thus, there may be slight discrepancies when one converts from the precordial electrocardiographic leads to the horizontal plane of the vectorcardiogram.

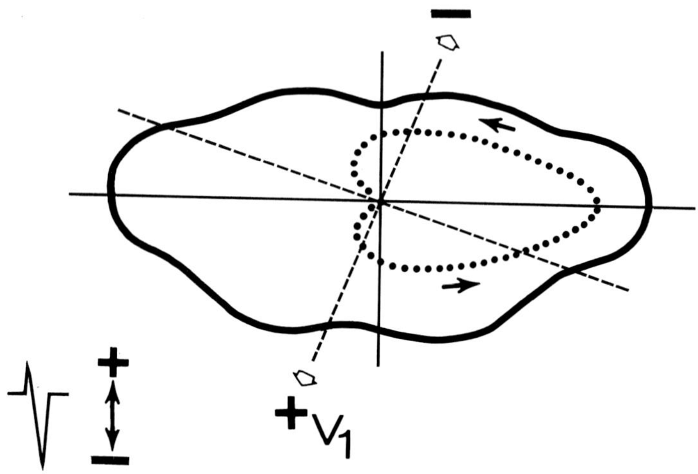

Figure 50. The method of converting from the horizontal plane of VCG to the precordial electrocardiographic leads is analogous to that described in Figure 48. For example, if we draw a line from lead V_1 through the E point, and then erect our perpendicular, we inscribe the ECG configuration of lead V_1. In this illustration, there is a small positive R wave followed by a deep negative S wave, reflecting the greater amount of negative QRS forces in lead V_1 as it views the normal adult horizontal plane vectorcardiogram.

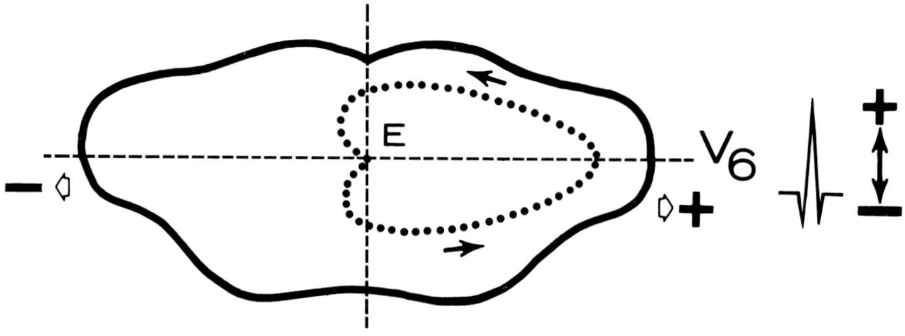

Figure 51. To determine the V_6 scalar electrocardiogram from the horizontal plane vectorcardiogram, draw a line from V_6 through the E point and erect a perpendicular at the E point. As lead V_6 sees the QRS loop, it is a small initial negative Q wave followed by a tall positive R wave and a small negative S wave.

is a photograph of this movement taken as if viewed from above. The sagittal plane* is divided into superior and inferior, and anterior and posterior, areas.

Most of the following discussion relates to the QRS loops of the vectorcardiogram, although the same principles hold for all waves. As the ECG electrode ''looks'' at the loop inscribed on the VCG, the individual ECG lead

*The right sagittal plane of the Grishman cube system is utilized in this book; the Frank lead system uses the left sagittal plane.

complex can be deduced in the following manner. A line is drawn from the ECG lead position to the E point of the VCG. A perpendicular is then drawn to this line, also passing through the E point. The area on the ECG lead side of the perpendicular lead is positive; the area away from the ECG lead is negative. As you go through the rest of this chapter, you should practice converting the VCG to individual ECG leads and vice versa. Figures 48–51 explain how this may be done.

THE NORMAL VCG

In the *neonate,* the initial (0.02 sec) QRS vector is anterior, inferior, and usually rightward (Figure 52). Premature infants may show more left ventricular forces than full-term infants. Mean QRS forces are rightward and may be either anterior or posterior; absence of terminal posterior QRS forces is often a subtle sign of right ventricular hypertrophy. In all three planes, the direction of inscription of the QRS loop is usually clockwise. Only rarely are figures of eight (7%) or clockwise rotation (5%) seen.

In the *infant,* after 30 hr of age the initial QRS forces are usually rightward, anterior, and superior (Figure 53). Initial leftward forces should be regarded as abnormal and may indicate pathologic degrees of right ventricular hypertrophy or conditions associated with anomalies of the conduction system, such as ventricular inversion (see discussion in Chapter 19).

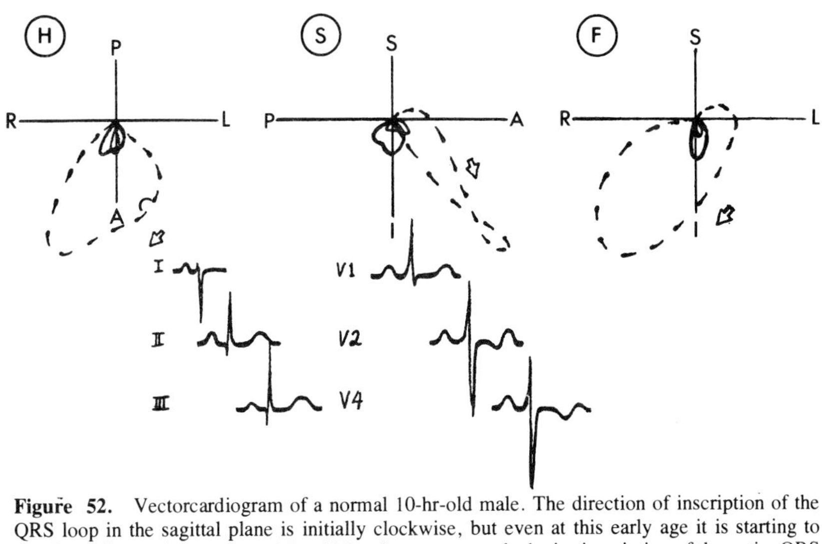

Figure 52. Vectorcardiogram of a normal 10-hr-old male. The direction of inscription of the QRS loop in the sagittal plane is initially clockwise, but even at this early age it is starting to develop a figure-eight pattern. After 48 hr of age, counterclockwise inscription of the entire QRS loop in the right sagittal plane is abnormal and indicative of a pathologic degree of right ventricular hypertrophy. The clockwise inscription of the QRS loop in the horizontal plane is normal at this age, as is the anterior shift of the T vector.

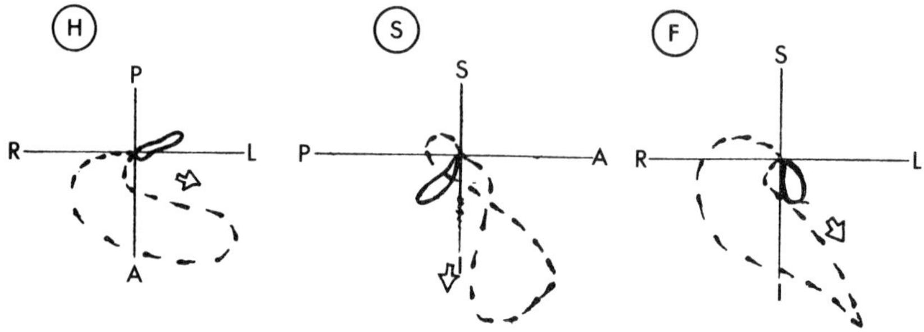

Figure 53. Typical vectorcardiogram of a normal 1-month-old child. The inscription of the QRS loop in the horizontal plane is still primarily clockwise and the QRS forces are predominantly anterior. Note, however, that the initial QRS forces are moving in a normal rightward and anterior direction, such that they inscribe a Q wave in V_6. Note that the T vector has shifted posteriorly—the normal position after 3 days of age.

In the horizontal plane, the direction of inscription of the QRS loop starts changing from pure clockwise to counterclockwise almost immediately after birth. By 1 month of age, only 18% of horizontal QRS loops are still inscribed completely clockwise, and by 2 or 3 months only 5% still are (Figures 54 and 55). After 3 months of age, pure clockwise rotation of the QRS loop in the horizontal plane should always be considered abnormal, and suggests right ventricular hypertrophy. The terminal QRS forces may return anterior to the E point prior to 1 year of age, but after this age such a loop suggests right ventricular hypertrophy.

In *normal older children,* the horizontal QRS loop is always inscribed in the counterclockwise direction. The direction of inscription in the frontal plane may be either clockwise or counterclockwise (Figure 56).

Usually, most of the QRS loop is oriented inferiorly, but there may be superiorly oriented terminal forces. The T loop is concordant (oriented in the same direction as the main portion of the QRS loop); that is to say, the angle normally formed by the mean T and QRS forces (QRS-T angle) is 45° or less. Angles wider than this are abnormal, when found in more than one plane.

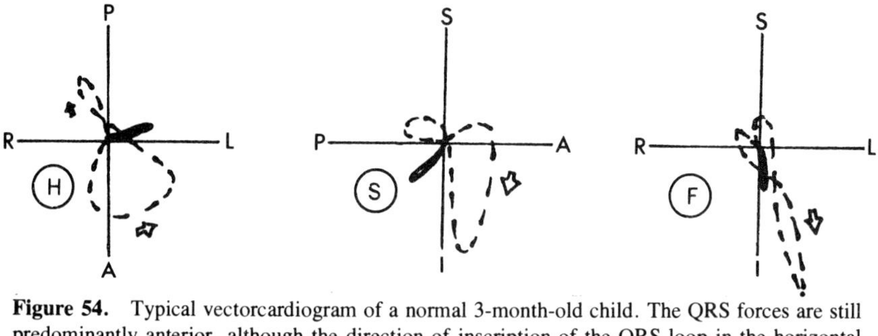

Figure 54. Typical vectorcardiogram of a normal 3-month-old child. The QRS forces are still predominantly anterior, although the direction of inscription of the QRS loop in the horizontal plane has changed to counterclockwise.

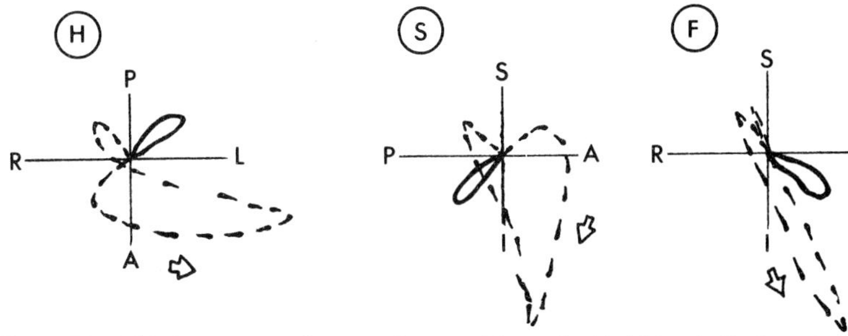

Figure 55. This is a vectorcardiogram of a normal 8-month-old child—similar in many respects to the vectorcardiogram of a normal 3-month-old child in Figure 54. The relatively anterior position of the QRS forces is the normal finding in preschool children.

In interpreting the vectorcardiogram, consider it as potentially abnormal if any of the following is found:

1. QRS-T angle is greater than 45° in two or more planes after 1 week of age.
2. Initial QRS forces are not anterior, rightward, and superior after 4 days of age.
3. Direction of inscription of QRS loop is predominantly clockwise in the horizontal plane after 3 months of age.
4. Direction of inscription of QRS loop is entirely counterclockwise in right sagittal after 2 days of age.
5. T vector is anterior after 3 days of age.
6. Magnitude of QRS forces is greater than 0.9 mV leftward, or 0.4 mV anteriorly or posteriorly.

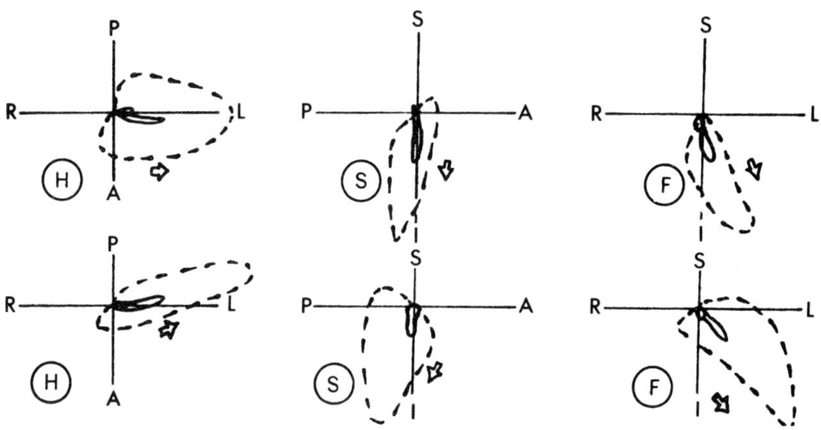

Figure 56. Vectorcardiograms of two normal adult males, one with clockwise and the other with counterclockwise inscription of the QRS loop in the frontal plane.

7. QRS loops are bizarre and contorted rather than clean and open or figure-eight in shape.
8. Mean P, QRS, and T vectors are not in the left inferior quadrant.

THE ABNORMAL VCG

The P Loop

After the first few days of life the P loop is found in the left and inferior quadrant, usually close to the isoelectric line dividing anterior from posterior (Figure 57). Normally, it is the smallest of the three loops emanating from the E point.

With enlargement of the right atrium, the P loop becomes longer and moves toward the right and inferior quadrant. This accounts for the tall, narrow P waves recorded in leads II, III, aVF, V_1, and V_2 in right atrial enlargement.

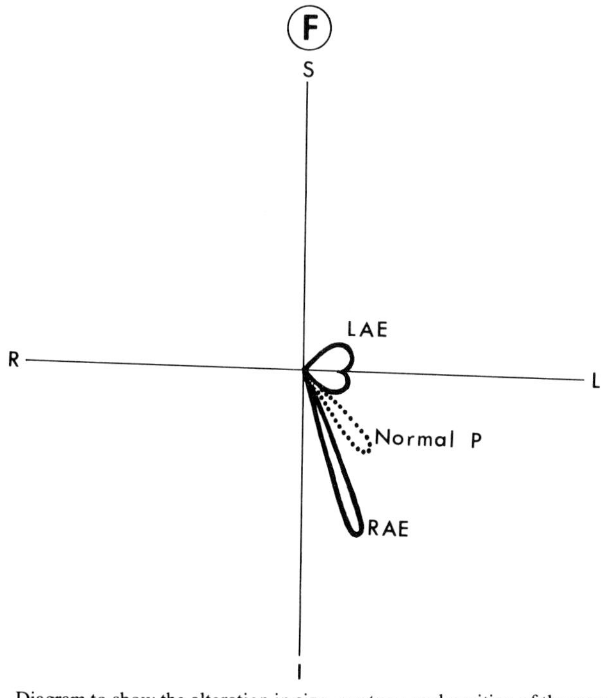

Figure 57. Diagram to show the alteration in size, contour, and position of the normal P loop of the vectorcardiogram in the presence of right and left atrial enlargement. In right atrial enlargement, the P loop remains narrow, but increases in amplitude and moves toward the right inferior quadrant with increase in size of the right atrium.

Left atrial enlargement causes a shift of the P loop toward the left superior quadrant and a notched "valentine" contour.

In left atrial enlargement, the P loop becomes broad and notched like a valentine and migrates toward the left superior quadrant. In this position, the characteristic P waves of left atrial enlargement are best seen in leads I, II, V_5, and V_6.

Ventricular Hypertrophy

In discussing ventricular hypertrophy, one must be aware of the normal position of the ventricles. The right ventricle is more anterior than rightward, and the left ventricle more posterior than leftward (Figures 58 and 59). Thus, an increase in the anterior QRS forces usually indicates right ventricular hypertrophy. Alternatively, an anterior shift of QRS forces may indicate a decrease in left ventricular activity resulting from either a congenital disorder (such as hypoplasia of the left ventricle) or left ventricular myocardial disease (such as a posterior myocardial infarction).

Conversely, an increase in posterior QRS forces may indicate left ventricular hypertrophy, hypoplasia of the right ventricle, or an anterior myocardial infarction (Figures 58 and 59).

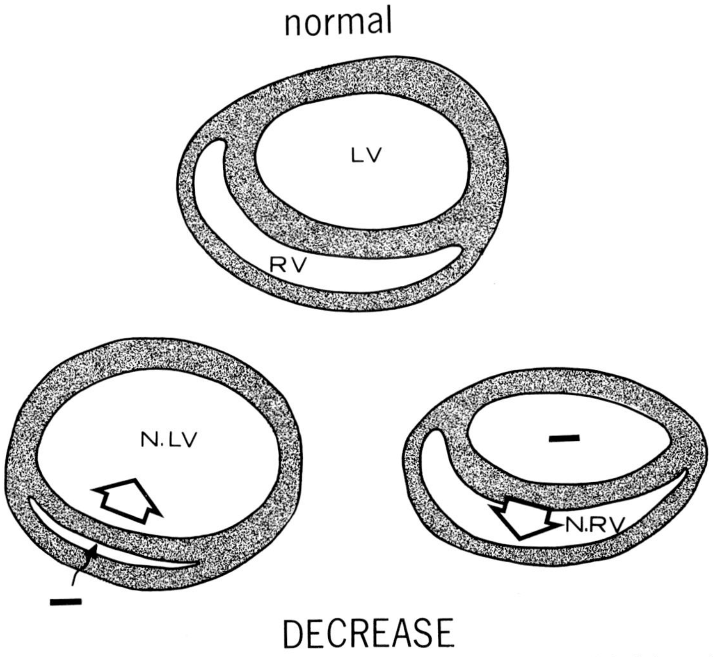

Figure 58. In the normal heart, the right ventricle is primarily anterior, and the left ventricle is predominantly posterior (upper middle). A decrease in right ventricular activity (lower left) results in an imbalance of electrical forces, causing an excess in the posterior direction even when the left ventricle is normal (N. LV). Conversely, a decrease in left ventricular activity (lower right) results in accentuation of the normal right ventricular forces (N. RV) so that the resultant vector is shifted anteriorly.

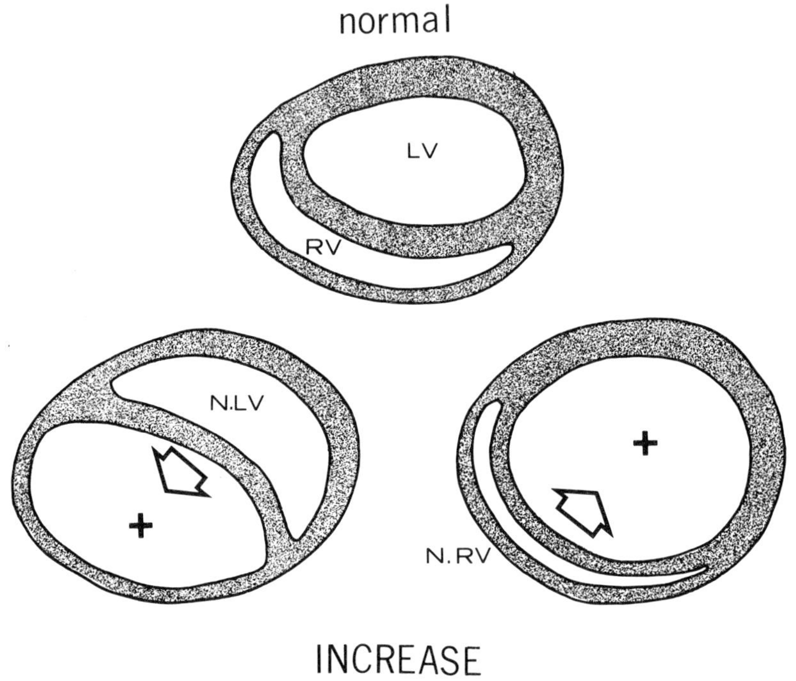

Figure 59. The electrical forces may also be imbalanced by an increase in size of one ventricle. Thus, right ventricular hypertrophy will cause the mean vector to move anteriorly, and with left ventricular hypertrophy the electrical forces will shift posteriorly.

Left Ventricular Hypertrophy The mean QRS forces shift leftward, posteriorly, and either inferiorly or superiorly (Figure 60). The QRS loop in the horizontal plane is inscribed counterclockwise, whereas the direction of the QRS loop in the sagittal plane is clockwise. The frontal plane QRS loop inscription is variable, but is usually counterclockwise or in a figure-eight pattern.

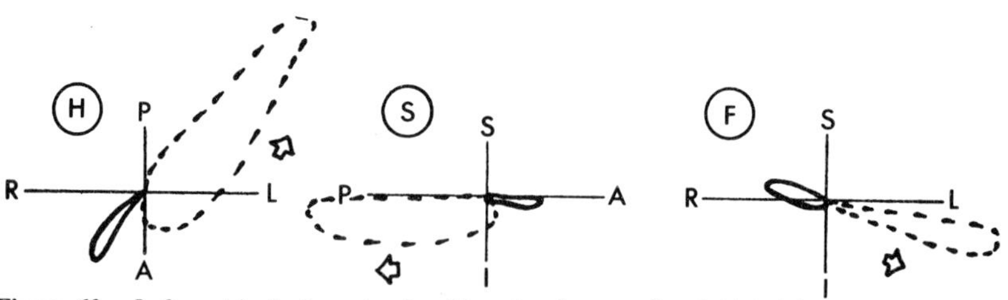

Figure 60. Left ventricular hypertrophy. Note the absence of an initial rightward and anterior QRS force, resulting in the absence of a Q wave in V_6, an important point in the diagnosis of left ventricular pressure overloading (see Figure 40). The mean T vector is opposite to the main body of the QRS loop (discordant) in all planes, producing negative T waves in the left precordial leads.

Left ventricular pressure overloading results in a decrease or absence of initial rightward and anterior QRS forces, decreasing the Q wave in the left precordial leads (Figure 60). Often the QRS loop is located more posteriorly than leftward. Then the shift from normal is best appreciated by noting the increase in the S wave in leads V_1 and V_2 rather than an increase in the height of the R wave in lead V_6. This is apparent, since V_1 views predominantly from anterior to posterior, while V_6 views from left to right (Figure 61).

The T loop may be small in relation to the size of the QRS loop, producing flattening of the left precordial T waves (Figure 62). The ST segment and the T wave may be opposite to the mean QRS vector, producing ST segment depression and T wave inversion in the left precordial leads (Figures 60 and 62).

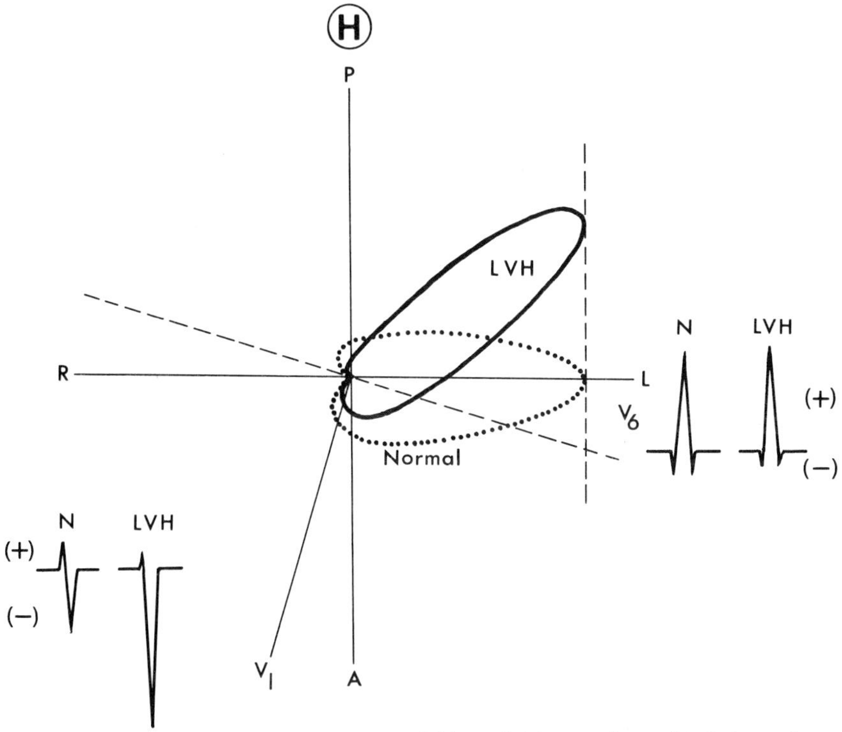

Figure 61. The vectorcardiogram is very useful in explaining certain empirical observations that are well known to the skilled electrocardiographer but difficult for the beginner to understand. One of these is that left ventricular hypertrophy is often best diagnosed by noting an increase in the size of the S wave in V_1, rather than an increase in the size of the R wave in V_6. The above diagram shows that with left ventricular hypertrophy the QRS loop may only move posteriorly, and may not increase its leftward voltage. Anterior and posterior shift can be noted by lead V_1, and thus the posterior displacement of the QRS loop causes an increase in the negative (S) wave in lead V_1. Concomitantly, lead V_6 can note only rightward and leftward shifts. Since the leftward extension of the QRS loop does not change (vertical dashed line), the R wave in V_6 remains the same height.

Left ventricular volume overloading results in increased initial rightward and anterior QRS septal forces, producing deep Q waves in leads I and V_5–V_7. The increased leftward orientation of the QRS loop also increases the size of the R wave in the left precordial leads. Although it maintains its normal orientation, the T loop often becomes symmetrical and increases in amplitude (Figure 62).

Right Ventricular Hypertrophy With moderate and severe right ventricular hypertrophy, the mean QRS forces are displaced to the right, anteriorly, and inferiorly (Figure 63). Reversal of the normal direction of the inscription of at least the terminal portion of the QRS loop, i.e., from counterclockwise to clockwise in the horizontal plane, is universally seen. Severe right ventricular hypertrophy causes rightward, posterior, and even superior shift of the QRS forces (Figure 64). In lesser degrees of right ventricular

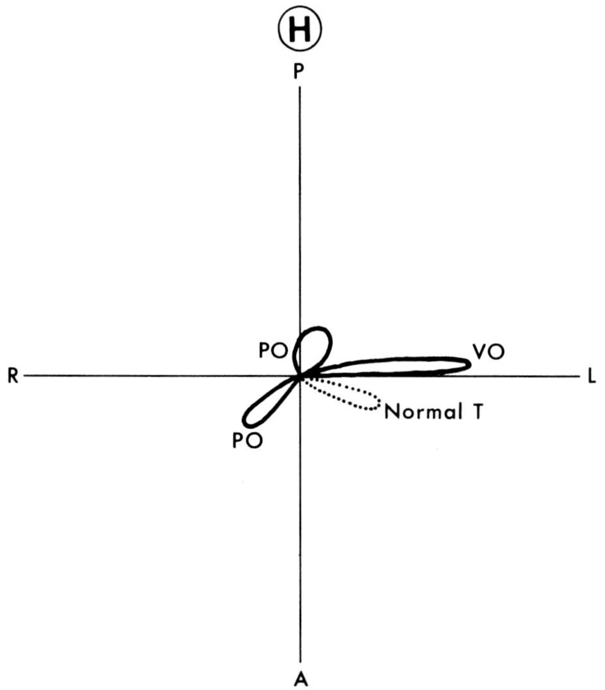

Figure 62. Diagram showing the alteration in size, contour, and position of the T loop in the vectorcardiogram with left ventricular pressure or volume overload.

Volume overload increases the amplitude of the T loop, but the width and position of the loop change relatively little. Thus, the length-width (L:W) ratio is increased from the normal values of about 3.0 to around 5.0.

With the pressure overload, the T loop becomes "fatter." It decreases in amplitude and increases in width, thereby decreasing the L:W ratio, often to around 1.0. The position of the T loop may remain concordant with the QRS loop, or it may become discordant and be noted on the right side of the E point.

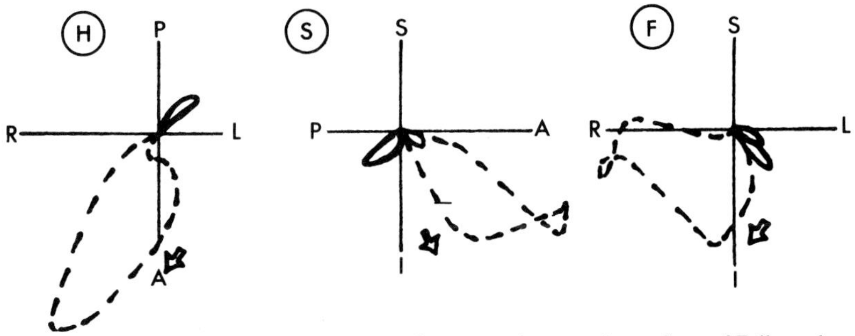

Figure 63. Severe right ventricular hypertrophy as seen in cyanotic tetralogy of Fallot, where right ventricular systolic pressure is approximately equal to left ventricular systolic pressure. Note the reversal from normal of inscriptions of the QRS loops in the horizontal and right sagittal planes. The mean QRS forces show a shift rightward, anteriorly and inferiorly.

hypertrophy, the direction of inscription of the QRS loop may be normal, although its position is more anterior than usual. Anterior shift of the T loop causing positive T waves in the right precordial leads may be the only manifestation of mild right ventricular hypertrophy. The QRS loop in this situation is normal.

Right ventricular pressure overloading often produces an initial leftward QRS force. The major QRS forces are rightward, anterior, and increased in amplitude, producing tall R waves in the right precordial leads. The T vector moves posteriorly and grows in size with further increases in right ventricular pressure (Figure 63). There may also be a posteriorly oriented ST vector, causing negative ST segments in the right precordial leads.

Right ventricular volume overloading results in larger than normal terminal QRS forces directed to the right and anteriorly. Such terminal QRS forces often reverse directions and may show a mild degree of slowing. These loops often produce an rSR′ pattern in the right precordial leads, although the

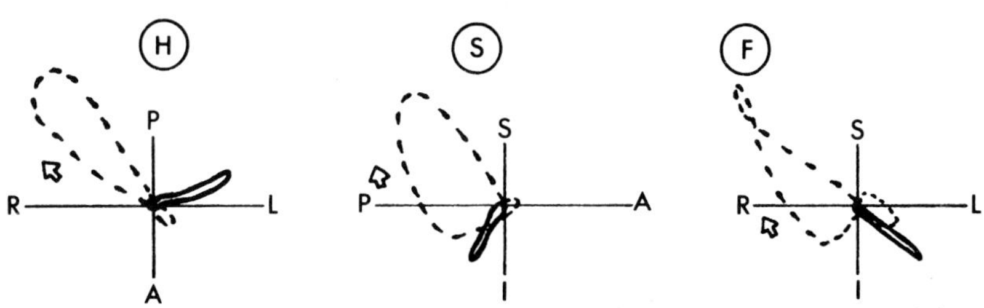

Figure 64. Severe right ventricular hypertrophy displaces the electrocardiographic QRS forces further rightward and even posteriorly and superiorly, with discordancy of T waves. Note that the abnormal directions of inscription of the QRS loops in the horizontal and right sagittal planes are the same as those seen in the previous figure. This type of horizontal plane vectorcardiogram, because of its posterior position, would produce dominant S (negative) waves in the right precordial leads. Such a paradox is explained easily by the vectorcardiogram.

height of the R′ waves is usually much less than that of the R wave seen with pressure overloading (Figure 65).

Combined Ventricular Hypertrophy Combined ventricular hypertrophy may be diagnosed whenever evidence exists for increased activity of both the right and left ventricles. Examples of such vector patterns are shown in Figures 66 to 69. Essentially, this diagnosis is suggested if the QRS loop occupies more right ventricular territory than normal while occupying significant left ventricular territory, or if the direction of inscription of the QRS loop suggests left ventricular predominance. Careful inspection of the figures should make these points clear.

The T Wave

After the first few days of life, the T wave normally lies in the left and inferior quadrant. Before 8 years of age, it is also directed posteriorly, causing negative T waves in the right precordial leads (Figures 54 and 55). After this age, the T vector moves to a more anterior position, and may be negative, diphasic, or positive in the right precordial leads.

The T wave is normally of long duration and appears as many dots bunched closely together. The normal length:width ratio is about 3. When the length:width ratio falls below 2.5, the T wave contour is abnormal and looks "fatter" (Figure 62). The contour and direction of inscription of the T wave are essential factors in the proper interpretation of most vectorcardiograms.

Bundle Branch Block

Left bundle branch block alters initial, middle, and terminal QRS forces so that they are widely divergent and oriented to the left, posteriorly, and either superiorly or inferiorly (Figure 70). The middle and terminal QRS forces appear as dots very close together, indicating slower than normal conduction and depolarization. The QRS complex lasts more than 0.12 sec. Inscription of the QRS loops may be counterclockwise in all planes, but in the horizontal

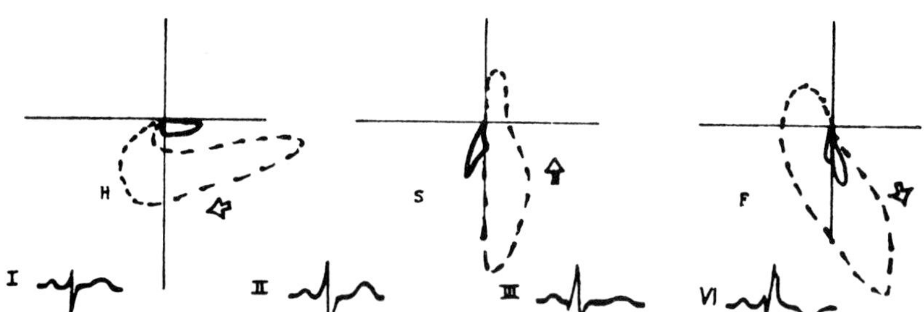

Figure 65. Right ventricular hypertrophy of a mild degree. This QRS pattern is frequently seen in an atrial septal defect of the foramen ovale type. Right ventricular systolic pressure may be expected to range around 40 mm Hg. Note particularly the rSR′ pattern produced in lead V_1 by the horizontal plane QRS loop, a frequent finding in volume overload of the right ventricle.

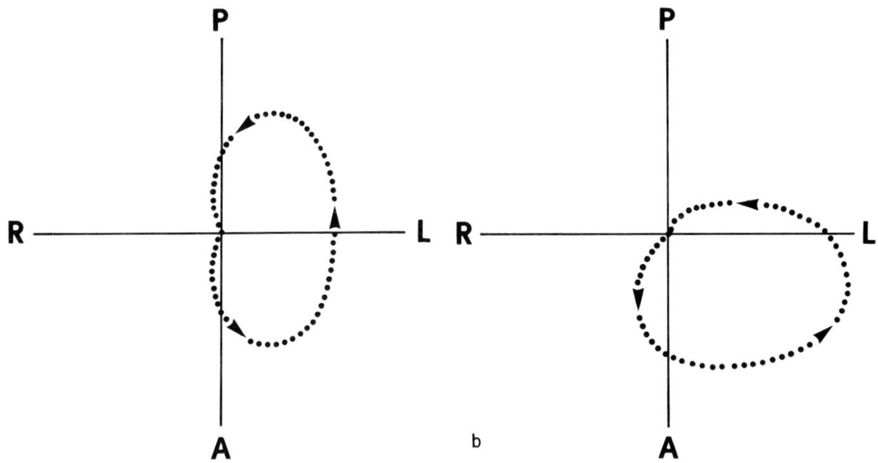

Figure 66. (a) The greater than normal anterior QRS forces indicate right ventricular hypertrophy. The larger than normal posterior forces indicate left ventricular hypertrophy, as do the leftward orientation and normal counterclockwise inscription of the QRS loop. (b) The pattern on the right is similar, although a greater portion of the "fat" QRS loop lies anteriorly and leftward. These large anterior forces indicate right ventricular hypertrophy. Because the QRS loop is predominantly leftward and has a normal counterclockwise inscription, additional left ventricular hypertrophy is suggested.

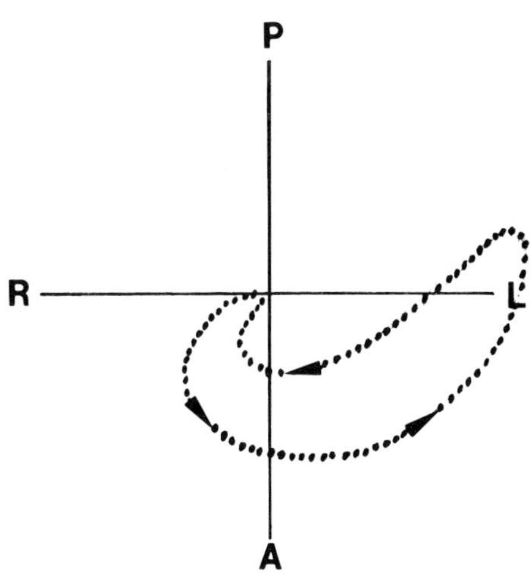

Figure 67. Right ventricular hypertrophy is indicated by the anterior position of the QRS loop with a reversed (clockwise) inscription of the terminal position. Additional left ventricular hypertrophy is suggested by a large initial rightward and anterior segment (causing large Q waves as V_6 views the loop), and the predominant leftward and normally inscribed (counterclockwise) main portion of the QRS loop.

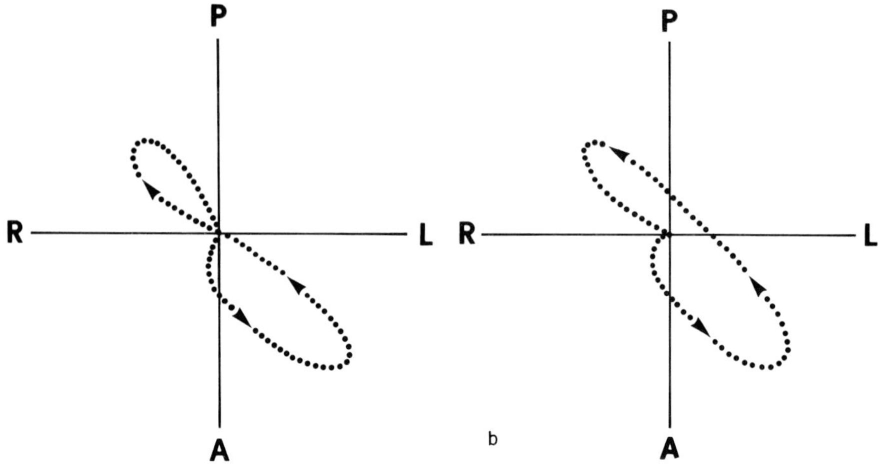

Figure 68. (a) The large leftward and normally (counterclockwise) inscribed QRS loop indicates left ventricular hypertrophy, whereas the large terminal rightward and posterior loop with reversed (clockwise) inscription indicates additional right ventricular hypertrophy. (b) The QRS loop pattern on the right is similar, with the only difference being that the large terminal rightward and posterior QRS loop has a normal direction of inscription. Both of these patterns will produce large diphasic QRS complexes in the mid-precordial leads.

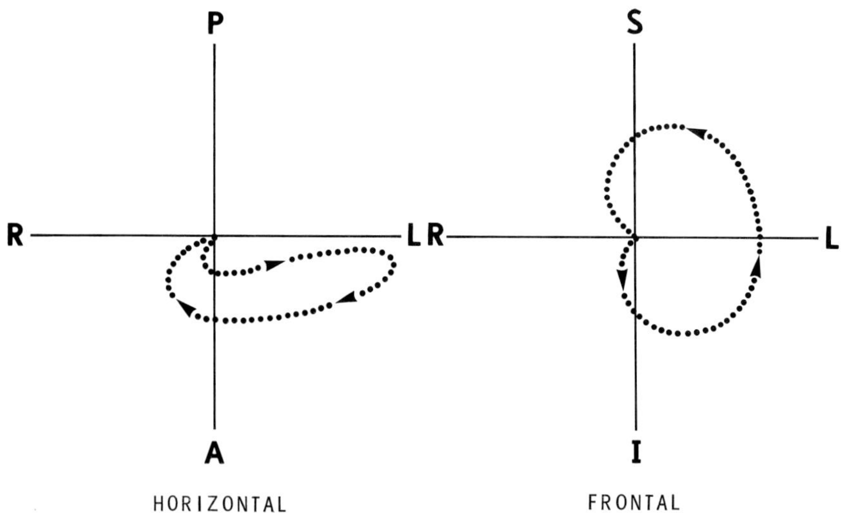

Figure 69. In this biventricular hypertrophy pattern, both horizontal and frontal plane loops are utilized to make the diagnosis. The horizontal plane QRS loop clearly shows right ventricular hypertrophy, with the entire loop being anterior and the inscription clockwise, and having a large terminal rightward and anterior segment. However, when the horizontal plane QRS loop shows a clockwise-inscribed right ventricular hypertrophy pattern, the frontal plane QRS loop is almost always also inscribed clockwise. When the frontal plane QRS loop is inscribed counterclockwise, this discordancy suggests additional left ventricular hypertrophy, particularly when the terminal portion is superiorly oriented.

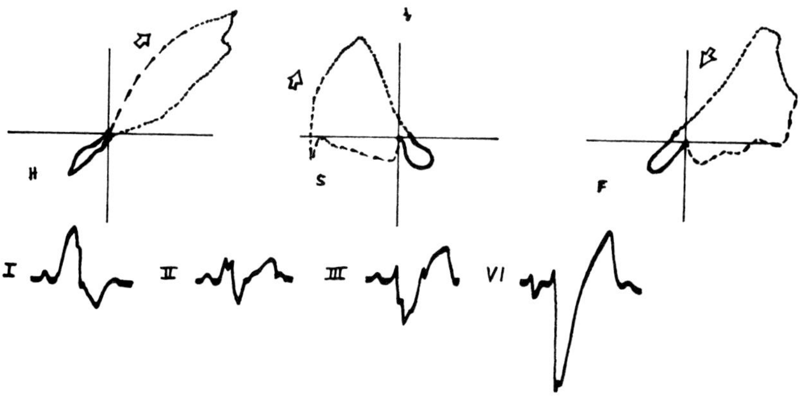

Figure 70. Left bundle branch block. Note the marked slowing and distortion of the mid- and terminal portions of the QRS vector loops. The QRS loop is inscribed in a reverse fashion from normal in the horizontal plane. The slowed conduction and depolarization causes the dots that are normally inscribed at every 2.5 msec to be so close together that they appear to be a single solid line.

plane it is often clockwise or figure eight. T loops are abnormal in shape and opposite in direction to the main QRS forces (discordant). The terminal portion of the QRS loop often fails to return to the starting point and produces an ST vector.

Right bundle branch block alters only the terminal QRS forces (Figure 71). Such terminal slowing of the QRS loop manifests itself as a large terminal appendage oriented rightward and anteriorly. As in left bundle branch block, the dots in this terminal appendage are close together, indicating slower conduction, which results in an increase in QRS duration. In the

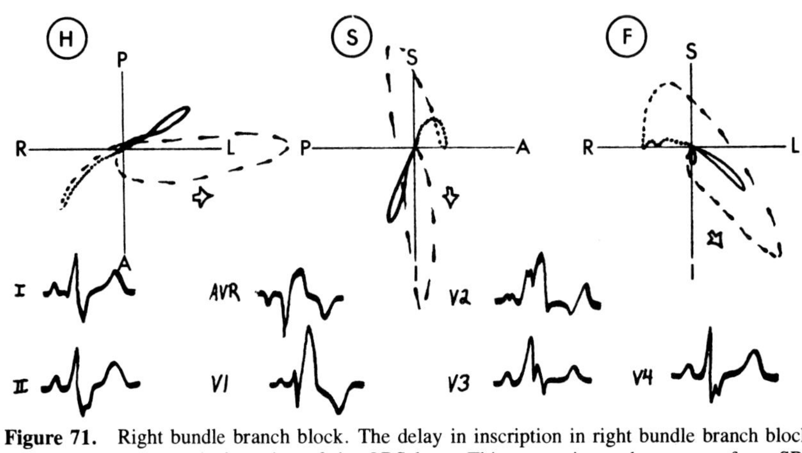

Figure 71. Right bundle branch block. The delay in inscription in right bundle branch block occurs during the terminal portion of the QRS loop. This vector is another cause of an rSR′ pattern in lead V_1, the R′ being secondary to the slowed terminal rightward and anterior portion of the QRS loop.

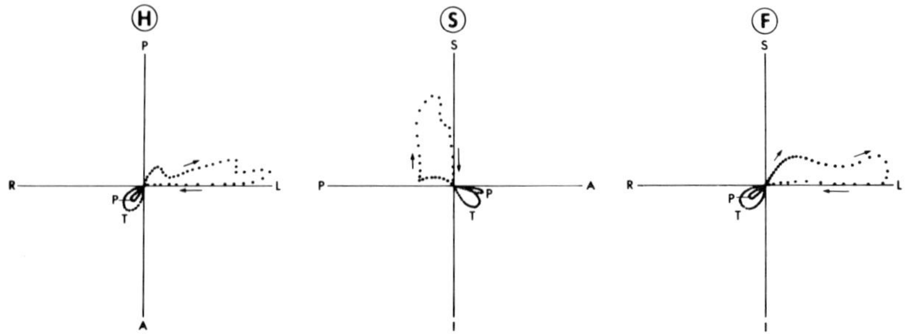

Figure 72. Diagram to show the vectorcardiographic hallmark of the Wolff-Parkinson-White (WPW) syndrome. This was redrawn from a vectorcardiogram taken on an 18-month-old girl with Ebstein's anomaly of the tricuspid valve. Note the initial slowing of the QRS loop in all planes, manifested by the dots placed close together. This is akin to the slow slurred onset of the QRS complex on the ECG, often called the "delta" wave. This particular WPW pattern mimics left bundle branch block.

horizontal plane, the direction of inscription of the terminal appendage may be either clockwise or counterclockwise. The T loop is usually increased in amplitude and discordant to the terminal appendage.

A posteriorly oriented, relatively small rightward and superior terminal appendage with only moderate slowing probably indicates right ventricular conduction delay. It may also be a normal variant.

Wolff-Parkinson-White or Preexcitation Syndrome

This syndrome exhibits a short P-R interval, prolonged QRS duration initated by a slower, slurred "delta" wave, and secondary ST segment and T wave changes. The vectorcardiographic hallmark of the WPW syndrome is slowing of the initial portion of the QRS loop, akin to the delta wave of the QRS complex in the ECG (Figure 72). It is caused by preexcitation of a portion of the ventricular musculature. This early but slow depolarization may take a variety of pathways, causing some WPW complexes to mimic right, and others left, bundle branch block.

BIBLIOGRAPHY

Benchimol, A., and Desser, K. B. 1975. Advances in clinical vectorcardiography. Am. J. Cardiol. 36:76–87.

Elliott, L. P., Taylor, W. J., and Schiebler, G. L. 1963. Combined ventricular hypertrophy in infancy. Vectorcardiographic observations with special reference to the Katz-Wachtel phenomenon. Am. J. Cardiol. 11:164–172.

Ellison, R. C., and Restieaux, N. J. 1972. Vectorcardiography in Congenital Heart Disease. W. B. Saunders Company, Philadelphia.

chapter 9

X-RAY EXAMINATION

Roentgenographic criteria for determining enlargement of cardiac chambers were formulated from studies of acquired lesions of the heart. Acquired lesions present a distinct advantage in evaluation and diagnosis—the physician knows that the pathology was superimposed on a basically normal heart. When dealing with congenital heart disease, no such guarantee exists. Any vessel or chamber may be in an anomalous position, diminutive in size, or entirely absent. Pathologic features secondary to a basically abnormal heart are more difficult to interpret.

GENERAL FEATURES

To evaluate the thoracic roentgenogram properly, the physician must develop a systematic approach. Before concentrating on the heart, evaluate the entire roentgenogram. The temptation to begin by analyzing the cardiovascular structures must be resisted. Certain specific features should be analyzed first, because they are often vital to a proper interpretation.

First, the films should be evaluated for rotation and for the degree of x-ray exposure. Second, extracardiac findings, skeletal abnormalities, and location of liver, stomach, and heart should be looked for. The third step consists of a step-wise analysis of the individual cardiac chambers and great vessels. Finally, the type and nature of the pulmonary vasculature are analyzed. Only after these steps are performed is the information ready to be assembled and utilized in a differential diagnosis schema.

Proper positioning of the patient may be detected by noting whether or not the two clavicles are symmetrical. Film quality strongly influences interpretation. Over- or underexposure leads to errors, particularly in the evaluation of pulmonary vasculature. Similarly, expiration distorts the cardiopulmonary silhouette and makes interpretation difficult. If a film shows improper positioning of the patient, if it is over- or underexposed, or if deep expiration has taken place during roentgenography, then the physician may need to have the film repeated.

In our opinion routine cardiac fluoroscopy is not warranted in infants and

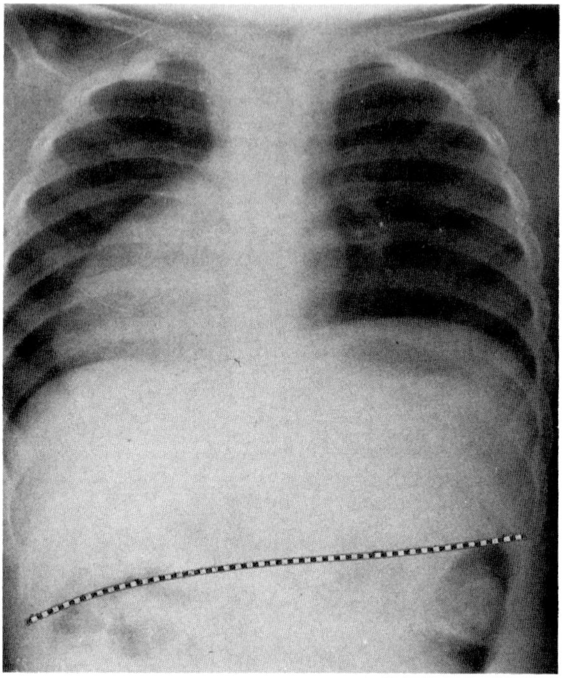

Figure 73. PA film of thorax and upper abdomen in a 1-year-old cyanotic child with multiple cardiac anomalies and absent spleen syndrome. Note that the cardiac apex and the stomach are on opposite sides. Furthermore, the liver shadow is abnormal. The lower edge of the liver, denoted in the photograph by the dotted line, extends across the entire abdomen, with a greater than normal amount on the left side of the body. Thus a plain film of chest and abdomen in a cyanotic child may be diagnostic for asplenia.

children. The amount of information garnered usually does not justify the radiation required. A limited fluoroscopic examination conducted by a highly skilled individual may be of value in some circumstances, for example, in the determination of the side of the aortic arch or the presence of a vascular ring.

ABDOMEN

In a proper chest film, the upper portion of the abdomen is included. Normally, the gastric air bubble is on the left, and the major portion of the liver is on the right, sloping upward toward the left. When equal amounts of the liver are on both sides and the lower margin of the liver forms a horizontal line, absent spleen syndrome (asplenia) should be suspected (Figure 73), especially if the cardiac apex or stomach is abnormal in location.

CHEST CAGE

The chest cage, including the spine and sternum, must be carefully analyzed. The spine may be straighter than normal ("straight back syndrome"), contain

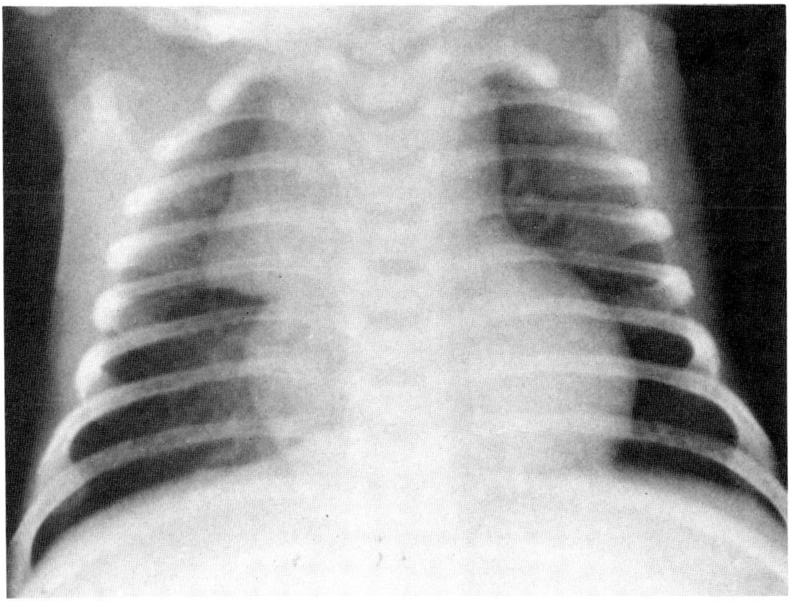

Figure 74. Prominent thymic shadow in a newborn infant. The sharp angle of the right border of the cardiac shadow, called the "sail sign," clearly identifies this as the thymus. (There is also some consolidation seen in the right lung, which was the reason for obtaining the x-ray).

abnormal vertebrae, or show kyphoscoliosis. The chest cage may have an increased anterior-posterior diameter with relatively flat diaphragms. This chest cage appearance is common in large left-to-right shunts.

The sternum and its associated ribs may show pectus excavatum or pectus carinatum deformities. The bones themselves may be abnormal (as in Hurler syndrome) and can provide a vital clue to the diagnosis of the cardiovascular problem.

Careful note should be made of the ribs, both the anterior and posterior portions. Distortion of the normal rib cage pattern occurs with congenital anomalies. Following thoracic surgery, one may note absence of a portion of a rib, a regenerated rib, and either narrowing or widening of the intercostal spaces. Wire sutures in the sternum are seen after a midline sternal splitting incision or a transverse incision that has crossed the sternum. Next, the thymic shadow should be evaluated. Many instances of apparent cardiomegaly on posteroanterior chest x-rays prove to be a prominent thymus gland. Especially in infancy, a large thymus may obscure the great vessels and distort the cardiac outline, making analysis difficult. A large thymus sometimes produces a bump on the right heart border, which is a helpful clue (Figure 74).

LUNGS

Many patients with significant heart disease have associated pulmonary disease. Pneumonitis, pleural fluid, and atelectasis are particularly common. Left lower lobe atelectasis should be carefully sought behind the heart shadow, because it is often missed.

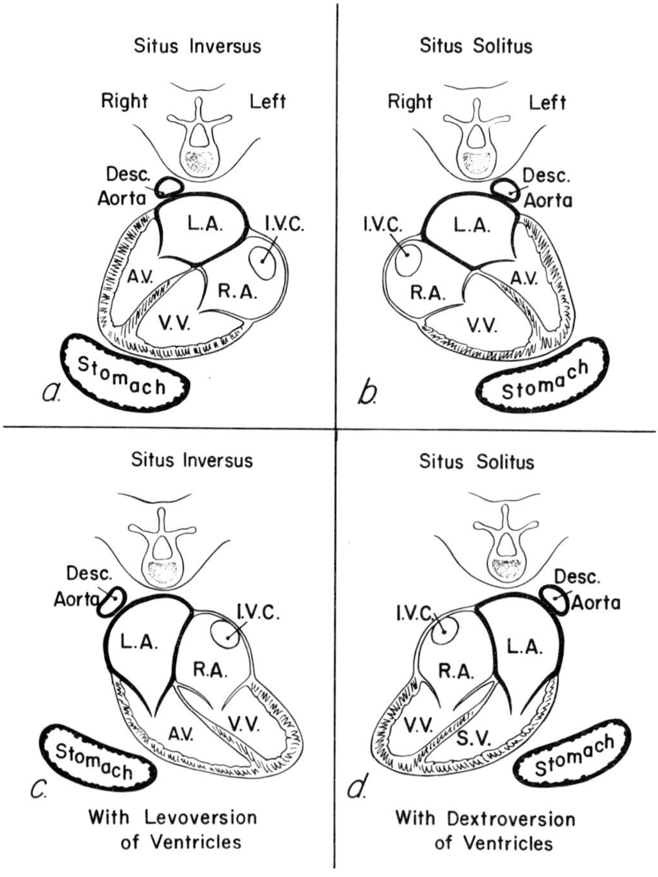

Figure 75. Schematic diagram of determining the situs, or position, of the heart by noting the side of the aortic knob and the gastric air bubble. These structures normally lie on the same side. Each of the two main positions, situs solitus (normal) and situs inversus, may be associated with the cardiac apex on the opposite side. (a) situs inversus, (b) situs solitus, (c) situs inversus with levoversion, and (d) situs solitus with dextroversion.

Key: LA = left atrium, RA = right atrium, IVC = inferior vena cava, SV = systemic ventricle, VV = venous ventricle.

PULMONARY VASCULATURE

An important feature in interpretation is the radiographic appearance of the pulmonary vasculature. The physician must first decide whether it is normal or abnormal. If abnormal, is the vasculature increased or decreased in prominence? If increased in prominence, is this secondary to left-to-right shunting or to pulmonary venous obstruction?

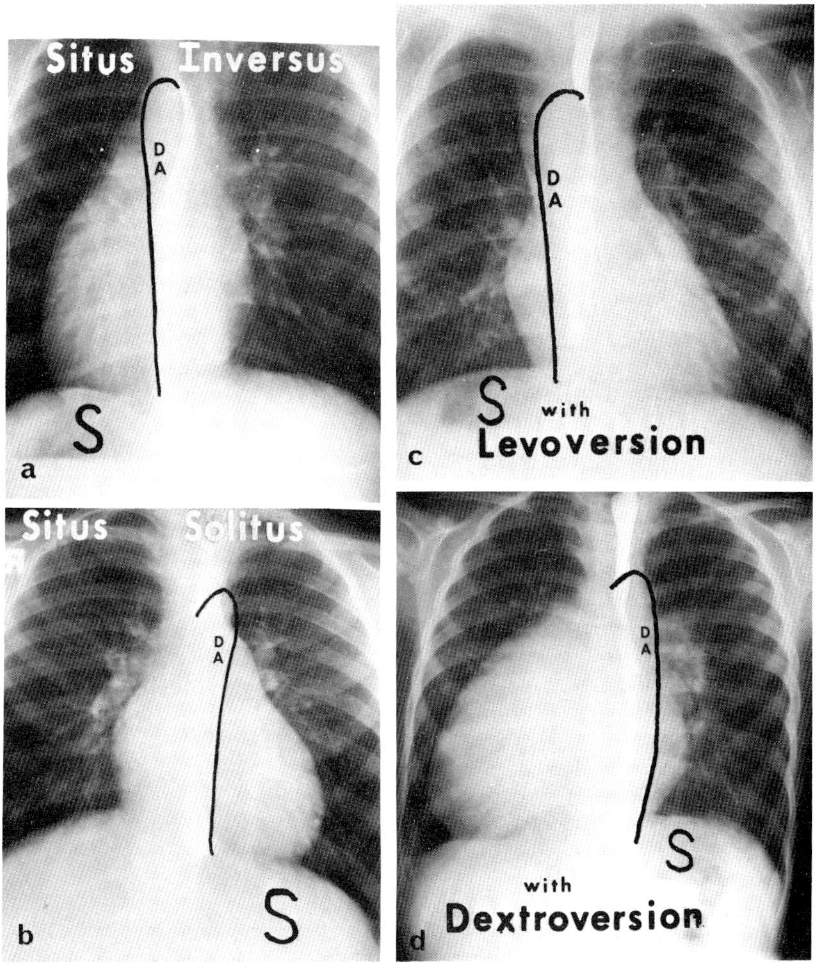

Figure 76. PA films of the chest demonstrating the four main kinds of cardiac position. (a) situs inversus, (b) situs solitus, (c) situs inversus with levoversion, and (d) situs solitus with dextroversion.

Key: S = stomach air bubble, DA = descending arch of aorta. (From Elliott, L. P., Jue, K. L., and Amplatz, K. 1966. A roentgen classification of cardiac malpositions. Invest. Radiol. 1:17.)

CARDIAC POSITIONS

Since the position of the heart and associated structures is vital to interpretation, this should be determined prior to evaluating the individual great vessels and cardiac chambers. In the normal (situs solitus) heart, the arch of the aorta, the left atrium, and the gastric air bubble are all on the left side (Figures 75 and 76).

The *situs solitus* heart has two patterns: 1) *normal,* with the cardiac apex on the left, and 2) *dextroversion,* with the cardiac apex turned varying degrees to the right. In the normally positioned heart, the incidence of congenital cardiac defects is around 1%, whereas with dextroversion an associated congenital cardiac malformation is nearly always present. Most common among such anomalies is congenitally corrected transposition with either a ventricular septal defect and/or pulmonic stenosis.

Situs inversus is a mirror-image of the normal position, with the heart, the aortic arch, the left atrium, and the gastric air bubble on the right. Two variations also occur in the situs inversus heart: 1) *complete* mirror-image or situs inversus heart, when the cardiac apex is to the right side, and 2) situs inversus *with levoversion,* when the cardiac apex is on the left. In the complete situs inversus heart, the incidence of associated congenital anomalies is 3% to 5%; in situs inversus with levoversion, the incidence of associated cardiac anomalies again approaches 100%. When rotation is superimposed on either the situs solitus or situs inversus heart, it must be presumed that there is an associated cardiac anomaly until proven otherwise.

The presence of a right-sided stomach together with a left-sided aortic arch and apex suggests polysplenia syndrome. Most such individuals have absence of the hepatic segment of the inferior vena cava with azygos continuation. This may often be detected by noting the greatly enlarged arch of the azygos vein, which forms a smooth, rounded shadow as it enters the superior vena cava.

THE CARDIOVASCULAR SILHOUETTE

The structures that contribute to the normal cardiac silhouette are shown in Figures 77 and 78. The four views of the standard cardiac examination are the posteroanterior (PA) view, the lateral view, the right anterior oblique (RAO) view, and the left anterior oblique (LAO) view. *The reader should acquaint himself thoroughly with these figures before reading further.*

The barium-filled esophagus is an important landmark in detecting cardiovascular abnormalities. The esophagus is in intimate contact with the aortic arch and descending thoracic aorta, the left main stem bronchus, and the left atrium. Of these, the aortic arch normally produces the deepest and most

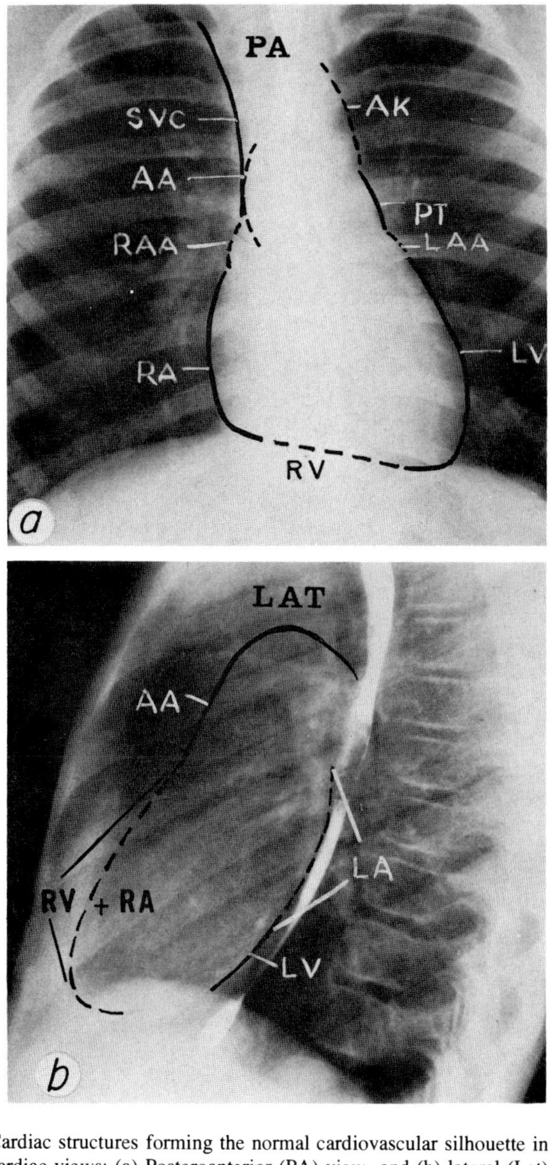

Figure 77. Cardiac structures forming the normal cardiovascular silhouette in two of the four conventional cardiac views: (a) Posteroanterior (PA) view, and (b) lateral (Lat) view.

Key: SVC = superior vena cava, AA = ascending aorta. RA = right atrium, RV = right ventricle, LV = left ventricle, LAA = left atrial appendage, PT = pulmonary trunk, AK = aortic knob, and LA = left atrium. (From Elliott, L. P., and Schiebler, G. L. 1965. X-ray diagnosis of congenital cardiac disease. Postgrad. Med. 37.)

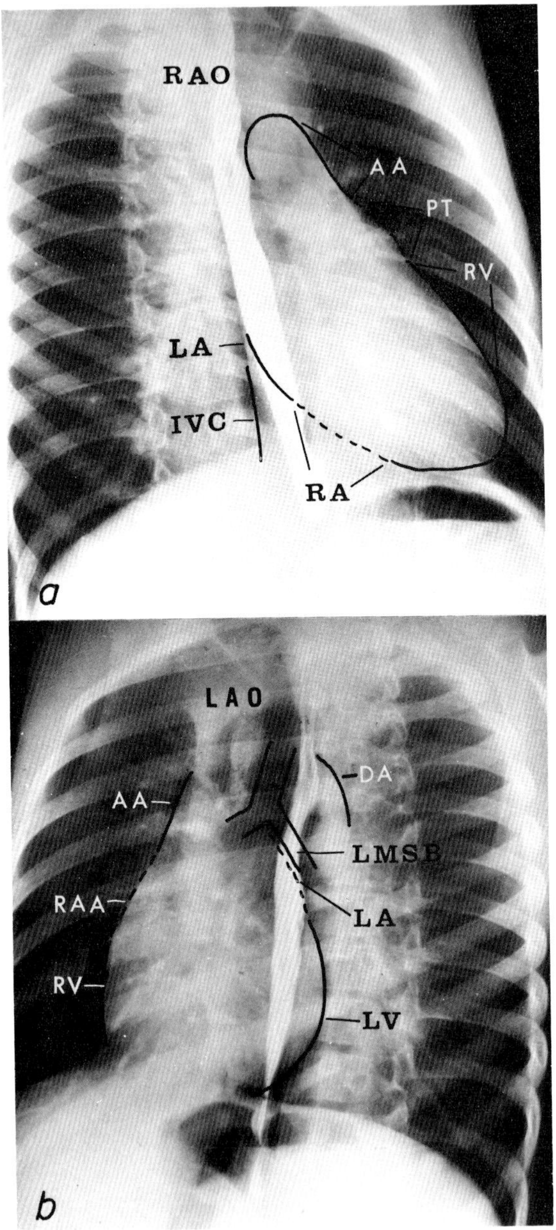

Figure 78. Cardiac structures forming the normal cardiovascular silhouette in the (a) right anterior and (b) left anterior oblique views. Abbreviations as in Figure 77.

Key: IVC = inferior vena cava, DA = descending thoracic aorta, and LMSB = left main stem bronchus. (From Elliott, L. P., and Schiebler, G. L. 1965. X-ray diagnosis of con genital cardiac disease. Postgrad. Med. 37. A-87.)

constant impression, a concave indentation to the left as seen in the PA and RAO views.

Left Atrium

Normally the left atrium lies slightly above the right atrium. The left atrium is centrally placed and does not form any part of the cardiac contour in the PA view. The left atrial appendage is a superior and leftward extension of the body and forms a short inconspicuous border between the pulmonary trunk and left ventricle. In the RAO and lateral views, the left atrium forms the midposterior position of the cardiac silhouette and is intimately related to the esophagus and left main stem bronchus. In the LAO view, the left atrium also lies adjacent to the left main stem bronchus.

Of the four cardiac chambers, enlargement in the left atrium is easiest to detect. Moreover, this chamber is by far the most important with regard to the functional and anatomic interpretation of cardiac disease. Left atrial enlargement is caused by increased volume secondary to either excess blood flow into the atrium or obstruction of outflow from the atrium. Excess blood fills the left atrium when there is a left-to-right shunt distal to the mitral valve, a right-to-left shunt through the foramen ovale, or an incompetent mitral valve that produces regurgitation from the left ventricle. Left atrial enlargement also occurs when there is difficulty in emptying, as in mitral stenosis or with a thick noncompliant left ventricle.

Left atrial enlargement (Figure 79) is indicated by: 1) elevation and bowing of the left main stem bronchus, best seen in the LAO view; 2) prominence of the left atrial appendage, largely in rheumatic heart disease; 3) deviation of the barium-filled esophagus to the right and posteriorly; and 4) a dense double contour seen in the middle of the cardiac shadow that outlines the inferior margin of the LA (downward displacement of this line indicates left atrial enlargement).

Right Atrium

The right atrium is an oval structure that forms the right heart border in the PA view and approximately the upper third of the heart border in the LAO view (Figure 80). The right atrial appendage, a superior and medial extension of the atrial body, varies considerably in size and may sometimes overlie the outflow tract of the right ventricle.

The causes for right atrial enlargement are similar to those described above for left atrial enlargement. Tricuspid regurgitation, Ebstein's anomaly of the tricuspid valve, and hypoplastic right ventricle all produce right atrial enlargement. Because it is difficult to diagnose isolated right atrial enlargement from plain films, this subject is discussed below under "Right Heart Enlargement."

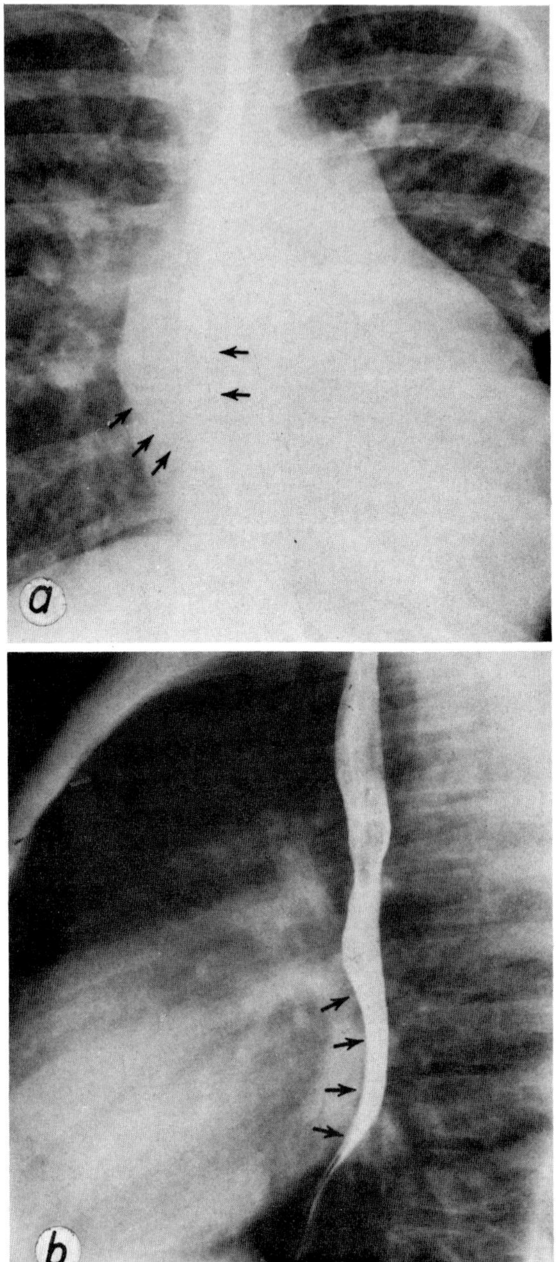

Figure 79. Left atrial enlargement. (a) PA view, deviation of the barium-filled esophagus to the right (horizontal arrows) and the dense double contour (oblique arrows). (b) Lateral view, posterior deviation of the barium-filled esophagus (arrows). (c) RAO view, posterior deviation of the barium-filled esophagus (arrows). (d) LAO view, shows elevation of the left main stem

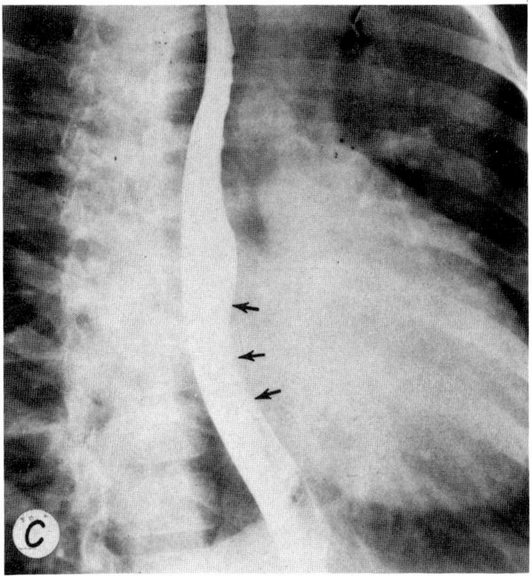

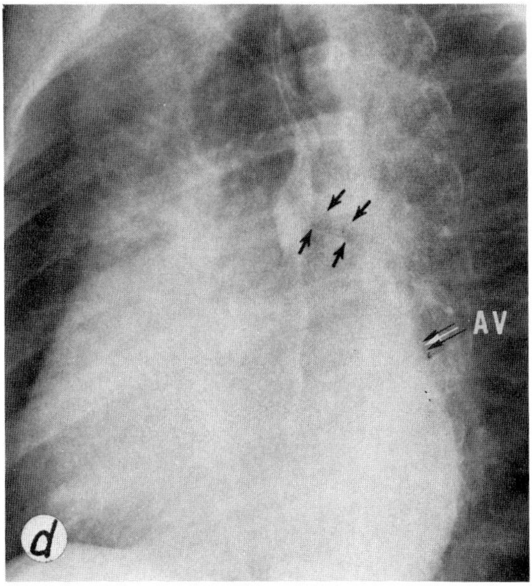

bronchus (arrows). An additional sign is an abnormal degree of density between the left main stem bronchus and the left atrioventricular (AV) groove (tip of black and white arrows). (From Elliott, L. P., and Schiebler, G. L. 1968. X-Ray Diagnosis of Congenital Cardiac Disease. Courtesy of Charles C Thomas, Publisher, Springfield, Ill.)

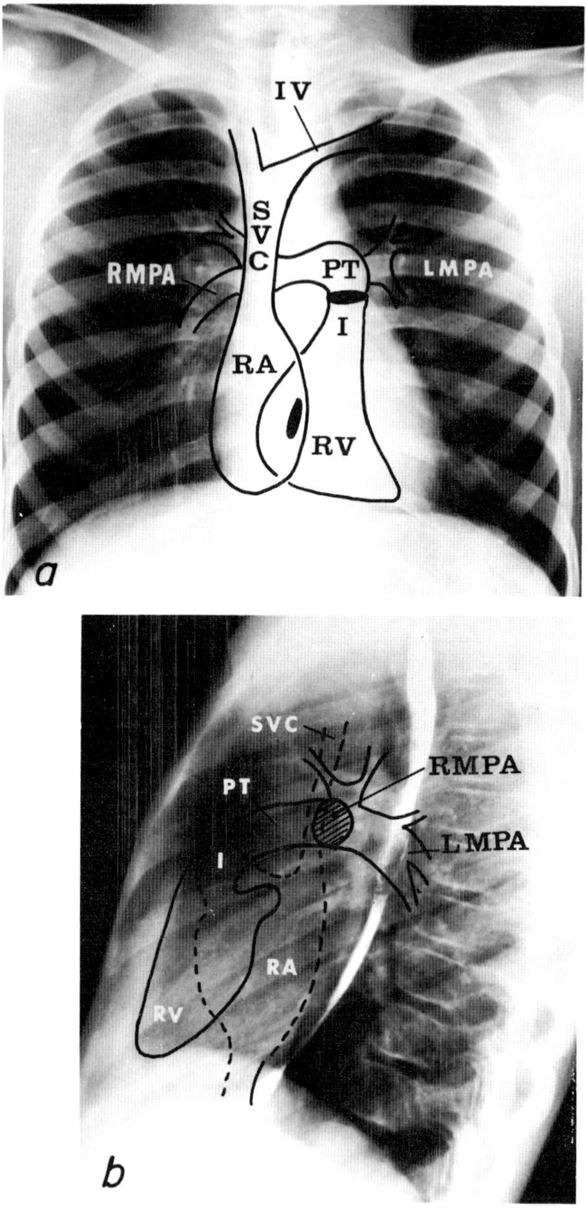

Figure 80. Schematic drawing of the right-side cardiac chambers and vessels superimposed on the normal thoracic roentgenogram. (a) Posteroanterior view; (b) lateral view. Abbreviations as in Figure 78.

Key: IV = innominate vein, RMPA = right main pulmonary artery, LMPA = left main pulmonary artery, I = right ventricle infundibulum. The lower dark circular area represents the tricuspid valve; the upper one, the pulmonary valve. (From Elliott, L. P., and Schiebler, G. L. 1965. X-ray diagnosis of congenital cardiac disease. Postgrad. Med. 37:A-87.)

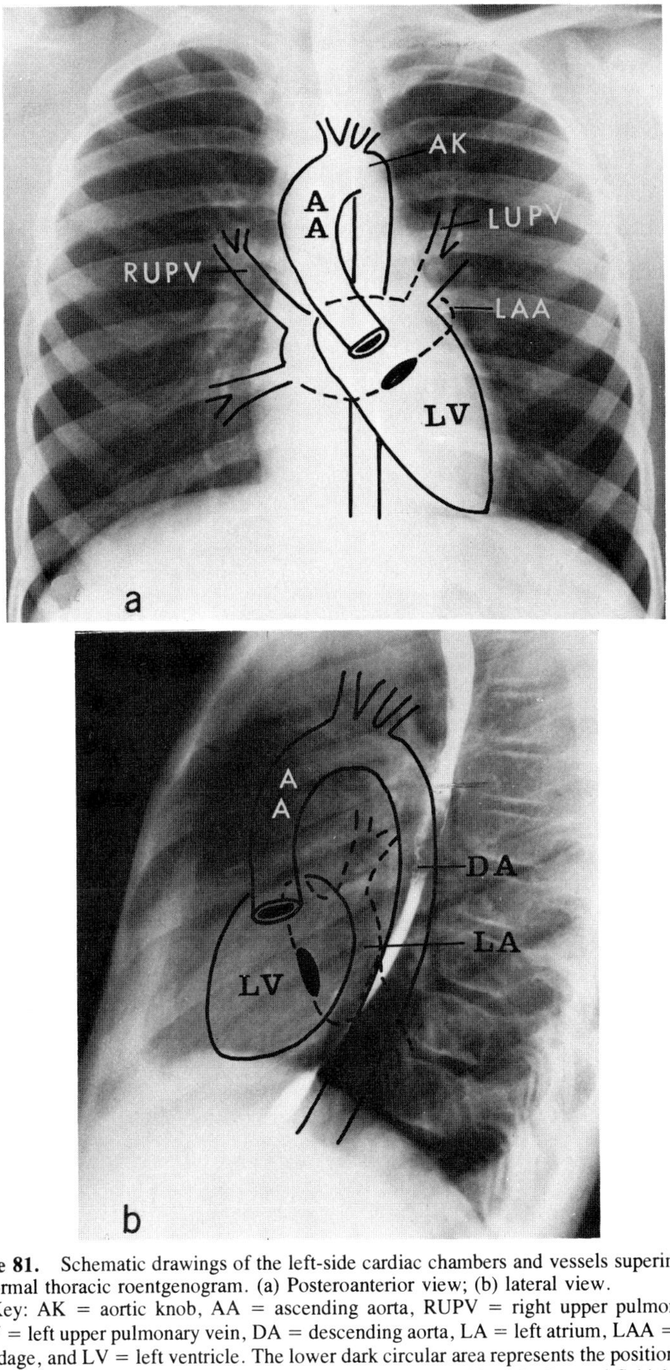

Figure 81. Schematic drawings of the left-side cardiac chambers and vessels superimposed on the normal thoracic roentgenogram. (a) Posteroanterior view; (b) lateral view.

Key: AK = aortic knob, AA = ascending aorta, RUPV = right upper pulmonary vein, LUPV = left upper pulmonary vein, DA = descending aorta, LA = left atrium, LAA = left atrial appendage, and LV = left ventricle. The lower dark circular area represents the position occupied by the mitral valve; the upper one, the aortic valve. (From Elliott, L. P., and Schiebler, G. L. 1965. X-Ray diagnosis of congenital cardiac disease. Postgrad. Med. 37:A-91.)

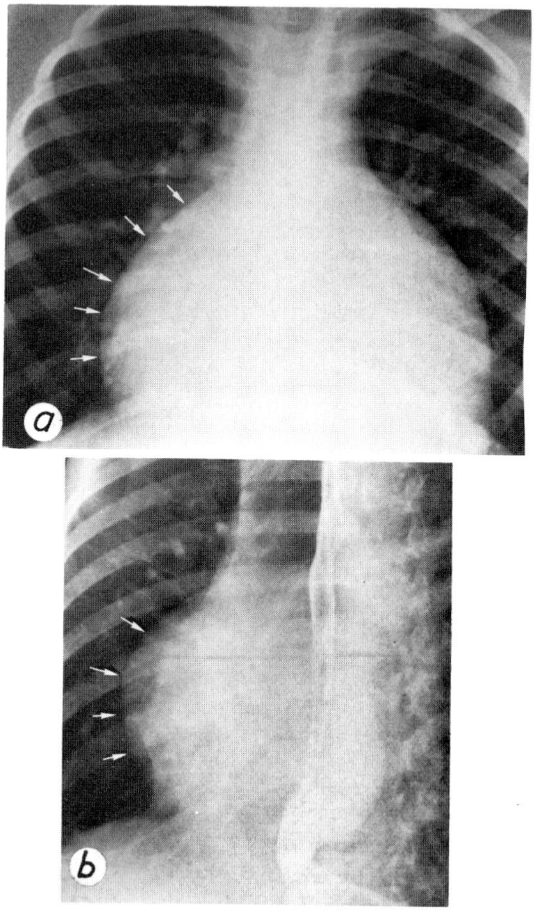

Figure 82. Right heart (right atrial and right ventricular) enlargement. (a) PA view, the right heart border (arrows) is abnormally convex, extending too far to the right. (b) LAO view, the anterior (right heart border) is abnormally convex. (c) Lateral view, there is an increased density (arrows) in the retrosternal space secondary to enlargement of the right atrial appendage. (d) Another LAO view showing abnormal right heart. In this patient, both the left and right ventricles are enlarged. However, the diagnosis of left ventricular enlargement cannot be ascertained radiologically in the presence of the right heart enlargement. (From Elliott, L. P., and Schiebler, G. L. 1968. X-Ray Diagnosis of Congenital Cardiac Disease. Courtesy of Charles C Thomas, Publisher, Springfield, Ill.)

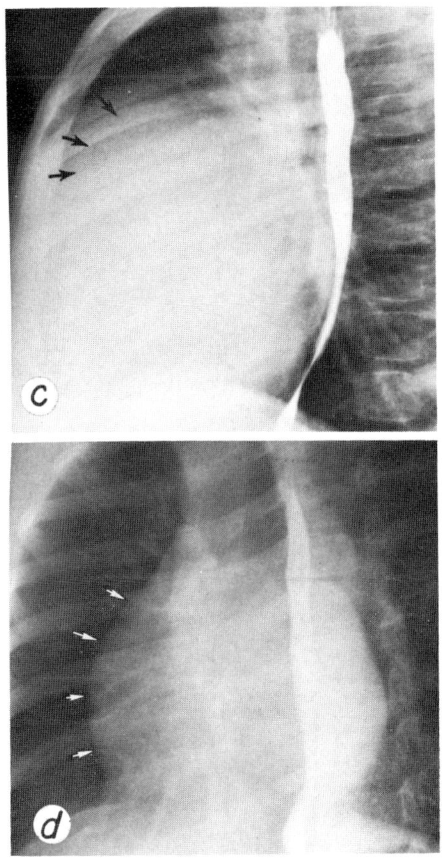

Figure 82. *continued*

The Ventricles

Normally the *right ventricle* is located more anteriorly than rightward and the *left ventricle* more posteriorly than leftward (Figures 80 and 81), but we refer to the ventricles as right and left to avoid needless confusion. The right ventricle is divided into an inflow portion, or body, lying directly below the tricuspid orifice, and an outflow portion, or infundibulum, lying between the body and the pulmonic valve.

Significant left-to-right shunting or valvar regurgitation causes primarily dilatation of the ventricular chamber, whereas ventricular outflow obstruction causes hypertrophy. (Dilatation is an increase in chamber or vessel volume without significant increase in thickness of the chamber or vessel wall. Hypertrophy implies enlargement of the mass, thus increasing the thickness of the chamber or vessel wall without increasing the capacity. Enlargement is a nonspecific radiologic term describing an increase in size of a part of the heart in response to either dilatation or hypertrophy.) Isolated hypertrophy of either ventricle is sometimes difficult to diagnose radiologically and is characterized more by change in shape of the cardiac silhouette than by increased size.

Right Heart Enlargement Right atrial and right ventricular enlargement are considered under the general term right heart enlargement. It is difficult, if not impossible, to assess the true size of the right atrium and the right ventricle from plain films. The cardiac contour classically ascribed to right ventricular enlargement may occur with only right atrial enlargement. Furthermore, when there is right ventricular enlargement, the right atrium is almost invariably enlarged as well. Fortunately, the correct diagnosis rarely depends solely upon determining whether it is the right ventricle or the right atrium that is enlarged.

In the PA view, the lower half of the right heart border tends to be more convex than in a normal heart and extends higher before meeting the superior vena cava (Figure 82a). The left side of the cardiac silhouette is usually formed by the right ventricle and the pulmonary trunk. The indentations normally seen between the aortic knob and the pulmonary trunk or between the pulmonary trunk and the left ventricle are obliterated. Usually the left ventricle is pushed posteriorly. An enlarged pulmonary trunk with an enlarged cardiac silhouette strongly suggests right heart enlargement.

The *LAO* view is superior to all other views in detecting early right heart enlargement. Moderate to marked convexity of the upper right (anterior) heart border where the outline of the ascending aorta meets the shadow of the right atrial appendage suggests right heart enlargement (Figure 82b,d).

Only when the right heart is gigantic does it appear behind the barium-filled esophagus in the RAO view. However, the right ventricular outflow tract may form an abnormal convexity in the anterior heart border.

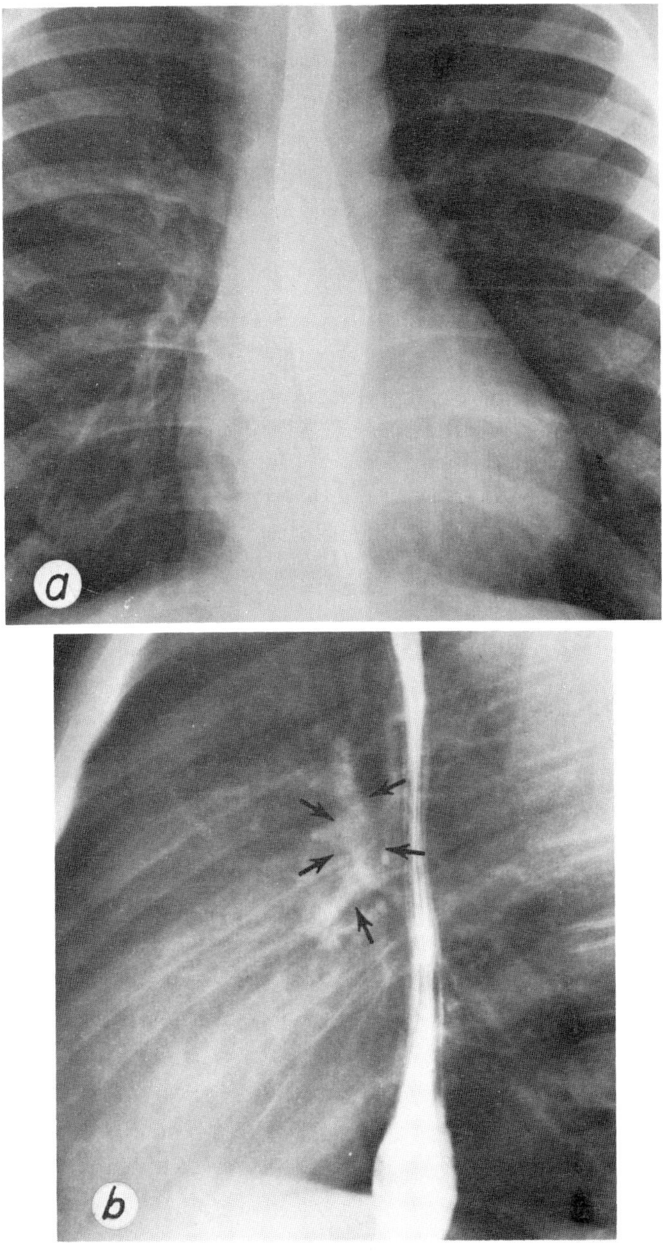

Figure 83. Decreased pulmonary vasculature. (a) PA view. (b) Lateral view. Characteristic of decreased vasculature is the hypoplastic appearance of the right and left hila, as well as a decrease in size of the intrapulmonary vessels. The lateral view (b) shows a small hilum outlined by arrows. (From Elliot, L. P., and Schiebler, G. L. 1968. X-Ray Diagnosis of Congenital Cardiac Disease. Courtesy of Charles C Thomas, Publisher, Springfield, Ill.)

In the lateral view, normally, only the lower part of the anterior surface of the right ventricle touches the sternum. With dilatation, particularly of the right ventricular infundibulum or right atrial appendage, the superior aspect of the retrosternal space is completely radiopaque (Figure 82c). This sign is vastly overrated and not as valuable as signs of right heart enlargement in the LAO view. Obliteration of the retrosternal space may also be due to an enlarged right atrial appendage or a normal heart in a patient with a narrow anterior-posterior diameter of the chest.

Right ventricular hypertrophy causes concentric thickening of the ventricular wall, which results in little, if any, actual enlargement (Figure 82b). It may, however, produce an unusual rounding of the cardiac contour. In many situations, without additional radiologic signs of heart disease (e.g., an enlarged pulmonary trunk) right ventricular hypertrophy may be missed.

Left Ventricle Normally posterior to the right ventricle (see Figure 81), the left ventricle is usually pear shaped in both PA and lateral views, with its apex resting on the diaphragm. The left ventricle forms the left heart border in the PA view and the lower posterior border in the lateral view.

Dilatation of the left ventricle produces an elongated heart with the apex pointed downward in the PA view (Figure 83). In the PA view, the left cardiac border is prominent, accentuated by the concavity present in the region of the pulmonary trunk.

In the LAO view, the posterior wall of the left ventricle appears bulky and globular and projects downward over the spine (Figure 84). Isolated left ventricular enlargement is characterized by the right or anterior border assuming a straight contour. Of the four cardiac views, the LAO is the best for detecting left ventricular enlargement, partly because this view also allows evaluation of the right heart.

When the heart border extends behind the barium-filled esophagus in the lateral view, left ventricular enlargement is probable. However, a cardiac shadow extending behind the esophagus may be due to a normal left ventricle displaced posteriorly by right ventricular enlargement, a giant-sized right atrium caused by severe tricuspid insufficiency, such as is found in Ebstein's anomaly of the tricuspid valve, or pericardial effusion.

Figure 84. (a) Left ventricular enlargement. (b) Normal-sized heart with left ventricular configuration. This pattern suggests hypertrophy in patients under 40 years of age. Note the abnormal ascending aorta—strong indirect evidence that the left ventricle is hypertrophied. (From Elliott, L. P., and Schiebler, G. L. 1968. X-Ray Diagnosis of Congenital Cardiac Disease. Courtesy of Charles C Thomas, Publisher, Springfield, Ill.)

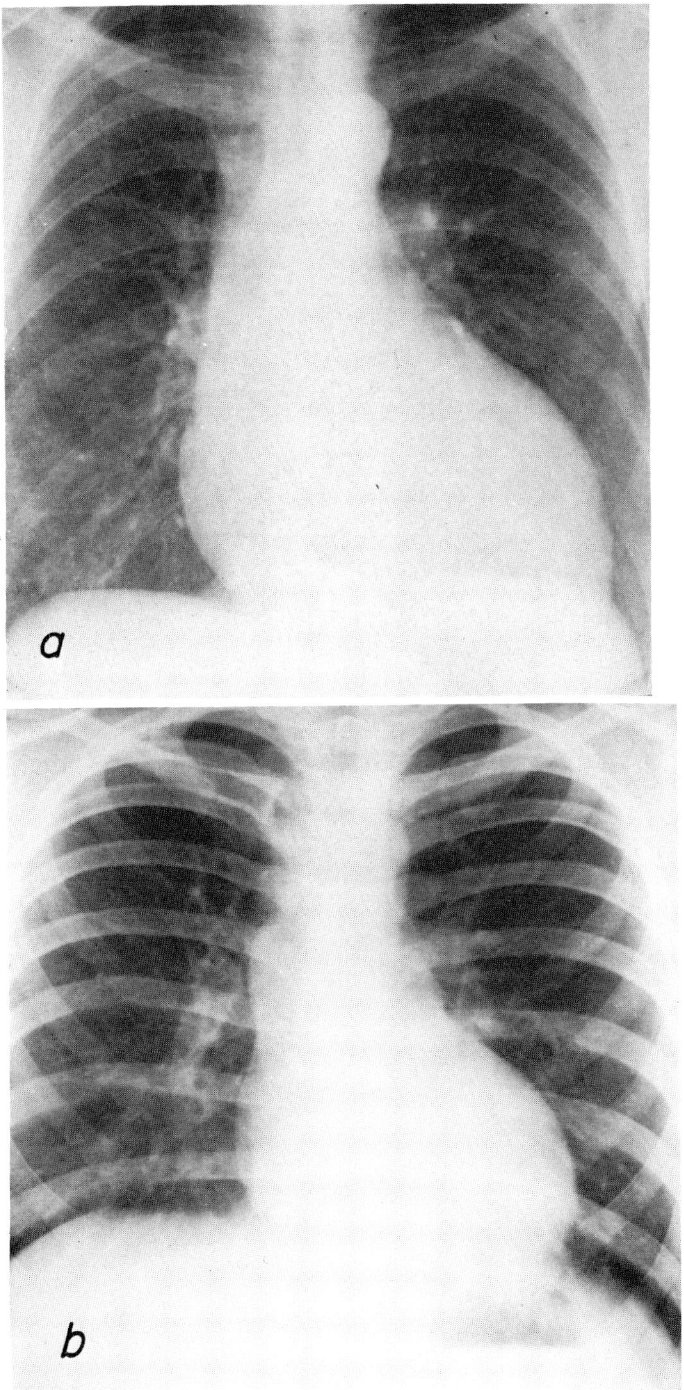
a
b

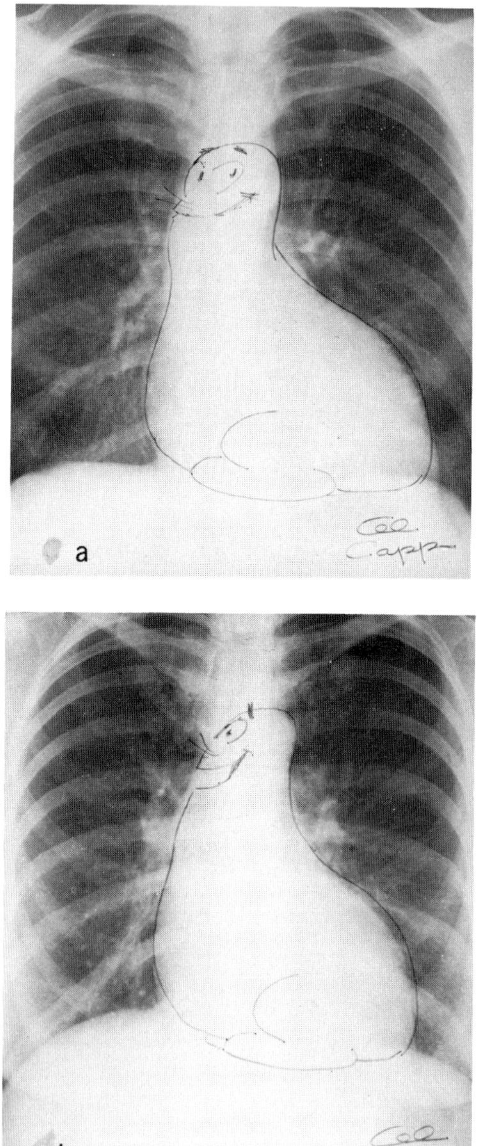

Figure 85. Drawing of a Shmoo on PA film of a patient with left ventricular enlargement (a) and a patient with left ventricular hypertrophy (b). These were done through the courtesy of Mr. Al Capp to dramatize the likeness of left ventricular disease to the configuration of the Shmoo. (Adapted from Elliott, L. P., and Schiebler, G. L. 1968. X-Ray Diagnosis of Congenital Cardiac Disease. Courtesy of Charles C Thomas, Publisher, Springfield, Ill.)

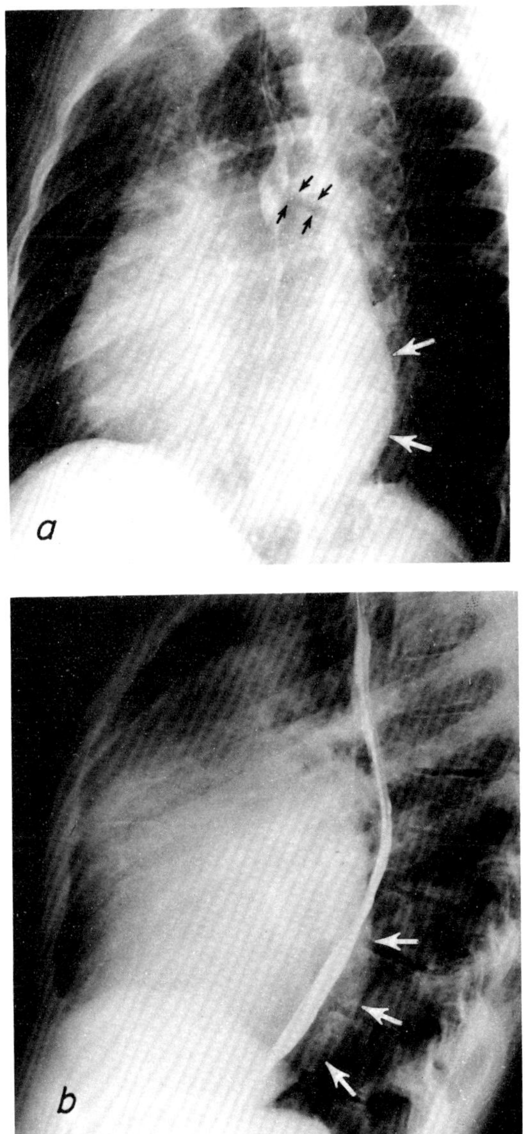

Figure 86. Left ventricular enlargement. (a) LAO view. White arrows indicate the enlarged left ventricle projecting beyond the spine. Note that the right or anterior heart border is normal, being in a straight line with the contour of the ascending aorta. Black arrows show the elevated left main stem bronchus secondary to left atrial enlargement. (b) Lateral view in the same case showing the enlarged left ventricle projecting posteriorly to the barium-filled esophagus. This is not a reliable sign unless right heart enlargement has been ruled out. (From Elliott, L. P., and Schiebler, G. L. 1968. X-Ray Diagnosis of Congenital Cardiac Disease. Courtesy of Charles C Thomas, Publisher, Springfield, Ill.)

Left ventricular hypertrophy per se does not usually result in an enlarged cardiac silhouette. The cardiovascular silhouette may assume the ''Shmoo'' configuration (Figure 85). In a young child, this configuration without enlargement of the total silhouette is nearly pathognomonic of left ventricular pressure overloading, resulting from coarctation of the aorta or aortic valve stenosis.

In difficult cases, left ventricular hypertrophy is probable when the ascending aorta is prominent, whereas right ventricular hypertrophy is probable when the pulmonary trunk is prominent. When both ventricles are enlarged, left ventricular size may be difficult to ascertain. On the other hand, an enlarged right ventricular component is usually detectable in all situations. The ECG is usually superior to the thoracic roentgenogram in detecting the left ventricular component of combined ventricular enlargement.

The Great Vessels

Thoracic Aorta In older children, the right lateral border of the ascending aorta may form part of the cardiovascular silhouette (Figures 81 and 86). The ascending aorta is clearly defined in the LAO view, where it forms the upper anterior portion of the cardiovascular outline. The transverse aortic arch forms a smooth, rounded bulge—the aortic knob—in the uppermost left margin of the cardiac shadow to the left of the upper thoracic spine.

In children, the aortic knob frequently produces a convex impression of the left side of the trachea and of the barium-filled esophagus. A normal or left aortic arch is seen coursing along the left side of the trachea, and can be seen descending through the chest along the left side of the spine. If the aortic arch is not clearly defined, its location may be determined by noting the position of the trachea. The trachea is located to the right of the midline when the aortic arch is left-sided and to the left of the midline with a right aortic arch. In a right aortic arch, the descending aorta may be seen along the right spinal border (Figure 87). The transverse aortic arch courses to the right of the trachea. This causes the aortic knob to appear at the right side of the spine, leaving a clear space on the left. The normal tracheal and esophageal impressions are reversed. The superior vena cava is often deviated to the right.

The *aortic valve* is an intracardiac structure that is inferior and medial to the pulmonic valve and overlies the thoracic spine. In the lateral view the aortic valve lies in the center of the heart shadow (see Figure 81).

In congenital cardiac lesions, the most common abnormalities of the aorta are:

1. Post-stenotic *dilation* of the ascending aorta secondary to aortic valvar stenosis. The thoracic roentgenogram shows the ascending aorta to have an increased curvature to the right and anteriorly seen best in the PA and LAO view (see Figure 86).

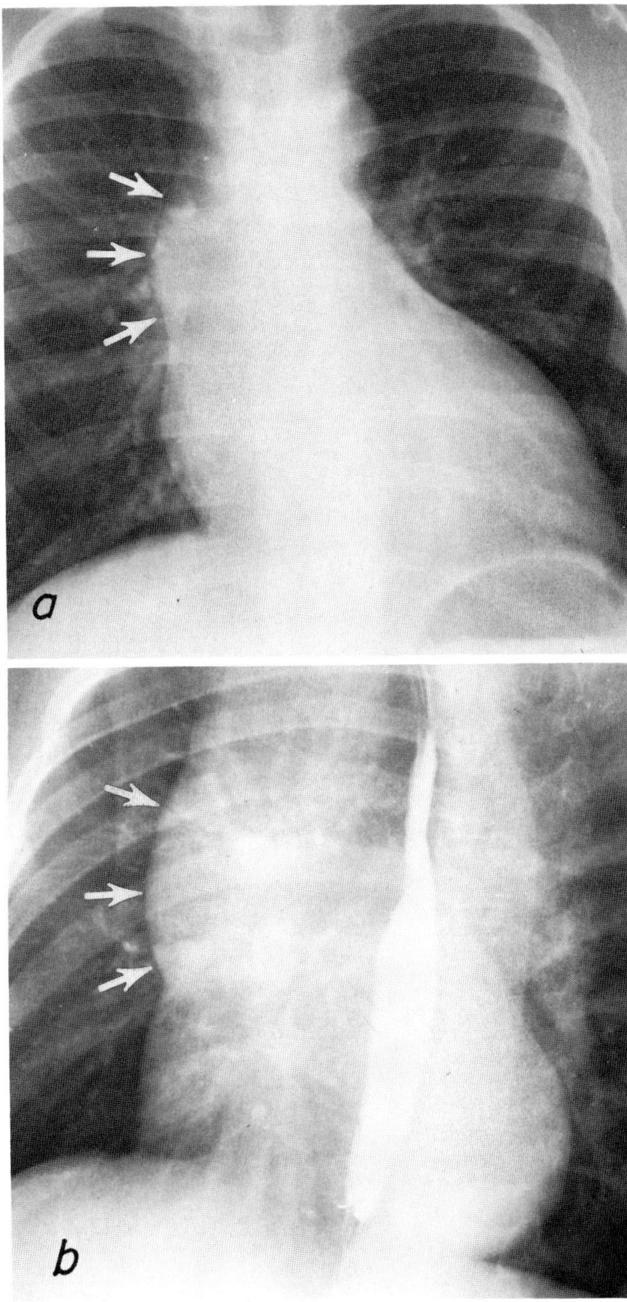

Figure 87.— Prominent ascending aorta (arrows) in the PA (a) and LAO (b) view. Note the straight right heart border below the prominent aorta in the LAO view. (From Elliott, L. P., and Schiebler, G. L. 1968. X-Ray Diagnosis of Congenital Cardiac Disease. Courtesy of Charles C Thomas, Publisher, Springfield, Ill.)

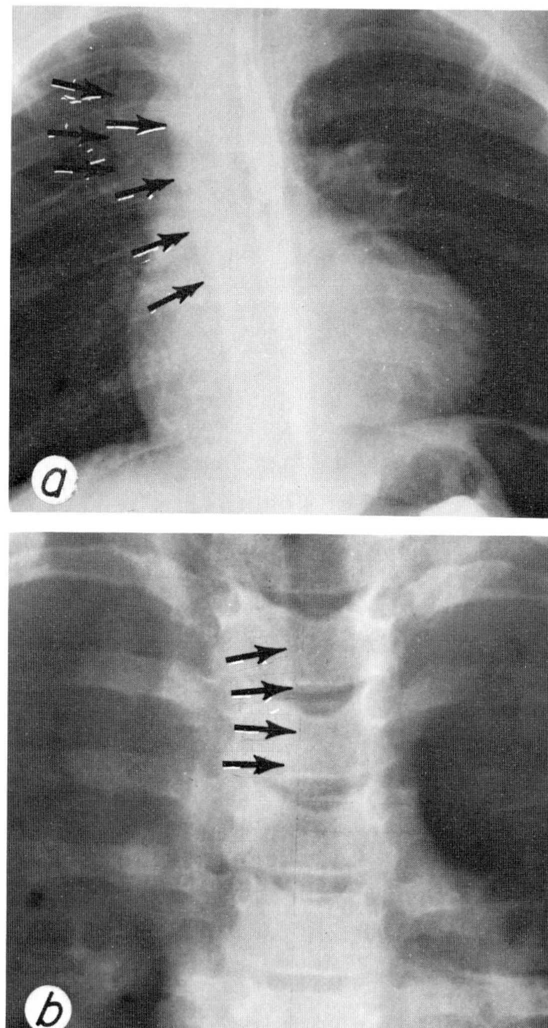

Figure 88. Right aortic arch. (a) PA view showing the superior vena cava (white arrows), which is pushed rightward by the right aortic arch. The inner black arrows outline the descending thoracic aorta on the right. There is a clear space on the left. (b) Close-up anteroposterior view of the trachea, which reveals a concave deformity on its right side (arrows). This is the most reliable sign of a right aortic arch. (Adapted from Elliott, L. P., and Schiebler, G. L. 1968. X-Ray Diagnosis of Congenital Cardiac Disease. Courtesy of Charles C Thomas, Publisher, Springfield, Ill.)

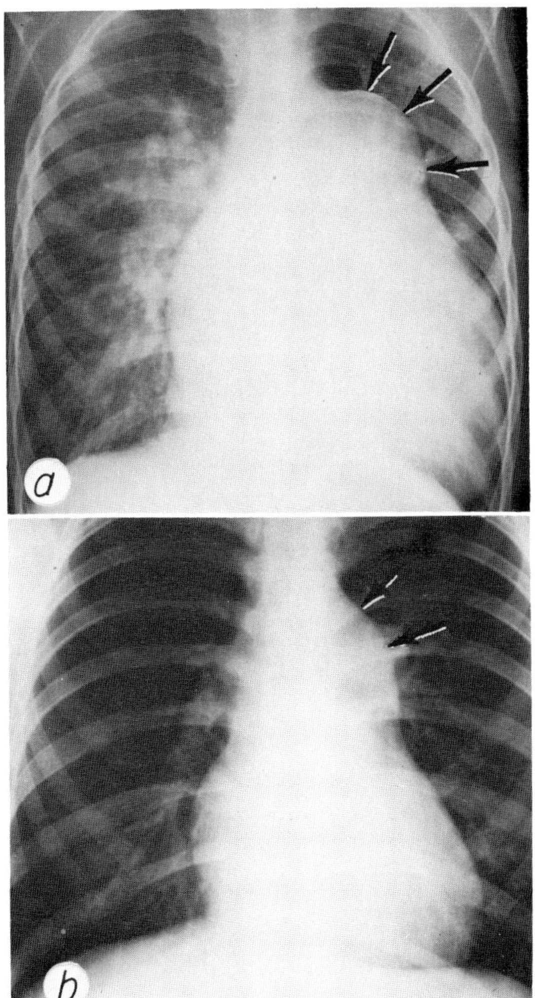

Figure 89. Enlargement of the pulmonary artery (a) with a left-to-right shunt (PA view) and prominent hilar and intrapulmonary vessels; (b) in pulmonic valve stenosis. Arrows show isolated prominence of the pulmonary trunk. The right hilar and intrapulmonary vessels are normal in size. (From Elliott, L. P., and Schiebler, G. L. 1968. X-Ray Diagnosis of Congenital Cardiac Disease. Courtesy of Charles C Thomas, Publisher, Springfield, Ill.)

2. Prominence of the ascending aorta and aortic knob may occur with patent ductus arteriosus, coarctation of the aorta, or truncus arteriosus.
3. In patients with a large intracardiac right-to-left shunt and pulmonary artery bed hypoplasia, the aorta is also often enlarged.
4. In a case of congenital heart disease with a *right aortic arch,* look at the vascular markings. If these are *increased,* suspect truncus arteriosus. If they are *decreased,* consider cyanotic tetralogy of Fallot. In both of these conditions, a right aortic arch occurs in 25%–30% of cases. Abnormal great vessels arising from the aortic arch occur most frequently in tetralogy of Fallot and coarctation of the aorta.

Pulmonary Trunk The *pulmonic valve* is not part of the cardiac silhouette, but is situated in the left, superior, and anterior aspect of the base of the heart at a level higher than that of the aortic valve (see Figures 80 and 81). The pulmonic valve is located at the periphery of the heart, as opposed to the aortic valve, which lies within the heart.

In the PA view, the pulmonary trunk normally forms a straight or slightly convex line at the left upper heart border between the left atrial appendage and the aortic arch (see Figure 77). In the RAO view, the pulmonary trunk forms a smooth, midly convex line directed posteriorly from the upper anterior aspect of the cardiac shadow (see Figure 78).

Enlargement of the pulmonary trunk, and usually of the left main pulmonary artery as well, may be present in: 1) normal individuals, especially adolescents; 2) idiopathic dilatation of the pulmonary artery; 3) pulmonic valvar stenosis (post-stenotic dilatation); 4) increased pulmonary blood flow, as in left-to-right shunts; or 5) pulmonary artery hypertension (Figure 88).

Abnormal Pulmonary Vasculature

When the physician decides that the pulmonary vasculature is abnormal, he must then decide whether it is increased or decreased. If increased, this may be secondary to a left-to-right shunt, pulmonary venous hypertension, or, on rare occasions, enlarged bronchial arteries.

Interpretation of pulmonary vascular markings is often difficult, particularly when they are nearly normal. The same observer may differ in his interpretation on successive days. Furthermore, the criteria for normal vascularity change with age. For example, when the vascular markings appear "normal" in the neonate, they are probably increased; when they appear "increased" in the adolescent, they are probably normal.

In the PA view, most of the middle and lower aspects of the right and left hilar densities are formed by the right and left main pulmonary arteries, respectively (Figures 89 and 90). The left hilar density is more difficult to evaluate in the PA view, because of superimposition of the pulmonary trunk, and is best evaluated in the LAO and lateral views.

The upper portion of the hilar densities (particularly the right hilar) is formed by the upper lobe pulmonary veins, as well as the pulmonary arteries. Normally, the right hilum assumes the shape of a Y turned on its side. The vascular structures that form both hila are sharply marginated. The cartilaginous bronchi form only a small portion of the normal hila. Often an individual artery can be seen on the end adjacent to the bronchus and is normally equal to or slightly smaller in diameter than the bronchus.

The right main pulmonary artery arises at a sharp angle from the pulmonary trunk (see Figure 80). The left main pulmonary artery is, in effect, a continuation of the pulmonary trunk and courses directly posteriorly and slightly to the left between the angle formed by the trachea and the left main stem bronchus. The direct posterior course of the left main pulmonary artery is best demonstrated in the LAO view.

The intrapulmonary arteries extend in a tree-like manner from the hilum into the lung, producing a distinct radiographic pattern called the vascular markings (see Figure 91). In contrast to systemic arteries, the branching

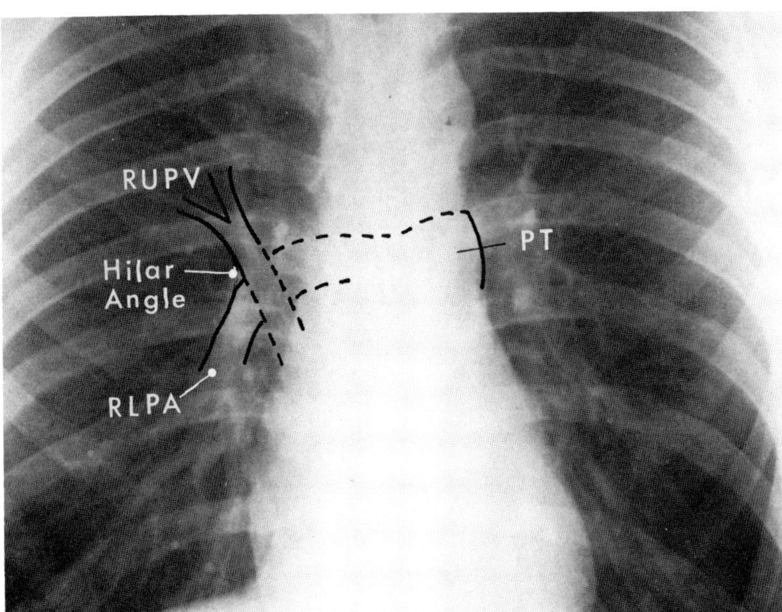

Figure 90. PA view showing the normal right hilar angle formed by the junction where the right upper pulmonary vein (RUPV) and the right lower pulmonary artery (RLPA) cross. PT = pulmonary trunk. In cases of pulmonary venous obstruction, the angle is obliterated by dilatation of the right upper lobe pulmonary vein. (Courtesy of Elliott, L. P., and Schiebler, G. L. 1968. X-Ray Diagnosis of Congenital Cardiac Disease. Courtesy of Charles C Thomas, Publisher, Springfield, Ill.)

pattern of the pulmonary arteries consists almost entirely of Y-shaped bifurcations, often clearly visible on the chest film.

The peripheral pulmonary veins play little part in producing the normal vascular pattern. In certain abnormal circulatory states, however, the pulmonary veins become prominent and contribute to prominence of the vascular pattern.

The roentgenographic signs of Table 11 and Figures 90 through 93 help to differentiate prominent pulmonary vasculatures that are secondary to left-to-right shunt lesions from those caused by pulmonary venous obstruction. Other examples of marked pulmonary venous obstruction are shown in Figures 129 and 202. Remember, however, that under certain conditions, such as a large left-to-right shunt in an infant with congestive heart failure, both arterial and venous markings may be prominent.

Bronchial Arteries Uncommonly, the pulmonary vasculature appears prominent secondary to an increase in flow through the bronchial arteries (Figure 94). Distinguishing prominent pulmonary arteries and veins from enlarged bronchial arteries may be difficult. Large bronchial arteries show a disorganized pattern and have a more stringy or reticulated appearance. The arteries themselves may produce small indentations in the barium-filled esophagus. All of the vessels are more nearly the same size. Also, the hilar

Table 11. Aids in differentiating two types of prominent pulmonary vasculature

	Left-to-right shunt[a]	Pulmonary venous obstruction
Pulmonary vessels	Prominent, discrete and well formed (Figure 92)	Hazy, diffuse, and poorly defined (Figures 92 and 93)
Bronchi in end view	Usually clear cut without dense peripheral cuff (Figure 94)	Slow thickened cuff of edema (Figure 93)
Hilar area	No hilar edema (Figure 94)	Hila are prominent and resemble a large indistinct mass (Figure 93)
Intrapulmonary vessels	Uniform distribution of prominent vessels, equal in upper and lower lobes (Figure 94)	Uneven distribution of prominent vessels, increase in size of upper lobe vessels as compared with lower lobe vessels (Figure 86)
Left atrial appendage	Rarely observed as a discrete bulge (Figure 92)	Often prominent (Figure 93), predominantly in patients with rheumatic mitral insufficiency

[a] These findings are predicated on the absence of left heart failure, since this increases pulmonary venous pressure and increases the difficulty of analysis.

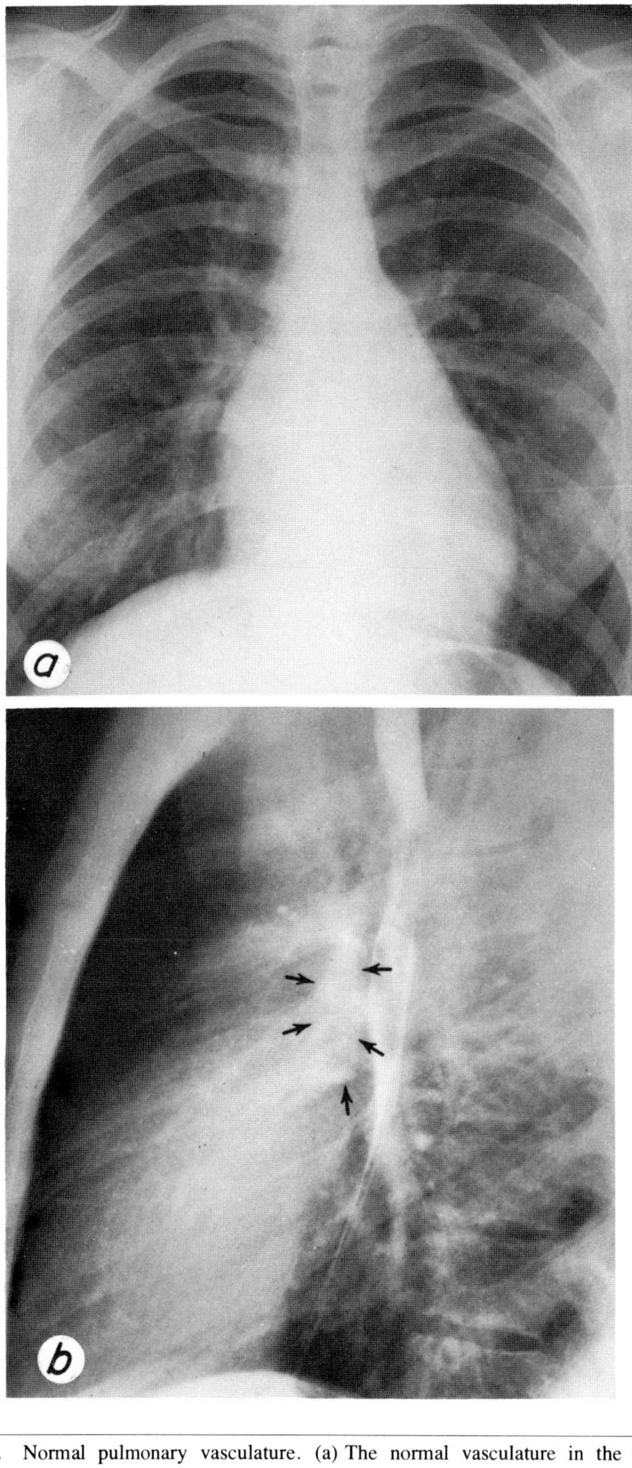

Figure 91. Normal pulmonary vasculature. (a) The normal vasculature in the PA view. (b) Lateral view showing the size and relative density of the normal hilum (arrows). (From Elliott, L. P., and Schiebler, G. L. 1968. X-Ray Diagnosis of Congenital Cardiac Disease. Courtesy of Charles C Thomas, Publisher, Springfield, Ill.)

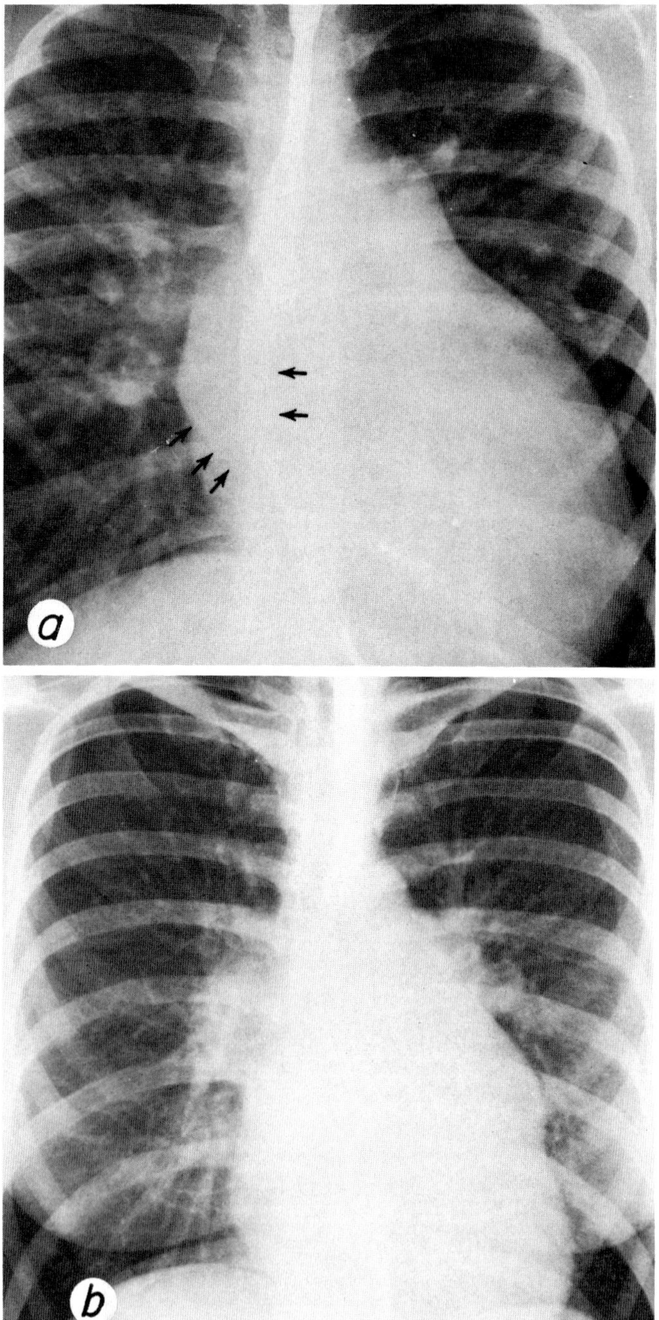
a
b

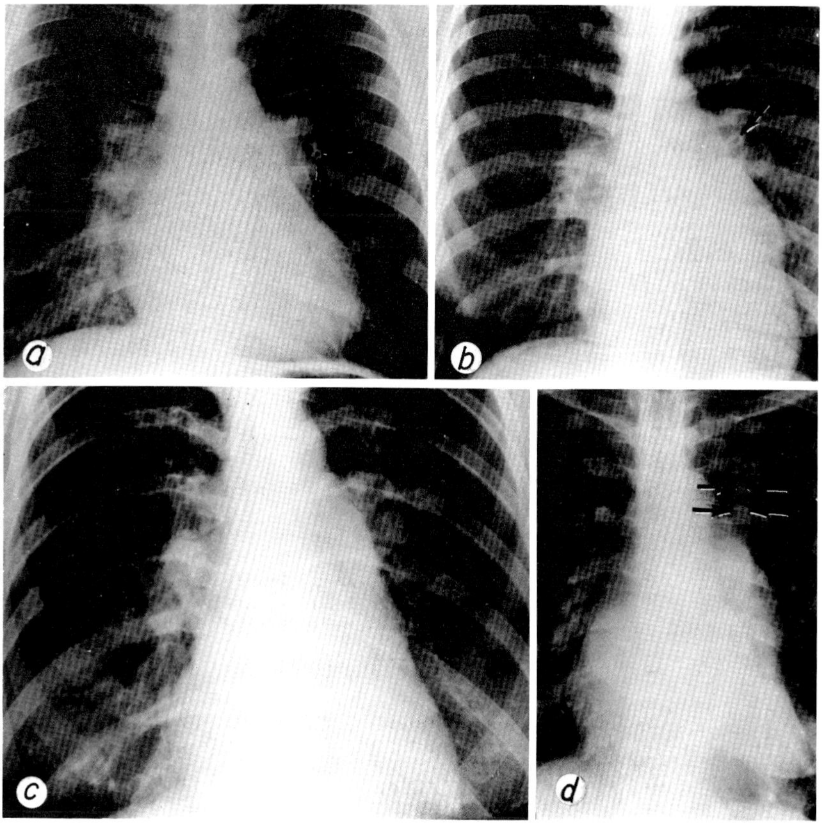

Figure 93. Pulmonary venous obstruction. PA views in four cases of mitral stenosis. (a) Arrows indicate a cuff of edema around a bronchus in the left hilum. (b) Arrow indicates a poorly defined bronchus with a large cuff of edema. (c) Note ill-defined hila and prominent upper lobe vessel. (d) Arrows outline an enlarged discrete left upper lobe pulmonary vein. (From Elliott, L. P., and Schiebler, G. L. 1968. X-Ray Diagnosis of Congenital Cardiac Disease. Courtesy of Charles C Thomas, Publisher, Springfield, Ill.)

structures are smaller than normal, and often inapparent in the lateral view. In addition, the pulmonic trunk is not seen.

Decreased Pulmonary Vascularity A decrease in the prominence of the hilar and intrapulmonary vessels is always associated with severe obstruction at or just below the pulmonic valve in conjunction with an intracardiac defect, allowing a right-to-left shunt at either the atrial or ventricular level

---

Figure 92. Two roentgenographic types of prominent pulmonary vascularity. (a) Secondary to a large left-to-right shunt. Arrows indicate a rightward displacement of the barium-filled esophagus, and the enlarged left atrial shadow within that of the right atrium (double contour). (b) Secondary to pulmonary venous hypertension in a case of mitral valve stenosis. (From Elliott, L. P., and Schiebler, G. L. 1968. X-Ray Diagnosis of Congenital Cardiac Disease. Courtesy of Charles C Thomas, Publisher, Springfield, Ill.)

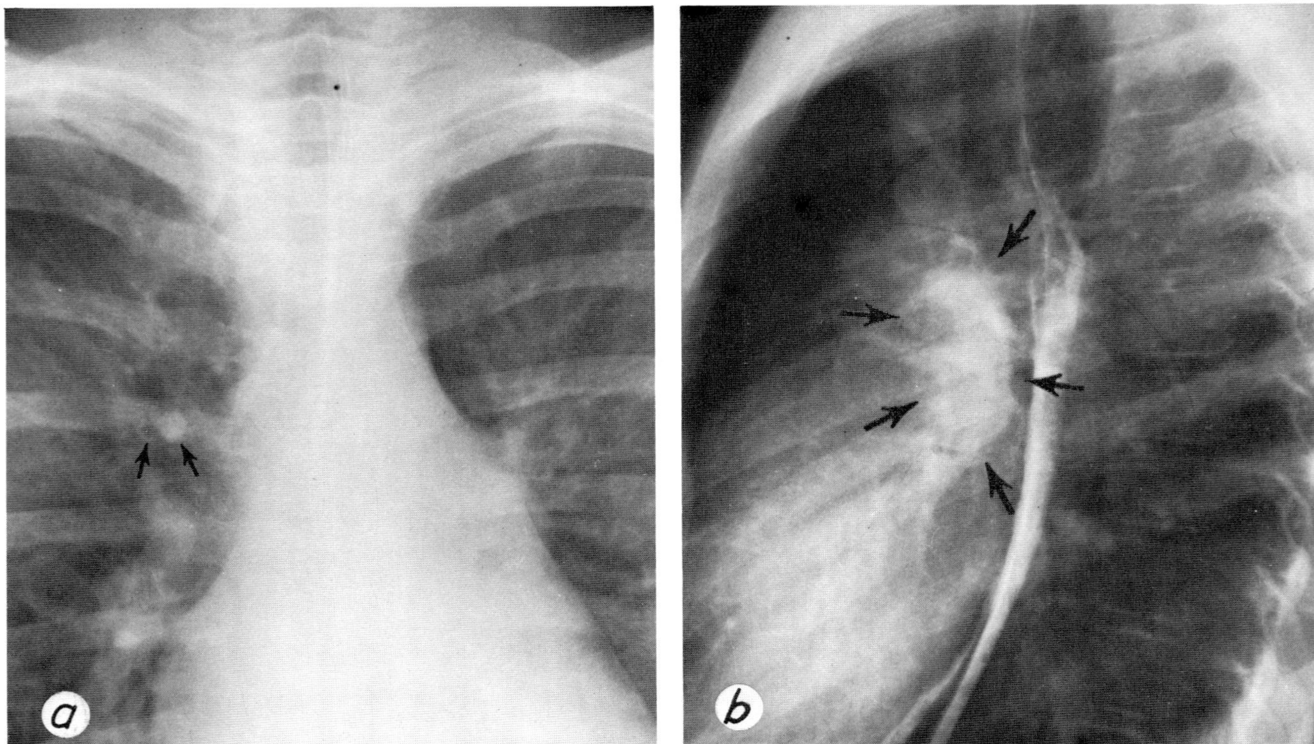

Figure 94. Prominent pulmonary vasculature of the left-to-right shunt type. (a) Close-up view showing the discrepancy between the bronchus (seen on end) and its larger companion pulmonary artery. (b) Prominent pulmonary vascularity, as seen in the lateral view. The hila, outlined by the arrows, appear enlarged and usually dense. (From Elliott, L. P., and Schiebler, G. L. 1968. X-Ray Diagnosis of Congenital Cardiac Disease. Courtesy of Charles C Thomas, Publisher, Springfield, Ill.)

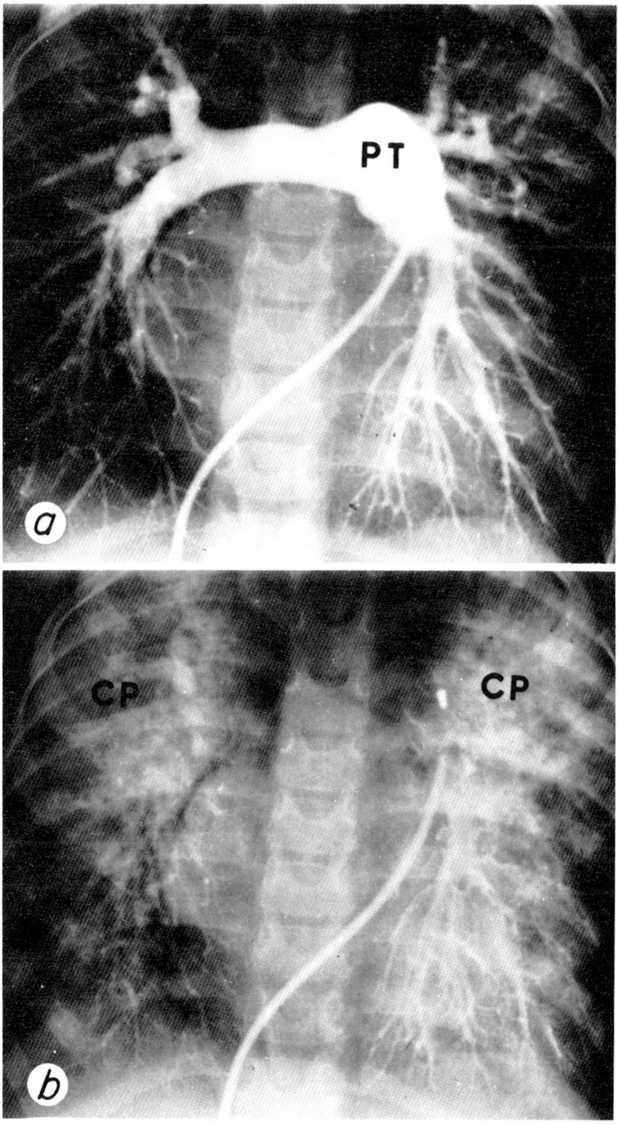

Figure 95. Pulmonary arteriographic findings in pulmonary venous obstruction. (a) Pulmonary arteries show dilatation and tortuosity of the upper lobe pulmonary arteries, whereas the lower lobe pulmonary arteries are relatively small. The flow through the upper lobe arteries is faster than through the lower lobe arteries. (b) This latter phenomenon is demonstrated best by the fact that the contrast media fills the upper lobe capillaries ("blush" appearance of the capillary phase, CP), sooner than the lower lobe capillaries. The pulmonary arteries in the lower lobes retain the contrast media longer and fail to show a capillary phase. These findings were noted in a case of endocardial fibroelastosis with left ventricular failure. Key: PT = pulmonary trunk. (From Elliott, L. P., and Schiebler, G. L. 1968. X-Ray Diagnosis of Congenital Cardiac Disease. Courtesy of Charles C Thomas, Publisher, Springfield, Ill.)

Table 12. Radiologic diagnosis of left-to-right shunt lesions[a]

Pulmonary vasculature	Left atrium	Aorta	Diagnosis
+	0	0	Shunt at atrial level
+	+	0	Shunt at ventricular level
+	+	+	Shunt at aortic level

[a] Key: 0 = normal size; + = enlarged or increased.

(Figure 95). In this situation, the hilar and the intrapulmonary vessels appear small, and the hilar vessels are less dense than normal. Both of these aspects are best appreciated in the lateral view.

Radiologic Diagnosis of Left-to-Right Shunts In patients with left-to-right shunts, one should first decide whether the shunt is at the atrial, ventricular, or great vessel level. Regardless of the site of the left-to-right shunt, there is an increase in pulmonary blood flow. Therefore, in all such shunts (provided that the pulmonary veins connect normally) there is an increased volume of blood entering the left atrium.

When the left-to-right shunt is at the atrial level, the left atrium discharges the excess blood into the right atrium. There is no enlargement of the left atrium, but the right atrium enlarges in response to the extra blood shunted into it.

In the case of shunts distal to the AV valves, the left atrium enlarges. Throughout ventricular systole (the period of maximal atrial volume), the left atrium contains excess blood entering from the overloaded pulmonary circulation. The left atrium must enlarge, since no septal defect is present to prevent the increased left atrial volume.

When the shunt is distal to the aortic valve (e.g., in patent ductus arteriosus), the ascending aorta enlarges to carry the excess blood flow. Table 12 schematizes these concepts.

BIBLIOGRAPHY

Elliott, L. P., and Schiebler, G. L. 1965. X-Ray diagnosis of congenital cardiac disease. Postgrad. Med. 37:A-87.

Elliott, L. P., and Schiebler, G. L. 1968. X-Ray Diagnosis of Congenital Cardiac Disease. Charles C Thomas Publisher, Springfield, Ill.

chapter 10

CARDIAC CATHETERIZATION: What, Who, and Why

HISTORICAL NOTES

The first measures of cardiovascular hemodynamics were by Rev. Steven Hales, who ascertained the pressures in the arteries and veins of conscious horses in 1733. By 1856, Chaveaux and Marey had designed and built a variety of special double lumen catheters, appropriate pressure transducers, and recording equipment. They measured pressures simultaneously in two chambers of the equine heart in order to determine the origins of cardiac sounds. We still use essentially the same type of catheter as that invented by Professor Marey. Although some advances have been made in the ease of recording pressures, current techniques are essentially those that he first used.

WHAT IS CARDIAC CATHETERIZATION?

Cardiac catheterization is a procedure in which one or more catheters are threaded into arteries and/or veins and then passed into the cardiac chambers and great vessels. The catheters themselves are made of finely woven dacron or a variety of extruded polyvinyl and polyethylene plastics. The catheters range in length from 50–150 cm and in external diameter from 1–4 mm. (The French size is three times this outside diameter; thus, a 6-F catheter is 2 mm O.D.)

Catheters come in a variety of shapes and have many special purposes. Some are designed primarily for measuring pulmonary artery wedge pressures, some for measuring pressures across a valve, and still others for angiocardiography. In addition, there are catheters that are preshaped for entering the renal arteries or coronary arteries, as well as catheters with special instruments at their tips for measuring intravascular pressure or sound, oxygen saturations, intracardiac or intravascular flow, or intracardiac electrograms.

How Cardiovascular Information Is Obtained

As the catheter progresses toward the heart, the pressure wave is transmitted along the fluid that fills it to a sensitive device that changes this mechanical energy in the catheter to electrical energy that can be recorded remotely (hence the name pressure transducer). These fluid-filled catheters are subject to a variety of artifacts, and if details of the pressure wave need to be recorded (e.g., the rate of change of pressure, *dp/dt*) manometer-tip catheters are preferred. Such catheters have tiny pressure transducers mounted at the tip and have sufficient fidelity to record not only pressures but also intravascular sounds. Their main drawbacks are expense and lack of variety of special shapes to enable easy placement in cardiac chambers.

Although Fick described the principle for measuring cardiac output in 1870, techniques for measuring oxygen saturation in the blood were not readily available until the development of the Van Slyke method in 1917 and of practical oximeters by Earl Wood in the late 1940s. These methods take advantage of the fact that the amount of oxygen contained in the blood on the right side of the heart and in that on the left side of the heart normally vary within rather small limits. Variations that exceed these normal limits are useful in diagnosing and quantifying intracardiac or intravascular shunting.

Another major method is that of indicator-dilution techniques, in which movement of the blood is tagged by rapid injection of an indicator into the blood at a specific location and sampling of the dye-blood mixture at another location. If the indicator is well mixed with blood and the subject's cardiovascular system shows no major shifts in flow patterns during the time of recording the curve, then these curves may be used to quantify flows and localize shunts in the subject.

Advantage may also be taken of special cardiac catheters to record intracardiac electrocardiograms. In recent years there has been a great deal of interest in recording the potentials from the bundle of His, as well as from the right and left bundle branches. These have proven to be useful in rationalizing the therapy of various arrhythmias.

New Information-Gathering Techniques

There are two areas where large-scale improvement may be expected—the estimation of left ventricular function and the development of noninvasive procedures, i.e., those that do not entail insertion of catheters into arteries or veins. The assessment of left ventricular function is complex because we need to quantify not only measures of contraction but also measures of relaxation. For example, in ischemic heart disease one may see localized areas of the left ventricle that do not move normally. An excellent discussion of the various noninvasive techniques involved in assessing left ventricular function may be found in Mason's article (see bibliography).

Noninvasive techniques include measurement of pulse wave velocity or systolic time intervals, analysis of carotid pulse tracings, etc., and are discussed by Meyer and Kaplan. The most promising of these techniques seems to be sonic reflectometry, or echocardiography (see Chapter 11). In this technique a narrow beam of high frequency sound waves (in the 1–15 mHz range) is passed through the skin and reflected in varying degrees by the body tissues. The amount of reflection depends on the differences in sonic properties at each interface. With this technique it is possible to measure the size of cardiac structures, follow the motion of the mitral valve, locate the mitral-aortic valve junction, calculate ventricular volumes, etc. Some of the more promising experimental machines rival the angiocardiogram in clarity of detail, without the hazards of radiation, catheterization, and injection of contrast media.

WHO SHOULD BE CATHETERIZED AND WHY?

Cardiac catheterization is useful in:

1. *Establishing the diagnosis,* particularly in complex cyanotic congenital heart disease.
2. *Hemodynamic evaluation,* i.e., quantifying the effect of the anomaly or lesion on the cardiovascular system.
3. Detailed *anatomic mapping;* this is primarily the purpose of angiocardiography.
4. Assessment of the results of *cardiac surgery.*

Cardiac catheterization solely for diagnostic purposes is rarely necessary except in patients with complex cyanotic heart disease, e.g., dextroversion with transposed great vessels. In most instances, an experienced cardiologist should be able to decide what the patient has and is therefore more concerned with the evaluation of the extent of the hemodynamic derangement or the exact anatomy.

The question of hemodynamic evaluation may arise in a child with a ventricular septal defect and high pulmonary pressures, when the decision on surgery depends on pulmonary resistance. Another common problem is assessing the severity and deciding the timing of surgery in a patient with aortic insufficiency. Our clinical guides to the severity of aortic stenosis are only fair and cardiac catheterization is usually needed to assess the need for and timing of cardiac surgery.

Similarly, the clinical diagnosis of tetralogy of Fallot is relatively easy to arrive at, particularly after the age of 4. (By then, three out of four patients with cyanotic heart disease will have tetralogy of Fallot.) For open heart repair, it is highly desirable to know the size of the pulmonic valve annulus so that the surgeon may be prepared to replace the pulmonic valve with a homograft if this seems desirable. Furthermore, a major branch of the right coronary artery crosses the outflow tract of the right ventricle in about 10% of cases, and the surgeon may then have to place his incision in other than the usual location. Still another example is the diagnosis of fixed fibromuscular subvalvar aortic stenosis, in which the length of the stenotic area may vary from a thin membrane located immediately below the valve to a long tunnel. Experience has shown that difficulty with surgery and the results thereof vary with the length of the affected area.

Following open heart surgery, the electrocardiogram is commonly altered by the presence of complete right bundle block, chest x-rays show either the effects of the surgery or a very slow regression of the abnormal findings, and there are often transient but confusing murmurs as the hemodynamic load changes. In many cases the total absence of a murmur and the return of all the laboratory findings to normal clearly indicate success of the surgery. However, in a substantial number of cases one or more findings are abnormal. We believe that most patients should be restudied to assess the extent of the return of the patient to normal, both for prognostic value and for guiding further management decisions.

WHEN SHOULD A PATIENT BE CATHETERIZED?

Since each cardiac catheterization should be designed to answer a clinical question, the selection of patients, as well as the timing, is based on the urgency of the need for a clinical answer. The basic question should be, "Will the type of detailed intracardiac and great vessel investigation possible by cardiac catheterization and angiocardiography aid in the management of this patient?" This is obviously an area that is impossible to discuss in a few sentences. Indeed, not all cardiologists will agree as to the need for cardiac catheterization in particular cases, and this philosophy will differ from center to center.

It should be abundantly clear by now that there is no such thing as a routine cardiac catheterization. Each catheterization must be specifically designed to answer the particular clinical questions involved. It is highly desirable to investigate as many areas of the cardiovascular system in as systematic a fashion as possible in order to detect findings not suspected clinically. While it is always preferable to do a "complete catheterization," the condition of the patient, as well as the nature of the clinical question being asked, may dictate that the procedure be shortened. A good plan is to first look for answers to vital clinical questions before going on to investigate other aspects of the cardiovascular system.

There are two special categories of patients that need to be discussed: the critically ill patient and the patient with trivial heart disease. It is our general philosophy not to reject patients who are critically ill if the differential diagnosis includes *a lesion that is operable* or if the data from the catheterization are vital to the *immediate management* of the patient. This means accepting some catheterization-related mortality, but we are convinced that this yields a better long-term salvage rate.

Patients with unusual innocent murmurs or trivial heart disease sometimes get mislabeled and the parents or patients are frightened into believing that there is serious heart disease present. Cardiac catheterizations are often helpful to "delabel" such patients. Telling the parents to "go home and forget about it" may not work if the child has been carrying a label of serious congenital heart disease for several years. Verbal reassurance that the patient does not have significant heart disease may not be as valuable as catheterizing the heart. In a number of instances we have had to catheterize adolescents who were interested in competitive sports when the team physician had refused to allow them to participate because of a murmur. Catheterization was used to prove that there were no significant abnormalities and to allow them to participate. While physicians should be reluctant to subject a patient to such a long, tedious, and expensive procedure, sometimes this may be the simplest way to prevent cardiac "cripples."

BIBLIOGRAPHY

Mason, D. T. 1972. In Yu N. Goodwin (ed.), Progress in Cardiology, Vol. I. Lea and Febiger, Philadelphia.

Meyer, R. A., and Kaplan, S. 1973. Non-invasive techniques in pediatric cardiovascular disease. In W. F. Friedman, M. Lesch, and E. H. Sonnenblick (eds.), Neonatal Heart Disease, pp. 235–261. Grune and Stratton, Publishers, New York.

chapter **11**

ECHOCARDIOGRAPHY

One of the most exciting diagnostic advances in cardiology has been the application of ultrasound. The principle of sonic reflectometry, to give its formal designation, is that sound is reflected at interfaces where the acoustical properties of the materials change. This is in marked contrast to roentgen rays, where the degree of radiopacity is determined primarily by the amount of water and mineral in the tissues. Since the cardiac muscle and the blood in the chambers are both composed largely of water, there can be no distinction between them on the chest x-ray. In contrast, sound waves are reflected at each boundary between blood and solid structures, such as the endocardium or cardiac valves.

Figure 96 shows a schematic of the application of a transducer for detecting these interfaces. The transducer has a piezoelectric crystal that is excited electrically so that it emits high frequency sounds, generally in the range of 1 to 30 MHz. The transducer can be designed to produce a well-collimated narrow beam or a cone-shaped wedge, depending on the particular application. In most systems the transducer is excited for a very brief time interval and then serves as the receiving element for over 99% of the time. The sound wave beam passes through the skin and the underlying tissue relatively unchanged until it reaches the first acoustical interface. Here a portion of the beam is reflected back toward the transducer and the remainder is passed through into the next layer of tissue. If the interface is bone or metal, virtually all of the sound energy is reflected back toward the transducer and little or none passes to the next layer. Air also causes a similar scattering of ultrasonic waves and nearly total reflection.

Since the speed of sound in water is known to be approximately 5 km/sec, it is possible to convert the time interval between reflections into distances. A word of caution may be inserted here—the speed of sound in water varies with temperature and with mineral impurities. Since the principle of sonic reflectometry is based on differences in acoustical reflection properties, it seems unlikely that the speed of sound in blood and in muscle will be exactly the same. Hence this assumption underlying diagnostic ultrasound leads to small, and as yet unknown, errors in measurements. A larger source

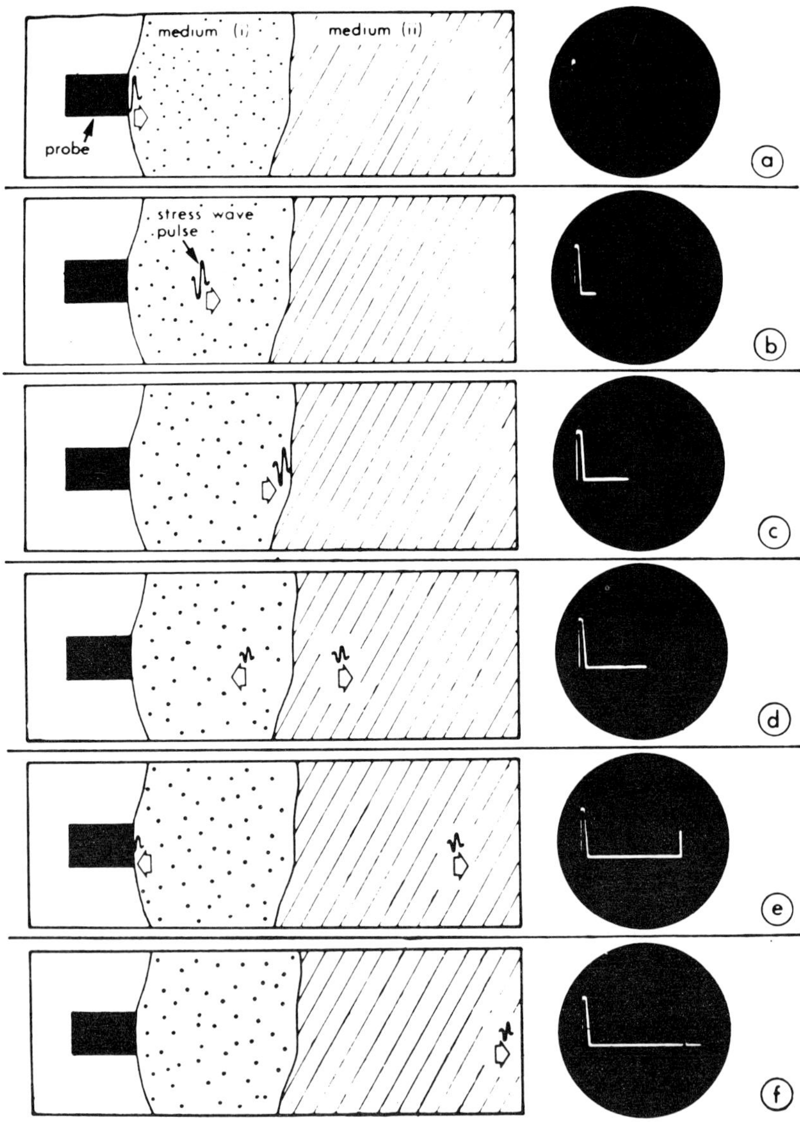

Figure 96. Basic principles of the pulse-echo system. The transducer probe sends a short burst of high-frequency sound waves into the first medium (i). When the boundary at the next sonically different medium (ii) is reached, a portion of the wave is reflected back toward the probe while the remainder continues to travel through medium ii.

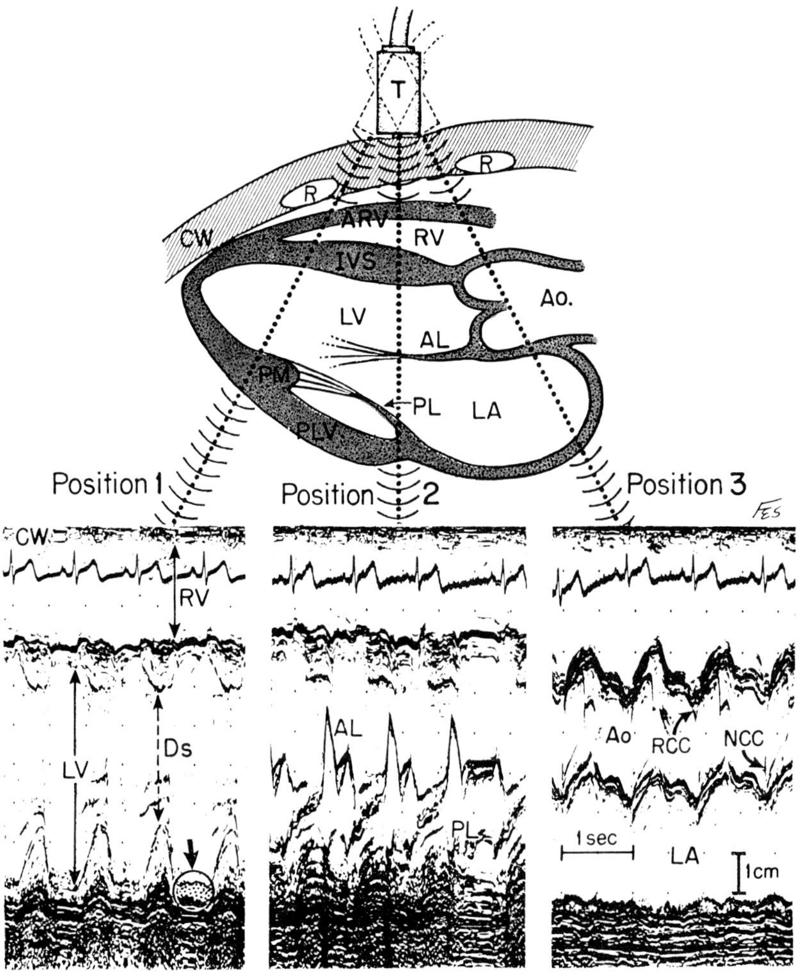

Figure 97. Schematic diagram through the longitudinal axis of the heart and the various pathways traversed by the ultrasonic beam. The corresponding one-dimensional echocardiographic pictures at the three different positions are actual recordings. Conventionally, motions toward the anteriorly placed transducer inscribe a positive deflection, while motions away from the transducer inscribe negative deflections. The single-headed arrow in position 1 points to the posterior left ventricular myocardial thickness (stippled area) bordered by the thin endocardium anteriorly, and the heavy black pericardial lung interface posteriorly. LV represents end-diastolic dimensions, and Ds represents the end-systolic dimensions. Position 2 illustrates the right ventricular borders anterior to the mitral leaflets, which are in the pathway of the beam. Horizontal time and vertical amplitude scales are drawn at the bottom of position 3. [Reproduced from Naggar, C. Z. 1977. Echocardiography: Its value to the clinician. Resident Staff Physician (July):95–111.]

of error is that the reflections are rarely as sharp as indicated on the schema of Figure 96. In general each surface reflects one major echo and two or more weaker echos on either side of the major echo. Fortunately, varying the controls available on the ultrasonic equipment allows one to suppress most of these secondary echos and to increase the degree of clarity and the distinctness of the desired echo.

In its usual application in cardiology, the technique is referred to as echocardiography. Figure 97 shows a cross-section of the heart and the application of a transducer in three common positions. Since the beam is narrow, it is necessary to move the transducer in order to examine all of the structures of interest.

It is far beyond the intent or scope of this chapter to discuss all the current applications of echocardiography. However, a few illustrations can point out some of the distinct advantages of the procedure. Figure 98 shows an echocardiogram of a normal aortic valve and a bicuspid aortic valve. Bicuspid valves demonstrate such eccentric shadows about 80% of the time. Echocardiography is also the diagnostic technique of choice for detecting asymmetrical septal hypertrophy (see Chapter 26). Figure 99 illustrates a typical echocardiogram in such a patient, whose interventricular septum is much thicker than the left ventricular free wall. A large ventricular septal defect often will show that the aortic root arises over the plane of the interventricular

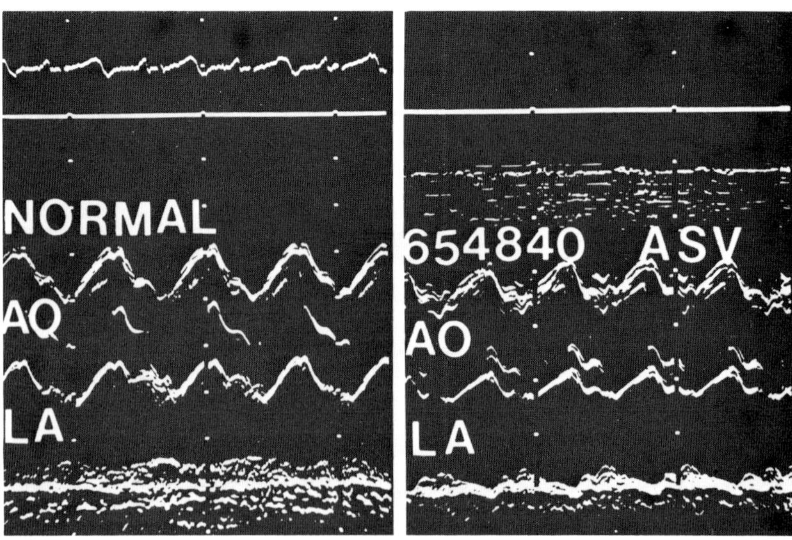

Figure 98. Echocardiogram of a normal heart through the region of the aortic root (left-hand panel), with a white line representing the aortic valve, which is located equidistant from the anterior and posterior aortic walls. On the right side the aortic valve is clearly closer to one wall (in this case the posterior), a finding commonly seen in bicuspid aortic valves.

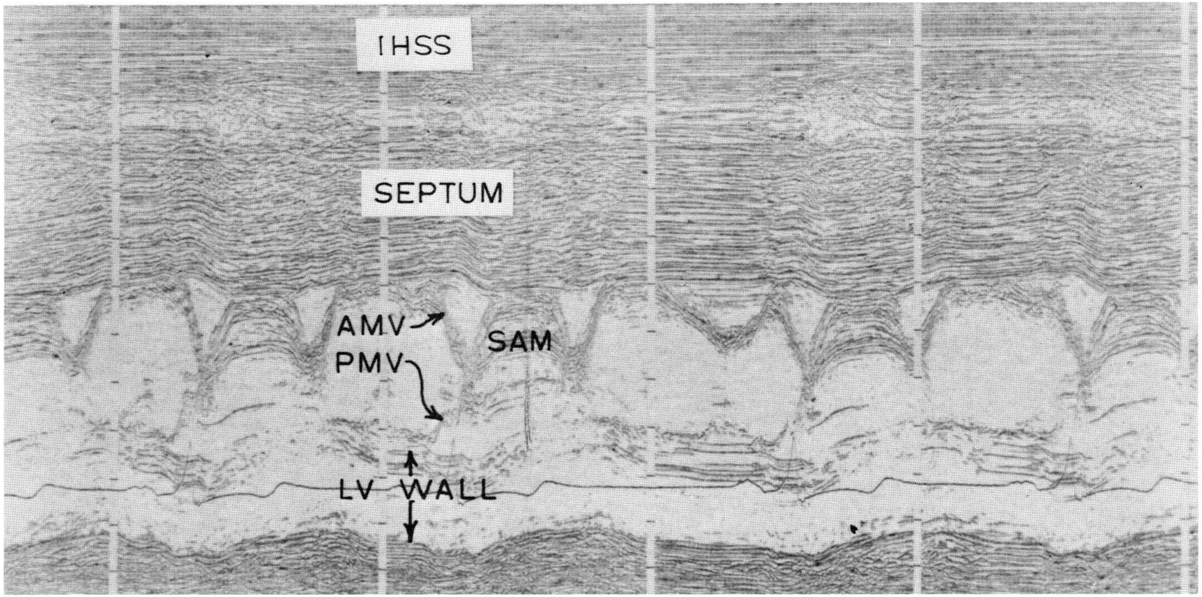

Figure 99. Asymmetrical septal hypertrophy is clearly demonstrated by the disproportionate thickening of the septum when compared to the free wall of the left ventricle. In contrast to the normal, the mitral valve moves anteriorly during ventricular systole; this is called systolic anterior motion and labeled SAM in the figure.

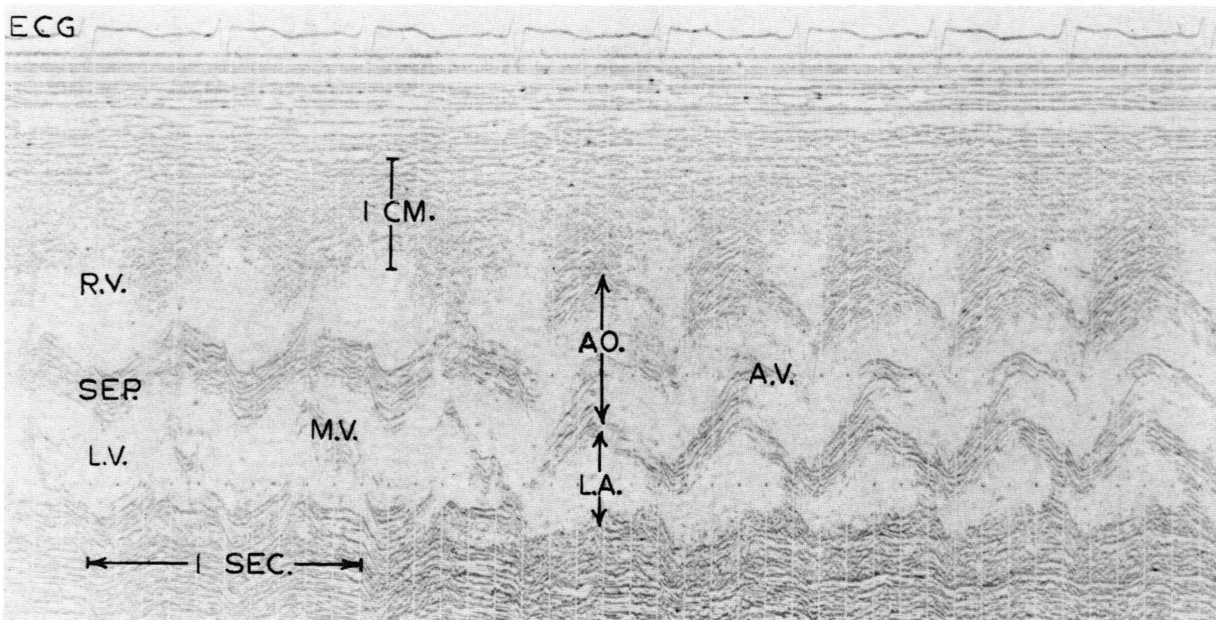

Figure 100. In a large ventricular septal defect, the aortic root (AO) may override the plane of the interventricular septum (SEP). Normally the anterior wall of the aortic root is continuous with the septum.

septum (Figure 100). This is due to the fact that there is free communication between the ventricles and the atria. Echocardiography is also now the preferred way of detecting pericardial effusion (see Figure 227). Another diagnosis that may be made relatively easily using echocardiography is prolapse of the mitral valve leaflets (see Figure 205).

SAFETY

In the amounts used in diagnostic echocardiography, the acoustical energy employed is less than 0.1% of the level at which biological damage has been detected. In contrast to x-ray or nuclear imaging, echocardiography appears to be completely safe. Thus repeated applications are possible without hazard to the patient. Furthermore, in many instances the diagnostic information obtained is superior to that obtainable from radiographic techniques.

FUTURE APPLICATIONS

The standard type of echocardiogram is motion-mode, or M-mode. All the illustrations in this chapter so far have been in this mode. Other exciting possibilities include employing an array of transducer crystals to obtain a picture more nearly resembling an angiocardiogram, and using a single transducer in a holder that allows it to be mechanically rotated rapidly through

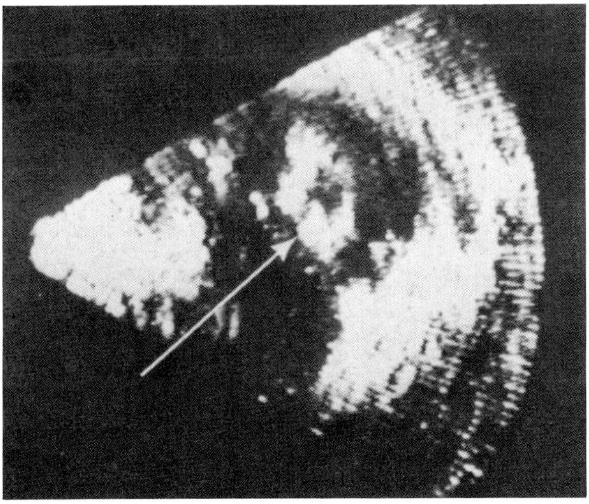

Figure 101. Scan through the mitral valve orifice in a patient with mitral stenosis. Note the narrowed mitral orifice. The arrow points to the thickened anterior mitral leaflet. (From Kisslo, J., von Ramm, O. T., and Thurstone, F. L. 1976. Cardiac Imaging Using a Phased Array Ultrasound System. Circulation 53:266. By permission of the American Heart Association, Inc.)

angles of up to 60° (sector scanning). Both the multiple crystal and sector scan views are displayed on a television monitor and recorded on a videotape recorder. At present the single still frames produced by these techniques lack the clarity of the M-mode scan (Figure 101). The display obtained by the recording or playback of the videotape is of far better quality.

One drawback to these new units is a cost that is several times higher than that of the conventional echocardiograph. Although these systems would seem to offer a great deal of promise for potential improvement, they are more complex in operation and maintenance than M-mode echocardiography.

Another interesting type of echocardiography has come to be known as contrast echocardiography. This is the injection of a small amount of cardio-green dye or similar liquid into a peripheral vein or, via a cardiac catheter, into a cardiac chamber. The resulting echos show a shower of reflections from tiny air bubbles caused by the injection. This is a useful technique during cardiac catheterization for detecting small shunts or for ascertaining the direction of flow through intracardiac valves.

SOME CAVEATS

The relatively low cost of M-mode echocardiographic units, as well as their safety, would seem to warrant wide-spread application of echocardiography. Indeed the question has been raised as to whether echocardiography will supplant electrocardiography, the chest x-ray, or even angiography. Experience has shown that the echocardiogram requires far more technician time to record than the usual electrocardiogram, and that the level of skill required for recording and interpretation is much higher. For example, it is often necessary for the physician to do the recording in order to know both the exact location and angulation of the transducer at the time that the recording is made.

Even casual perusal of the figures in this chapter suggests that the complexity of interpretation is much greater than that for the electrocardiogram or vectorcardiogram. Furthermore, it is our strong belief that the echocardiogram needs to be integrated into the total clinical picture, in the same way that the ECG, VCG, and x-ray are. Interpretation of the echocardiogram as an isolated laboratory procedure can lead to erroneous diagnoses. This is especially true in infants and young children, where the cardiac anatomy may be atypical. Obviously, ventricular inversion or cardiac malposition makes interpretation of the echocardiogram extremely difficult.

An example of such an error is illustrated in Figure 102. In this small infant a clinical diagnosis of truncus arteriosus was made. The initial echocardiogram showed what appeared to be two separate great vessels. After cardiac catheterization confirmed the clinical diagnosis of persistent truncus arteriosus, the echocardiogram was repeated by the cardiologist. As is evident in the figure, the correct diagnosis *could* be made by echocardiography.

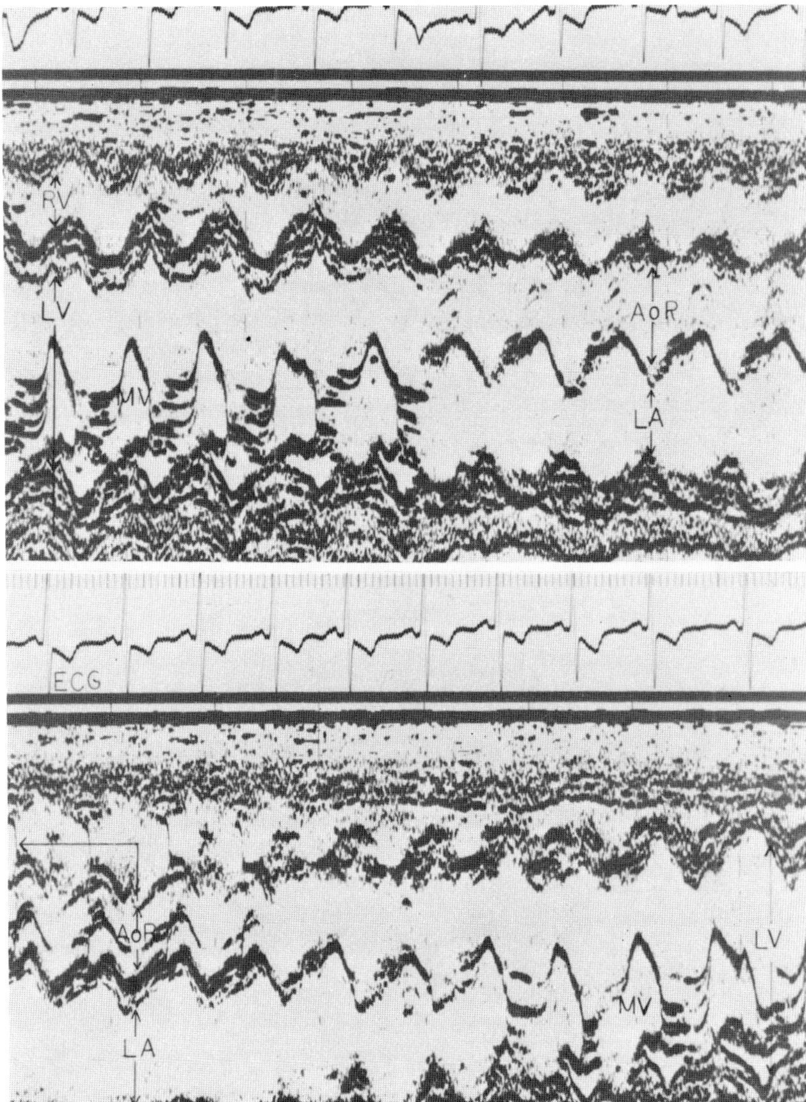

Figure 102. Echocardiogram of an infant with persistent truncus arteriosus, illustrating the difficulty of interpretation. (Top) Initially interpreted as showing a normal aortic root (AoR). Actually the anterior wall of the aorta lies against the chest wall and the echos are continuous with the anterior wall of the right ventricle (RV). (Bottom) Shows a valve leaflet (horizontal arrow) passing through the erroneously labeled anterior wall of the aorta, which is actually the truncal leaflets.

For these reasons we do not think that echocardiography should be considered part of the routine evaluation of children with cardiac problems. Echocardiograms should be obtained to answer specific questions. This technique appears to be most useful as a followup for patients who have been catheterized. In other words, we obtain an echocardiogram at the time of cardiac catheterization and then use subsequent echocardiograms to assess possible hemodynamic changes. Echocardiography is also useful as a check on the electrocardiographic diagnosis of left ventricular hypertrophy, since voltage criteria are so poor for establishing this diagnosis in children. It would appear to be valuable in examining first degree relatives of patients with documented asymmetrical septal hypertrophy. Echocardiography is also useful for following the changes in left atrial size in premature infants who are being treated for patent ductus arteriosus. There appears to be a good correlation between left ventricular pressure, wall thickness, and cavity size in patients with aortic stenosis. Although the echocardiogram is very useful in establishing diagnosis of pericardial effusion, we feel that its use should be reserved for the same institution in which the pericardiocentesis would be accomplished.

In sum, the complexities of interpretation and potential errors, often requiring that a cardiologist do the recording, and the time needed for recording would indicate that echocardiography will not be as widely applied a technique as the electrocardiogram. To maximize the value of the echocardiogram, it should be used in the context of a complete evaluation of the cardiovascular system by a physician skilled in the total assessment of heart disease in infants and children.

BIBLIOGRAPHY

Griffith, J. M., and Henry, W. L. 1974. A Sector Scanner for real time two-dimensional echocardiography. Circulation 49:1147–1152.

Kerber, R. E., Kioschos, J. M., and Lauer, R. M. 1974. Use of an ultrasonic contrast method in the diagnosis of valvular regurgitation and intracardiac shunts. Am. J. Cardiol. 34:722–727.

Sahn, D. J., Terry, R., O'Rourke, R., Leopold, G., and Friedman, W. F. 1974. Multiple crystal cross-sectional echocardiography in the diagnosis of cyanotic congenital heart disease. Circulation 50:230–238.

Solinger, R., Elbl, F., and Minhas, K. 1974. Deductive echocardiographic analysis in infants with congenital heart disease. Circulation 50:1072–1096.

ten Cate, F. J., Kloster, F. E., van Dorp, W. G., Meester, G. T., and Roelandt, J. 1974. Dimensions and volumes of left atrium and ventricle determined by single beam echocardiography. Br. Heart J. 36:737–746.

chapter 12

CONGESTIVE HEART FAILURE

INCIDENCE

Congestive heart failure secondary to congenital heart disease nearly always occurs during the first year of life. Congestive heart failure occurring after 1 year of age may follow cardiac surgery, anemia, infective endocarditis, or a similar complicating condition. An initial bout of failure between the ages of 5 and 15 years from a congenital malformation of the heart is exceedingly rare; congestive heart failure occurring at this time is usually due to an acquired lesion. In adults, long-standing cardiac overwork may result in fibrotic changes in the myocardium and ultimately in congestive heart failure.

MAJOR CAUSES

First Week of Life

The most common congenital malformation of the heart causing early congestive heart failure is the *hypoplastic left heart syndrome* (Chapter 28). In this syndrome, the left ventricle and ascending aorta are markedly hypoplastic, with the mitral and aortic valves severely stenotic or atretic.

Other causes of heart failure in the first week of life are coarctation of the aorta, complete transposition of the great vessels, and endomyocardial diseases, especially that caused by Coxsackie B myocarditis. Marked tricuspid insufficiency associated with pulmonary atresia with intact septum, Ebstein's anomaly, and myocardial dysfunction secondary to severe hypoxemic stress may also cause congestive failure. There are also several extracardiac causes of neonatal congestive heart failure:

1. A *large systemic arteriovenous fistula,* often located in the brain, or a large hemangioma of an organ (e.g., the liver) causes early congestive failure.

2. *Anemia,* especially secondary to hemolytic disease of the newborn (hydrops fetalis), may cause fulminating congestive heart failure. In twins, vascular connections in the placentae may allow transfusion of blood from one twin to the other; thus one will be born with a very low hematocrit.
3. Infants born with very *high hematocrit* (over 70%) from a maternal fetal transfusion or from the twin transfusion syndrome may present in congestive failure.
4. Infants of *diabetic mothers* may be born with grossly dilated hearts and other evidence of heart failure.

Remainder of the First Year

Complete transposition of the great vessels is one of the most common causes of congestive heart failure in the neonatal period. Infants with inadequate mixing of blood because of a small atrial septal defect or patent foramen ovale tend to get into difficulty early. Those cases of transposition that do not develop congestive heart failure until after 3 months of life have large shunts and enormous pulmonary blood flows.

Infants who initially develop congestive heart failure at about 2 or 3 months of life commonly have large pulmonary blood flows secondary to a left-to-right shunt. Since pulmonary vascular resistance is usually elevated for a short time after birth, these babies do not have such large pulmonary blood flows early in life. As pulmonary vascular resistance decreases, pulmonary blood flow increases and congestive heart failure ensues. There is some evidence that premature infants are born with lower pulmonary resistance than term infants; thus, those with left-to-right shunts tend to develop congestive heart failure earlier in life than full-term babies.

Disease-Related Causes

1. Seventy-five percent of *supraventricular tachycardia* occurs prior to four months of age. Tachycardia usually must last at least 24 hr before failure occurs.
2. From ages 1 to 15 years, *rheumatic carditis* is the most common cardiac cause of congestive failure.
3. Heart failure also may complicate acute *glomerulonephritis* in patients in whom severe hypertension, fluid retention, and interstitial pulmonary edema occur. Other more chronic forms of *renal disease* may also cause heart failure.
4. Primary myocardial diseases, such as *infectious myocarditis,* are less common than either rheumatic or renal diseases as causes of congestive heart failure.
5. *Anemia* may precipitate heart failure in a patient with congenital heart disease. Hemoglobin levels less than 6 g/dl may result in cardiac decompensation even in the absence of organic heart disease.

6. *Infective endocarditis* may cause congestive heart failure in a patient with an otherwise benign asymptomatic congenital heart defect. Indeed, if such an individual develops heart failure, either endocarditis or anemia is the most likely diagnostic choice.
7. Congestive heart failure secondary to *cor pulmonale* in childhood is most frequently seen in patients with cystic fibrosis. Surgical shunts from the ventricle of the brain to the right atrium, with chronic embolization to the lungs, may also cause cor pulmonale.

Surgical Causes

Following heart surgery, children who did not have congestive failure may develop it. This occurs most commonly in:

1. Patients who have had large systemic artery-to-pulmonary artery shunts (for example, a Waterston shunt) may develop excessive left ventricular volume overload and thus heart failure.
2. Postoperative patients whose surgery required substantial ventricular muscle resection (for example, repair of tetralogy of Fallot with severe infundibular obstruction), particularly if some residual right ventricular hypertension persists.
3. Surgically induced complete heart block.

DIAGNOSIS

In the first months of life, early recognition of congestive heart failure depends largely on subtle signs. Lethargy or fatigue during feeding, anorexia or vomiting, and failure to gain weight are common symptoms. The neonate may simply be irritable and described as cranky, colicky, or a restless sleeper. Since these symptoms are nonspecific, and indeed could be the harbinger of almost any childhood illness, they are easily overlooked.

There are three major signs of congestive heart failure that are, however, not necessarily all present in every patient. *Tachypnea,* a respiratory rate greater than normal for age, may present as a feeding problem; that is, the infant must stop and rest while feeding, because of the increased respiratory effort. Labored respirations may also be present, although not nearly as often. When seen, such difficulty in breathing suggests a large left-to-right shunt. *Tachycardia* is a valuable sign. A rate higher than that of the normal neonate is nearly universal in cases of congestive heart failure. *Hepatomegaly,* and less commonly splenomegaly, are important indicators of right heart failure. There are several other signs that may also be diagnostic:

1. Periorbital or facial *edema* is seen only with severe congestive failure. Dependent edema, ascites, and anasarca are late manifestations in infancy and usually occur as terminal symptoms. In infancy, these are most frequently seen with endocardial fibroelastosis; in older children, with

acute glomerulonephritis. Only rarely does one see overt pulmonary edema in infancy. Peripheral edema is common in premature infants, reducing its value as a diagnostic sign of heart failure.

2. *Rales* at the bases of the lungs are difficult to categorize, since they may be due to congestive heart failure or to a concomitant pulmonary infection, which is frequently present in these children.
3. In infants with a rapid heart rate, a *gallop rhythm* may be heard because of an accentuated summation sound in which S_3 and S_4 are superimposed on each other because of the shortening of diastole in tachycardia.
4. Extremities may be *cool and clammy,* with a pulse amplitude less than normal, indicating low cardiac output.
5. *Excessive sweating* has been noted in infants having congestive heart failure.
6. Some degree of *cardiomegaly* is present on roentgenographic examination. (Congestive heart failure with a small heart on x-ray can occur with severe pulmonary venous obstruction. Pulmonary venous congestion, with prominent hilar shadows and a fuzzy and indistinct pulmonary vasculature, is seen in this condition.)
7. Increasing *right atrial enlargement* may be noted in serial electrocardiograms.

In the older child and the teen-ager, the signs and symptoms of congestive heart failure are generally similar to those found in the adult.

Some diagnostic tips for specific lesions are:

1. In acute glomerulonephritis with hypertension, one may observe paroxysmal nocturnal dyspnea, a gallop rhythm, an accentuated aortic component of the second sound, and interstitial pulmonary edema with few or no rales. Rarely, these children present in fulminating pulmonary edema, with rales heard over both lung fields.
2. Patients with cyanotic tetralogy of Fallot rarely develop congestive heart failure. A cyanotic infant with congestive heart failure probably does *not* have tetralogy of Fallot, unless there is accompanying anemia, infective endocarditis, a previous operative shunt, or too rapid infusion of intravenous fluids.
3. Overt failure with *excellent pulses* suggests an aortic run-off lesion, particularly patent ductus arteriosus or truncus arteriosus.

THERAPY

Digitalis Therapy

We prefer to use the following dosages, which are slightly lower than recommended by others (Table 13). It is easier to give more digoxin later than to treat digitalis intoxication. Also, inadequate doses for some patients may

Table 13. Dosages of important anticongestive drugs

Drug	Age grouping	Dose	Route of administration
Digoxin (total digitalizing dose)	Premature	0.02 to 0.03 mg/kg	PO,IV
	0–2 years	0.04 to 0.08 mg/kg	PO,IV
	2+ years	0.02 to 0.03 mg/kg with a maximum of 2.5 mg	PO,IV
Digoxin (maintenance)	All	¼ of total digitalizing dose	PO
Ethacrynic Acid (Edecrin)	All	0.5 to 1.0 mg/kg per dose; can be repeated every 12 hr	IV
		10–20 mg/kg/day in three to four doses	PO
Furosemide (Lasix)	All	0.5 to 0.75 mg/kg per dose; repeat as necessary according to response; do not exceed 8 mg/kg/day	IV
		5–10 mg/kg per day in three to four doses	PO
Chlorthiazide (Diuril)	All	20–40 mg/kg/day in two or three divided doses; give intermittently	PO

cause toxicity in others, and an adequate dose in one patient may be inadequate for another.

In *infants and children,* we use digoxin exclusively. For infants, the total digitalizing dose of digoxin is 0.04 to 0.08 mg/kg. This is given in three divided doses, usually one-half initially and then one-quarter in 6 to 8 hr and the last quarter in another 6 to 8 hr. The total digitalizing dose may be given over a shorter time interval for severe failure.

In *premature infants,* with their immature renal function, the digitalizing dose of digoxin should be reduced to 0.02 to 0.03 mg/kg. We use the same dose orally and parenterally, although some authorities feel that the parenteral dose should be only 75% of the oral dose. *In the presence of severe congestive heart failure and edema, the route of administration should be intravenous.* In mild or moderate degrees of congestive heart failure, we prefer the oral route. Recent work has suggested that intramuscular administration should be avoided if possible.

In the *older child,* the total digitalizing dose is 0.02 to 0.03 mg/kg. When the child weighs over 50 kg, one should limit the total digitalizing dose to the adult dose, which is between 2.0 and 2.5 mg of digoxin.

Maintenance dosage is typically 25% of the total digitalizing dose, one-half of which is given every 12 hr. *Each patient is an independent experiment in digitalization, and dosage must be individualized according to patient response.* For best results when using digitalis, remember the following:

1. Have someone else check your dosage calculations.
2. Check the nurse's calculations and preparation.
3. Remember that individual variations are great.
4. Use the lowest effective dose.
5. The primary cause of digitalis intoxication is overdosage.
6. For severe congestive heart failure and edema, use intravenous administration.
7. Reduce dosage for premature infants.

Digitalis Intoxication *Cardiac manifestations,* most important in infants and children, include:

1. Ventricular arrhythmias: premature ventricular contractions; bigeminy, where ventricular complexes occur in pairs, usually one normal beat followed by a beat originating in an abnormal fashion (ectopic beat); or atrioventricular block, ranging from 2:1 to complete.
2. Exaggerated sinus arrhythmia.
3. Supraventricular block: paroxysmal atrial tachycardia with block, or nodal tachycardia.

ST segment changes and inversion of T waves merely show that there is some digitalis in the heart. By themselves, they indicate neither digitalis intoxication nor adequate digitalization.

Digitalis also affects other organ systems. Anorexia in infants or nausea and vomiting in older children may occur. These may be difficult to ascribe to digitalis intoxication in the absence of other findings. Drowsiness, headaches, mental confusion ("digitalis delirium"), and convulsions may occur. Impaired color vision, dilation of the pupils, optic neuritis, and even blindness have been reported. Urticaria, eosinophilia, and gynecomastia have also been reported.

A *low serum potassium* increases the likelihood of digitalis toxicity, even when only a low or average dose of digitalis has been given. This is most commonly due to:

1. Rapid diuresis following digitalization
2. Renal disease
3. Vomiting
4. Reduced dietary intake
5. Steroid therapy
6. Increased adrenal activity

High Ca^{2+} levels are thought by some authorities to increase the sensitivity of the myocardium to digitalis. Excretion of digitalis may be decreased by renal disease, which predisposes to digitalis intoxication.

Treatment of Digitalis Intoxication The primary steps in treatment are:

1. Stop digitalis.
2. Stop diuretics.
3. Monitor the ECG continuously.
4. Treat any arrhythmias that develop.
5. Measure serum electrolytes and administer potassium as necessary to keep potassium at high normal level.
6. Consider exchange transfusion.
7. Monitor serum digoxin levels (these may be useful, but usually cannot be relied on for acute management).
8. Decrease serum calcium (intravenous Versene has been recommended, but there is little experience with its use on children).

Summary of Digitalis Therapy

1. Definitely establish that the drug is needed for treatment of either congestive failure or arrhythmias.
2. Take an electrocardiogram prior to administration of digitalis to differentiate changes due to drug therapy from those due to disease.
3. The oral route is best for initiating digitalization. For patients with severe congestive heart failure, give digitalis intravenously.
4. The keystone in the management of congestive heart failure is administration of one of the digitalis preparations. In infants, if digitalis *alone* does not improve the congestive heart failure, do not expect the adjuncts of oxygen, diuretics, and a low-sodium diet to have any dramatic effect. Fortunately, most congestive heart failure in infancy and childhood can be controlled with digitalis alone.
5. Give the total digitalizing dose as one-half initially, one-fourth after 6 to 8 hr, and the last fourth 6 to 8 hr later. After digitalization is complete, one-eighth of the total digitalizing dose is given twice a day.

6. Take an electrocardiogram prior to the last digitalis dose to check for evidence of digitalis toxicity.
7. Relatively less digoxin is needed for premature infants.
8. In adolescents, the total digitalizing dose for adults (2.0 to 2.5 mg) is usually correct.

Use of Diuretics or Sodium and Water Restriction

A number of potent diuretics have been introduced in recent years and have achieved widespread use for pediatric patients with congestive heart failure. Two of these, furosemide and ethacrynic acid, were initially available only for parenteral use. A pediatric suspension is now available, but these drugs are significantly less effective orally. Both of these agents work by blocking sodium reabsorption in the renal tubules. They are powerful, rapid-acting drugs whose action is not affected by serum chloride concentration, and they are not nephrotoxic. Dosages are outlined in Table 13. The thiazade drugs are also useful, particularly for outpatients. Intermittent therapy (for example, every second or third day) can be used. Oral potassium supplementation is advisable with most diuretics because they increase urinary potassium loss. Aldosterone antagonists, such as spironolactone, retard potassium and hydrogen excretion even in the absence of the adrenals; hyperkalemia may occur with kidney disease or potassium supplementation.

In addition water and sodium intake may be restricted. It is better to maintain an adequate caloric and protein intake and give periodic diuretics than to persist with a low-sodium formula that the child refuses to eat. SMA-26 or Similac PM 60-40 contain approximately one-fourth of the amount of sodium in cow's milk (Table 14). These formulas are palatable to infants, and their use will ensure that caloric intake does not suffer.

Vasodilator Therapy

In recent years several different vasodilator drugs have been used in the treatment of congestive cardiac failure. These drugs have been used on the

Table 14. Sodium content of infant formulas

Preparation	Calories/ounce	Sodium (mEq/liter)
Human breast milk	22	7
Cow's milk	21	22–25
Evaporated milk	20	25–27
Enfamil	20	11
Similac	20	11
Similac PM 60-40	20	6.5
SMA-26	20	6.5
Lonalac	20	1.1

premise that a decrease in systemic arteriolar resistance improves cardiac performance and that this improved performance is accompanied by a reduction in myocardial oxygen demand. Acute congestive failure has been successfully improved by the use of intravenous vasodilator drugs, notably sodium nitroprusside. Oral agents such as nitrates and hydralazine have been of use in the management of chronic congestive heart failure. At the moment, there are little data available concerning the use of these agents in infants and children, with the exception of several articles concerning their use in the treatment of congestive failure following open heart surgery. It is likely, however, that this mode of therapy will become a more important part of the overall therapy of congestive heart failure in the pediatric age range within the next few years.

Other Therapeutic Steps

1. Placing the child in a *head-up position,* or in an isolette that folds in the center, somewhat similar to the cardiac bed of adults, is of great help.
2. *Oxygen with water mist* should be run into an isolette at a rate sufficient to keep the environmental oxygen concentration around 50%. The humidity should not be so high that water covers the inside of the isolette, drips onto the patient, or generally obscures a clear view of him.
3. Mild *sedation* is helpful to reduce restlessness. Morphine in dosage of 0.1 to 0.15 mg/kg is often helpful for severely cyanotic infants.
4. *Bronchopneumonia* coexists so frequently with congestive heart failure in infants and young children that it must always be considered. When present, it should be treated with appropriate antibiotics.
5. When frequent diuretics are needed, *adding potassium to the diet* will prevent hypokalemia. Electrolyte imbalances are not uncommon and serum electrolytes should be obtained at periodic intervals.
6. *Anemia,* particularly a hemoglobin less than 7 g/dl or a hematocrit less than 20%, may aggravate congestive failure. In these cases, packed cell transfusions in small doses may do far more than digitalis.

ETIOLOGIC DIAGNOSIS

In infants, early establishment of an etiologic diagnosis is vital. As soon as the condition of the patient permits, further diagnostic studies should be considered. Obviously, no definite length of time can be stated for early management of congestive heart failure. If there is little or no improvement in the clinical signs of congestive heart failure, diagnostic studies should be undertaken promptly rather than continuing to hope for improvement. This calls for all the art and experience of the physician. Our guideline is that it is better to do a few unrewarding studies than to lose a baby with an operable heart lesion through procrastination.

When the response to anticongestive measures has been less than optimal, the physician should suspect that the cardiac decompensation is not congestive in nature. Patients with coarctation of the aorta, mitral stenosis, or severe pulmonic or aortic stenosis often show only minimal response to medical therapy. The primary problem here is obstruction of blood flow and, although there may be an element of cardiac decompensation present, adequate relief depends on removal of the obstruction. Similarly, anemia must be corrected by transfusion or other therapy.

Pericardial tamponade often mimics congestive heart failure, even to the presence of "cardiomegaly." When a high suspicion exists, pericardiocentesis is indicated. Constrictive pericarditis can often be distinguished by a relatively small heart size that is out of proportion to the degree of ascites and venous distention. If significant pericardial effusion is present, digitalis is contraindicated, since slowing the heart rate may make matters worse. Pulmonary hypertension secondary to chronic lung disease (for example, cystic fibrosis) often shows only minimal improvement with digitalis.

Diseases of the endomyocardium, such as rheumatic myocarditis, viral myocarditis, and severe endocardial fibroelastosis, also often exhibit less than optimal benefit from digitalis. The diseased myocardium is often already contracting to the best of its ability and we are only "flogging a tired horse." Careful and persistent medical management will usually be rewarded by gradual improvement.

BIBLIOGRAPHY

Cohen, S. N., Doyle, E. F., and Rutkowski, M. M. 1973. Drug therapy of heart disease in pediatric patients. Am. Heart J. 86:133–137, 270–275.

Eichna, L. W. 1960. Circulatory congestion and heart failure. Circulation 22:864–886.

Kim, P. W., Krasula, R. W., Soyka, L. F., and Hastreiter, A. R. 1975. Postmortem tissue digoxin concentrations in infants and children. Circulation 52:1128–1131.

Krasula, R., Yanagi, R., Hastreiter, A. R., Levitsky, S., and Soyka, L. F. 1974. Digoxin intoxication in infants and children: Correlation with serum levels. J. Pediatr. 84:265–269.

Smith, T. W., and Haber, E. 1973. Digitalis. N. Engl. J. Med. 289:1010–1015, 1063–1072, 1125–1130.

PART II Congenital Heart Disease

Before turning to the specific cardiac anomalies of Part II, we would like to offer a few words of encouragement. When the field of pediatric cardiology is initially surveyed, one tends to be overwhelmed by the fantastic array of congenital cardiac malformations that are found, both alone and in combinations. Remember that over 85% of all cases of heart disease seen in children fall into ten categories (Table 15). Concentrate on learning the essentials of these lesions and, at least initially, forget the "rare birds."

Table 15. Incidence of the commonest cardiac anomalies in three university hospitals

	Keith (Toronto)	Krovetz (Gainesville)	Krovetz (Baltimore)
Total congenital heart cases	15,104	1,344	3,300
Ventricular septal defect	28%	26%	26%
Pulmonic stenosis, isolated	10%	8%	14%
Tetralogy of Fallot	10%	11%	11%
Patent ductus arteriosus	10%	11%	8%
Atrial septal defect (secundum)	8%	8%	9%
Aortic stenosis (discrete)	7%	5%	6%
Coarctation of the aorta	5%	6%	5%
Endocardial cushion defects	3%	7%	5%
Complete transposition of the great arteries	5%	5%	3%
Total anomalous pulmonary venous connection	1%	1%	1%
Totals	87%	88%	88%

chapter 13

ATRIAL SEPTAL DEFECT: Ostium Secundum

HISTORICAL NOTES

Morgagni, in 1765, was probably the first to record in detail a case of atrial septal defect (ASD). This anomaly then apparently went unmentioned until Louis described a large atrial septal defect in 1826. The first series of cases was reported by Rokitansky in 1875, when he described seven ostium secundum defects in his great work on defects of the cardiac septa.

Although Murray reported a possibly successful attempt to close a suspected atrial septal defect by an extracardiac suture technique in 1948, Bailey, in 1952, and Bjork Crafoord, in 1953, were the first to report large series of operations on atrial septal defects in which successful repairs were accomplished.

INCIDENCE

The relative incidence of atrial septal defects increases with age, because children with other severe defects die. After the second or third decade of life, it is the most commonly discovered cardiac anomaly. Atrial septal defects occur more often in females—as much as three to one over males in some series.

ETIOLOGY

Familial occurrence is not unusual, both in siblings and in multiple generations. Holt-Oram syndrome (ostium secundum atrial septal defect with skeletal malformations, particularly of the thumb and forearm) is transmitted in an autosomal dominant pattern. In other families the inheritance pattern is autosomal recessive. The incidence of congenital heart disease in other members of the family is about twice that in the general population. Neither maternal age nor birth rank seem to be important etiologic factors, and no specific teratogens have been identified.

PATHOLOGY

The most common type of atrial septal defect is the ostium secundum variety. This defect occurs in the region of the fossa ovalis and results from either an excessive size of ostium secundum or a deficiency of septum secundum, or both. Occasionally these defects extend inferiorly, reaching close to the inferior vena cava (Figure 103).

Sinus venosus defects occur in the superior, posterior portion of the atrial septum, closely related to (and sometimes extending into) the superior vena cava. Drainage of one or more of the pulmonary veins, particularly the right pulmonary veins, into the right atrium is nearly always present.

Defects in the inferior portion of septum primum, usually associated with a cleft mitral valve, are in fact a form of endocardial cushion defect, and are discussed in Chapter 14.

Prolapse of the mitral valve, sometimes with mitral insufficiency, frequently accompanies ostium secundum atrial septal defect. This combination is easily confused with ostium primum complex or rheumatic mitral insufficiency.

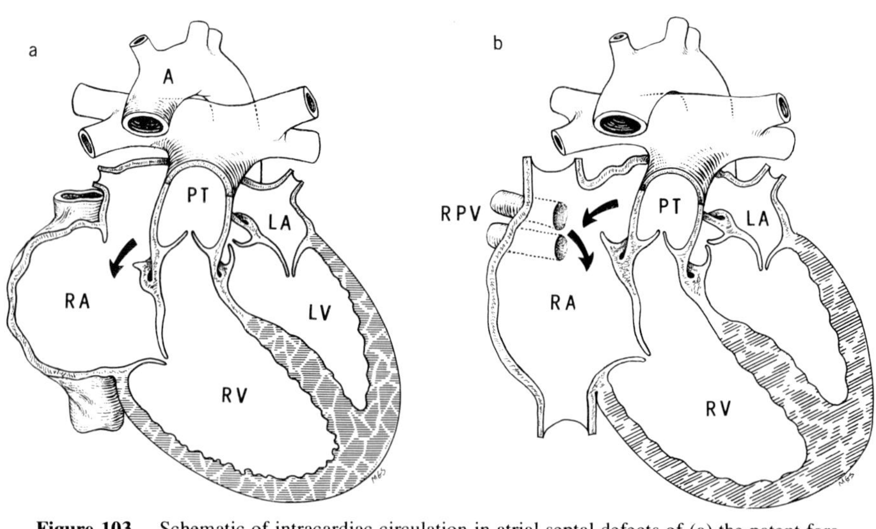

Figure 103. Schematic of intracardiac circulation in atrial septal defects of (a) the patent foramen ovale type and (b) the sinus venosus type with partial anomalous pulmonary venous connection. The arrows in both cases indicate the flow of pulmonary venous (arterialized) blood into the right atrium. (From Elliott, L. P., and Schiebler, G. L. 1968. X-Ray Diagnosis of Congenital Cardiac Disease. Courtesy of Charles C Thomas, Publisher, Springfield, Ill.)

HEMODYNAMICS

A left-to-right shunt in an uncomplicated atrial septal defect probably begins in infancy, but is usually not clinically apparent at that time. This is because the murmurs of atrial septal defect are not impressively loud, and wide splitting of the second sound is not always present in the infant with an atrial septal defect. Perhaps this is just as well, since an asymptomatic ASD in an infant does not require treatment but may nevertheless create parental anxiety.

ASD characteristically produces very large left-to-right shunts, with the pulmonary blood flow commonly being three to four times the systemic flow. The left-to-right shunt results in right heart volume overload, affecting the right atrium, the right ventricle, and the pulmonary arteries. Average left atrial pressure is only slightly higher than right atrial pressure (1 to 4 mm Hg), but this is sufficient to force large amounts of blood through a large defect.

Right ventricular systolic pressure is usually normal or only slightly elevated. Pressure differences of 10 mm Hg or more are common across the pulmonic valve as a result of increased pulmonary flow, and indeed create the usual systolic murmur. Pulmonic valve stenosis should be suspected as an additional anomaly when the pressure difference is larger than can be accounted for by the increased pulmonary blood flow.

Pulmonary vascular resistance is characteristically less than normal. Obstructive pulmonary vascular disease does not occur in the pediatric age range, but can occur in the older individual in whom a large shunt has been present since infancy. Affected adults may develop pulmonic insufficiency because of dilation of the pulmonic annulus, pulmonary vascular disease, or both.

CLINICAL FEATURES

Typically no significant symptoms are noted, even in infancy. Some degree of growth retardation, especially of weight, may occur with large shunts, as well as an increased susceptibility to respiratory infections.

Patients characteristically are acyanotic and have slender builds. Left chest prominence is due to right heart enlargement. A right ventricular lift is palpable, as is a prominent pulmonary artery pulsation. The first sound is normal, but occasionally may be split, with a prominent tricuspid component. There is a pulmonary systolic ejection murmur maximal in the second left intercostal space, transmitted widely over both lung fields. Wide, fixed splitting of the second sound throughout the respiratory cycle is a hallmark of ASD (Figure 104). Confirmation of the diagnosis by auscultation requires identification of an early to mid-diastolic murmur, superficial in quality, located at the lower left sternal border. A result of increased tricuspid valve flow, this murmur may increase with inspiration. Although its intensity is a rough indicator of the size of the left-to-right shunt, at times this murmur is difficult to hear because of its low pitch.

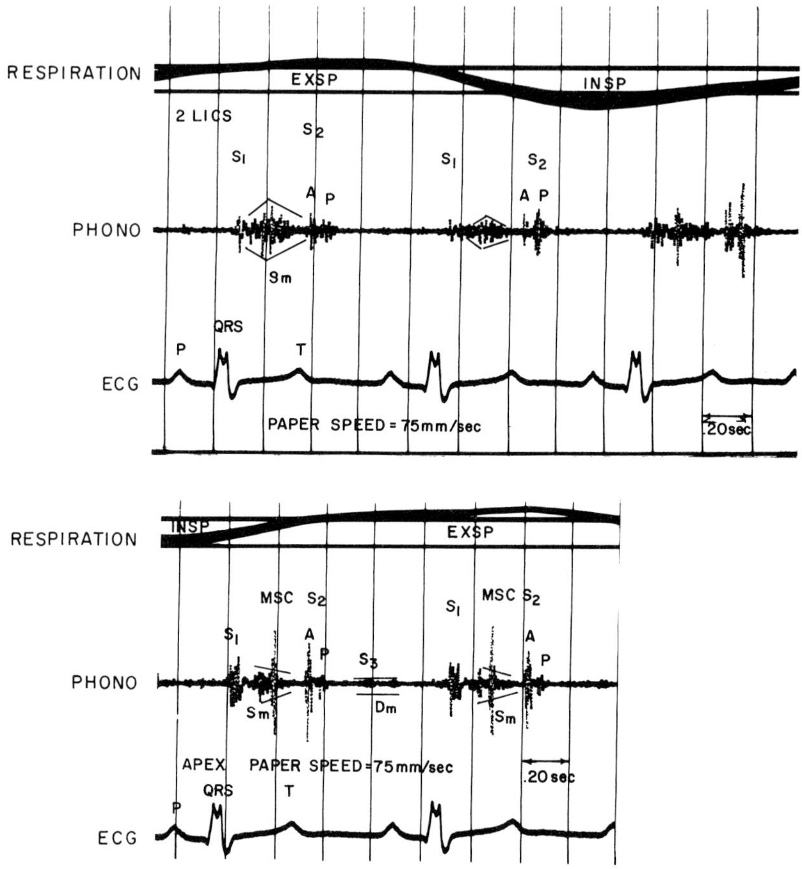

Figure 104. Phonocardiogram of a 12-year-old male with atrial septal defect illustrating the wide, fixed splitting of the second sound. The diastolic murmur at the apex is due to relative tricuspid stenosis.

A systolic thrill at the left base or in the suprasternal notch, with or without a pulmonic ejection click, indicates an abnormal pulmonic valve. An early to midsystolic click at the apex should be carefully sought in patients with ASD because of the frequently associated prolapsing mitral valve. Changes in the patient's body position, exercise, or a Valsalva maneuver can help to identify this sound. Sometimes a late systolic apical murmur of mitral insufficiency may be heard.

ROENTGENOGRAPHIC FEATURES

The most important features are: 1) increased pulmonary arterial blood flow; 2) a normal-sized left atrium; and 3) right ventricular and right atrial enlarge-

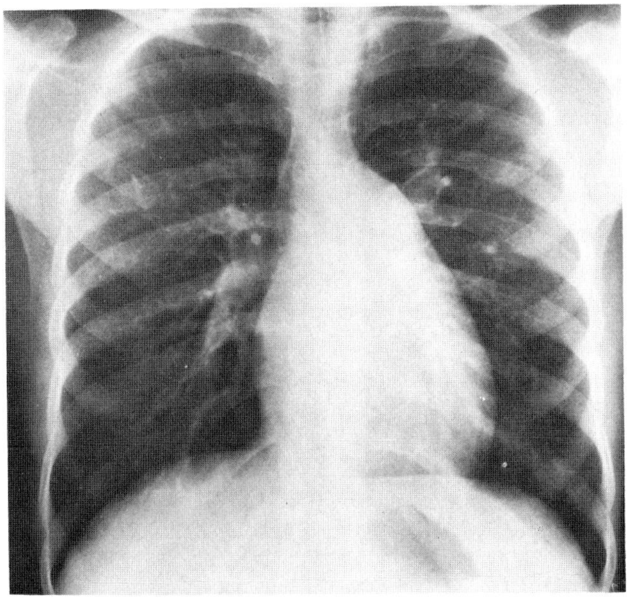

Figure 105. X-ray illustrating the increased pulmonary blood flow and enlargement of the main pulmonary artery in a 13-year-old male with atrial septal defect.

ment. The pulmonary artery is enlarged, but may be difficult to see because of a dilated right ventricular outflow tract. The aorta is normal in size (Figure 105). Careful attention should be paid to the skeleton because scoliosis may suggest the presence of a prolapsing mitral valve. The association of these two findings has been clearly established in the literature.

ELECTROCARDIOGRAPHY

An rsR′ pattern in right precordial leads and right axis deviation are common, and indicate moderately increased pressure and volume overloading in the right ventricle (Figure 106). Right atrial enlargement may be found in 15%–35% of electrocardiograms. The P-R interval is at the upper limits of normal or slightly prolonged for age and rate. Nearly 10% of patients will have left axis deviation rather than the usual right axis deviation, thus mimicking the findings of an endocardial cushion defect (see Chapter 14). In our experience, this finding is frequently associated with a prolapsing mitral valve.

The presence of an rsR′ in the right precordial leads is not due to right ventricular conduction delay or block, but to right ventricular hypertrophy. Evidence of this is that, following repair of an atrial defect, the R′ decreases, which would not occur if the right bundle were defective. Furthermore, as right ventricular pressure increases, the pattern may change to a pure R wave.

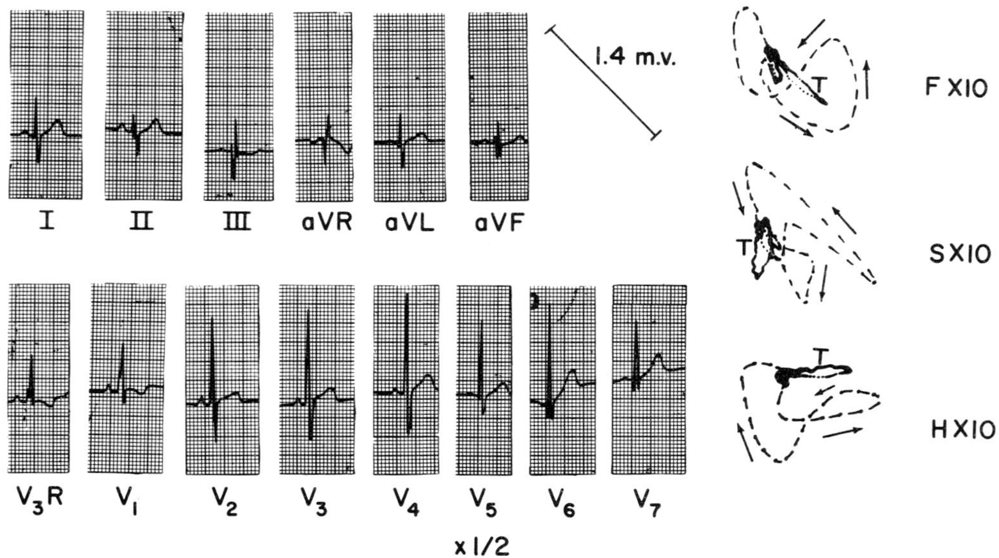

Figure 106. Electrocardiogram and vectorcardiogram of a 6-year-old female with atrial septal defect. An rSR′ or splintered R pattern in lead V_3R or V_1 is very common with this defect.

Finally, significant terminal conduction delay and terminal slowing, such as are seen in true right bundle branch block, are rarely seen in atrial septal defect.

DIFFERENTIAL DIAGNOSIS

Pulmonic stenosis, if mild, may be difficult to differentiate from ASD. The presence of a pulmonic click or a suprasternal notch systolic thrill suggests an abnormal pulmonic valve. In pulmonic stenosis, the second sound is widely split, but the pulmonic component moves with respiration and may be slightly reduced in intensity. A tricuspid flow murmur, the *sine qua non* of auscultatory diagnosis of ASD, is not present in pulmonic stenosis, and in mild cases the ECG may be normal or may show only an anterior shift of the T wave, producing upright T waves in right precordial leads.

Idiopathic dilatation of the pulmonary artery may cause similar findings on chest x-ray, but with its unimpressive auscultation and normal ECG it is easily distinguished from ASD.

Total anomalous pulmonary venous return may mimic ASD in infancy, especially when only minimal cyanosis is present.

Ostium primum ASD will show characteristic ECG findings as well as frequently demonstrating a murmur of mitral insufficiency. Differentiation of an ostium primum ASD from an ostium secundum ASD with a prolapsing mitral valve may be quite difficult on clinical grounds alone. An echocardiogram is sometimes helpful in making this distinction, but left ventricular angiography is usually required.

Partial anomalous pulmonary venous return without an ASD is extraordinarily rare. The only clinical clue is the observation that the second sound, although widely split in both, will vary appropriately with respiration in the presence of isolated partial anomalous pulmonary venous return. Definitive diagnosis usually can be made at cardiac catheterization by means of selective indicator-dilution curves.

Ventricular septal defect is seldom confused with ASD because the murmurs are quite different. Both can occur in the same patient, of course, and in these instances the clinical findings are generally dominated by the ventricular septal defect.

PROGNOSIS

Although a large atrial septal defect may rarely cause unremitting congestive heart failure and death in infancy, medical management will usually carry these patients to an age when open heart surgery can be more easily performed. Those children whose defects are not detected until after infancy rarely develop symptoms before 30 years of age. Even many years ago, in Abbott's series, the mean age of death in atrial septal defects was 40 years. If not surgically corrected, patients with large defects tend to develop increasingly severe symptoms, such as chronic congestive heart failure, dysrhythmias, or the Eisenmenger reaction.

Pulmonary hyper-resistance due to obstructive vascular disease does not occur in childhood or adolescence, but does complicate ASD in the adult. The murmur becomes less intense, the second sound less widely split, and the pulmonic component of the second sound louder. A murmur of pulmonic insufficiency may often be heard. Other suggestive features are severe right ventricular hypertrophy on ECG, a prominent jugular "a" wave, marked cardiomegaly, and congestive heart failure. Cyanosis may occur as a result of either congestive heart failure or a central right-to-left shunt.

Prognosis depends largely on the size of the left-to-right shunt. When it is small (less than 25% of pulmonary blood flow) and the right heart pressures are normal, life expectancy is most likely not affected and surgery is not indicated.

Spontaneous functional anatomical closure rarely occurs. When it does, it is probably related to an initially stretched foramen ovale rather than to closure of a true defect.

MANAGEMENT

Medical management appears to be the order of the day in infancy and childhood. We prefer to postpone surgery until the child reaches an age of 4–6 years. Our group performs open heart surgery in all patients whose left-to-right shunt exceeds 35% of pulmonary flow and in whom pulmonary resistance is less than systemic resistance. However, we recognize that using this size shunt as a dividing line is largely arbitrary.

Surgery usually consists of direct closure of the defect. When the defect is extremely large, a prosthetic patch may be needed. In the presence of anomalous pulmonary venous connection, reconstructive procedures must be performed. This often also requires a prosthetic patch, particularly for the sinus venosus type, when the right pulmonary veins enter the right atrium. Anomalous pulmonary veins are redirected to the left atrium by means of an appropriate diverting patch. In sinus venosus defects, the surgeon should exercise care to avoid damage to the sinoatrial node, a potentially distressing complication.

Operative mortality should essentially be that of thoractomy, anesthesia, and perfusion, i.e., less than 1%. When pulmonary hypertension, chronic congestive heart failure, and elevated right atrial pressure exist, the mortality is appreciably higher. Postoperative catheterization studies on 48 children showed complete closure in 46 and small residual shunts in the other two.

BIBLIOGRAPHY

Anderson, M., Lyngborg, K., Møller, I., and Wennevold, A. 1976. The natural history of small atrial septal defects: Long term follow-up with serial heart catheterizations. Am. Heart J. 92:302–307.

Besterman, E. 1961. Atrial septal defect with pulmonary hypertension. Br. Heart J. 23:587–598.

Evans, J. R., Rowe, R. D., and Keith, J. D. 1961. The clinical diagnosis of atrial septal defect in children. Am. J. Med. 30:345–356.

Hastreiter, A. R., Wennemark, J. R., Miller, R. A., and Paul, M. H. 1962. Secundum atrial septal defects with congestive heart failure during infancy and early childhood. Am. Heart J. 64:467–472.

Lee, Y., and Scherlis, L. 1962. Atrial septal defect. Electrocardiographic, vectorcardiographic and catheterization data. Circulation 25:1024–1041.

chapter 14

DEFECTS OF THE ENDOCARDIAL CUSHIONS

The earliest reference to an endocardial cushion defect is attributed to Méry, in 1700. However, it was not until 1846 that Peacock described the low placement of the atrial septal defect in this anomaly, and its common association with a ventricular septal defect and a cleft in the anterior leaflet of the mitral valve. Rokitansky, in an 1875 report of 10 cases, gave the first clear description of the ostium primum complex, i.e., an ostium primum defect with a cleft mitral valve. Rogers and Edwards, in 1948, pointed out that the ostium primum complex and the complete atrioventricular canal represent different degrees of severity of the same basic anomaly.

The characteristic electrocardiographic pattern of a superiorly oriented counterclockwise QRS vector was documented by Blount and Toscano-Barbosa in 1956. Early reports of surgery using hypothermia and occlusion were accompanied by a very high mortality. Following the introduction of cardiopulmonary bypass, Cooley and Kirklin, in 1956, reported surgical success in nine of 12 patients with endocardial cushion defects.

Among many recent authors who have contributed to understanding of these defects, Gian Rastelli stands out. Completed after Dr. Rastelli's death at age 36, the monograph on atrioventricular canal defects edited by Feldt gained its impetus and much of its substance from Rastelli, and will provide the interested reader with the most lucid and complete presentation of this group of heart defects.

INCIDENCE

Endocardial cushion defects comprise between 2% and 7% of all cases of congenital heart anomalies. There is a high degree of association of the complete form with the Down syndrome, which was seen in nearly one-half of our cases of complete AV canals. Interestingly, partial forms are uncommon in the Down syndrome.

PATHOLOGY

There are potentially three lesions (Figure 107):

1. A defect in the lower part of the atrial septum, called an ostium primum atrial septal defect.
2. A defect in the ventricular septum related primarily to the inflow portion of the right ventricle and both the inflow and outflow portions of the left ventricle.
3. Defects in those portions of the atrioventricular valves related to the atrial and ventricular septa, such as cleft anterior leaflet of the mitral valve, cleft septal leaflet of the tricuspid valve, and common anterior and posterior leaflets.

The classification proposed by Rastelli* has come into wide usage:

I. Incomplete forms (divided atrioventricular valves with no ventricular septal defect)
   A. Ostium primum atrial septal defect with cleft mitral valve
   B. Common atrium with abnormal atrioventricular valve
   C. Isolated cleft of anterior leaflet of mitral valve or septal leaflet of tricuspid valve

II. Complete forms (common anterior leaflet with ventricular septal defect)
   A. Anterior leaflet divided and attached to ventricular septum (Type A)
   B. Anterior leaflet divided and free floating (that is, not attached to ventricular septum) (Type B)
   C. Anterior leaflet undivided and free floating (Type C)

The *incomplete form* consists of an ostium primum atrial septal defect, in the lower portion of the atrial septum, and a cleft anterior leaflet of the mitral valve, with each component of this leaflet triangular in shape and equal in size. There may also be a defect in the septal leaflet of the tricuspid valve, but the ventricular septum is intact (Figure 108). This common pairing of defects, termed the ostium primum complex, accounts for approximately two-thirds of all patients with defects of the atrioventricular canal. The left ventricular outflow tract demonstrates a characteristic "swan's neck" deformity as a result of the displaced atrioventricular orifice. The attachment of the anterior

---

*Modified from Titus and Rastelli. 1976. In R. H. Feldt (ed.), Atrioventricular Canal Defects. W. B. Sanders Company, Philadelphia.

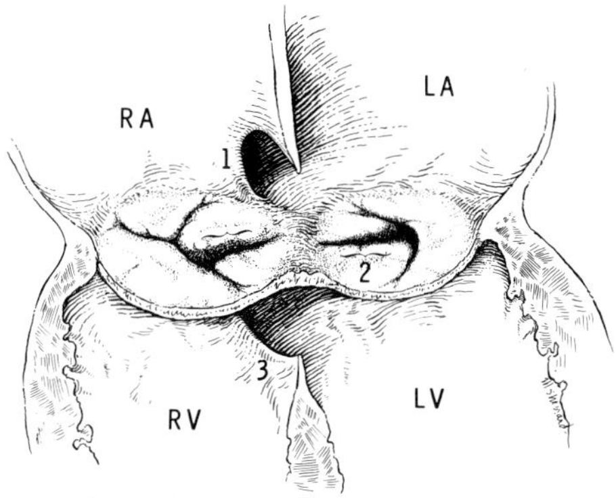

Figure 107. Three defects in the endocardial cushion that are of clinical importance may occur either singly or in combination. These are (1) a low-lying atrial septal defect, the so-called ostium primum, (2) a cleft in the septal leaflet of the mitral valve or the tricuspid valve, and (3) a relatively posterior ventricular septal defect. (From Elliott, L. P., and Schiebler, G. L. 1968. X-Ray Diagnosis of Congenital Cardiac Disease. Courtesy of Charles C Thomas, Publisher, Springfield, Ill.)

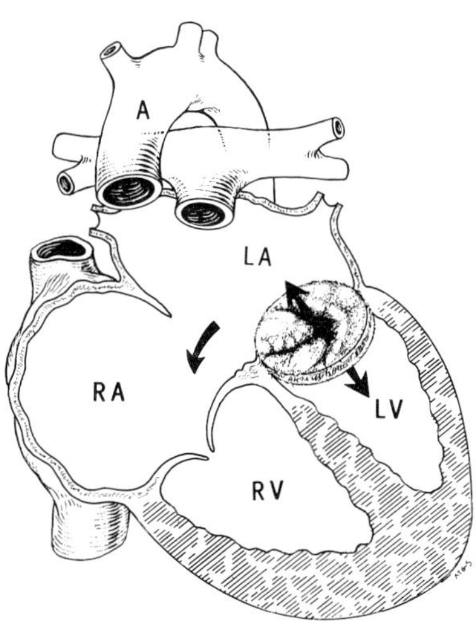

Figure 108. Schematic intracardiac circulation in endocardial cushion defect (ostium primum) with a cleft in the septal leaflet of the mitral valve. When the cleft causes regurgitation of blood from the left ventricle to the left atrium, a portion of this blood enters the right atrium. Thus, there is little or no stimulus for left atrial enlargement in the presence of an atrial septal defect, even in the presence of mitral insufficiency. (From Elliott, L. P., and Schiebler, G. L. 1968. X-Ray Diagnosis of Congenital Cardiac Disease. Courtesy of Charles C Thomas, Publisher, Springfield, Ill.)

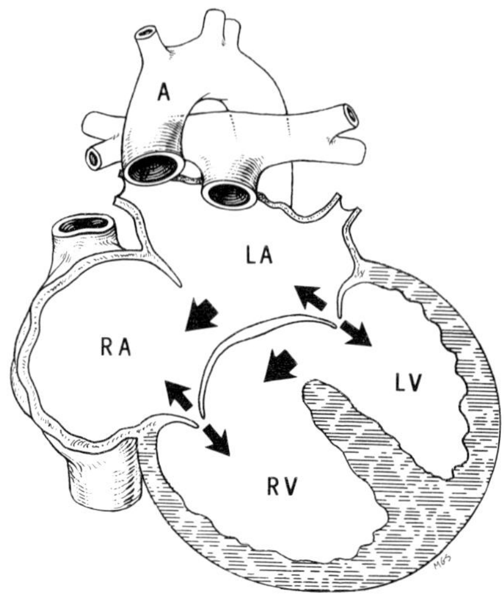

Figure 109. In the complete form of the endocardial cushion defect, all four anomalies are present. This results in a markedly inefficient heart. There is incomplete separation of venous and arterial blood, and both AV valves leak. (From Elliott, L. P., and Schiebler, G. L. 1968. X-Ray Diagnosis of Congenital Cardiac Disease. Courtesy of Charles C Thomas, Publisher, Springfield, Ill.)

leaflet of the mitral valve to the top of the ventricular septum prevents communication between the ventricles.

In the *complete form* of atrioventricular canal, a ventricular septal defect is present and the atrioventricular valve is common to both ventricles (Figure 109). The anterior common leaflet is usually divided, with each portion attached by short chordae to the ventricular septum (Type A). Less commonly, the divided anterior leaflet has no chordae to the ventricular septum, but instead has chordae from each portion going to a right ventricular papillary muscle (Type B). In the most primitive form of atrioventricular canal, fortunately the least common, the anterior leaflet is undivided and free floating (Type C).

INCOMPLETE ATRIOVENTRICULAR CANAL

Clinical Features

The clinical picture depends to a large extent on whether or not the cleft anterior leaflet of the mitral valve allows significant mitral regurgitation. Even though a cleft may be present, there may be little or no regurgitation and the main hemodynamic lesion is a left-to-right shunt at the atrial level. One may find few symptoms until later in life, the incomplete form thus mimicking the clinical picture of a secundum atrial septal defect. If mitral insufficiency is present, the direction of the regurgitant stream often is directly into the right atrium.

Physical findings are similar to those of a simple atrial septal defect (Chapter 13). A prominent right ventricular lift is felt parasternally, and often a pulmonary artery impulse is felt as well. There is rarely a thrill, but a systolic murmur resulting from excess pulmonary blood flow (Figure 110) is heard in the second left intercostal space. Occasionally, the murmur sounds like an innocent pulmonary ejection murmur. With high pulmonary flows, a diastolic murmur resulting from excess flow across the tricuspid valve is heard along the lower left sternal border. The second sound in the pulmonary area is widely split and remains so during the respiratory cycle. The pulmonic component of the second sound may be moderately increased. With severe pulmonary hypertension, it will be loud and banging.

If mitral insufficiency is significant, symptoms may occur early in life, including evidence of congestive heart failure in the infant or easy fatigability and frequent respiratory tract infections in the child. In these patients auscultation will demonstrate the high-frequency crescendo murmur of mitral insufficiency in addition to the systolic and diastolic murmurs resulting from the left-to-right atrial level shunt. This combination of systolic and diastolic murmurs often has a "push-pull" quality. The presence of additional apical diastolic sounds and murmurs depends on the degree of mitral insufficiency.

Roentgenographic Features

Pulmonary vascular markings are increased in proportion to the magnitude of the left-to-right shunt (Figure 111). A small or normal-sized aorta contrasts with a large pulmonary artery. There is no left atrial enlargement, unless there is mitral regurgitation, and the atrial defect is relatively small.

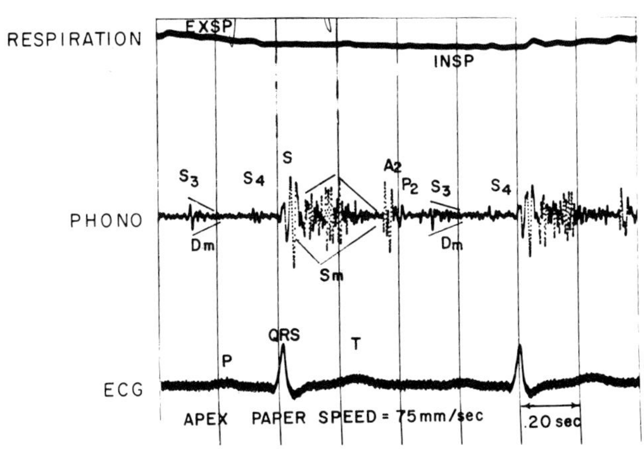

Figure 110. Phonocardiogram of a 36-year-old patient with ostium primum syndrome. Note the prominent diastolic murmur and the presence of an S_3 and an S_4.

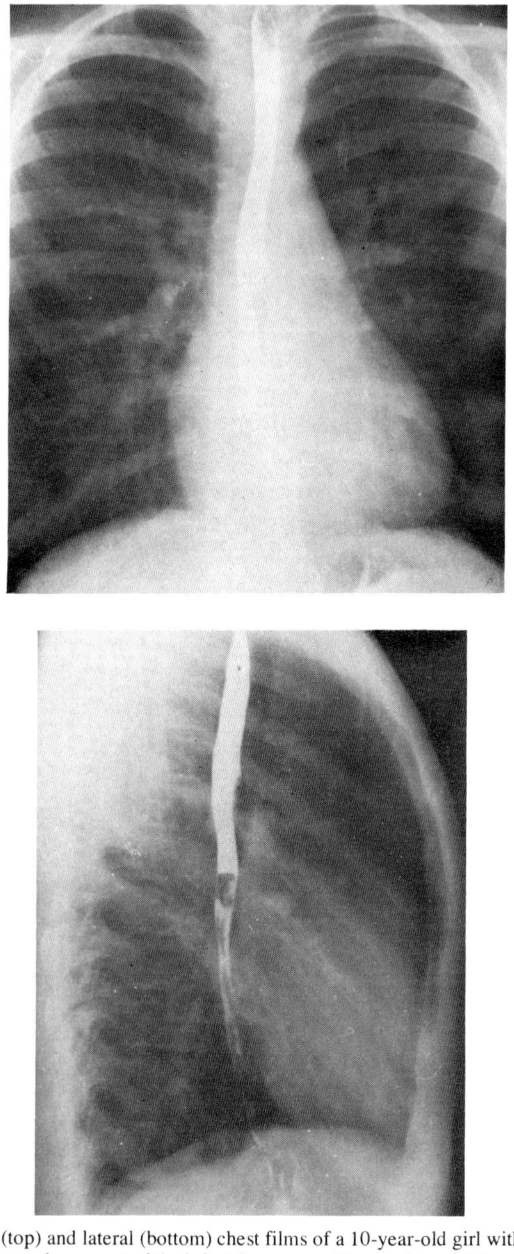

Figure 111. PA (top) and lateral (bottom) chest films of a 10-year-old girl with ostium primum complex. There is no enlargement of the left atrium even with mitral insufficiency, since the atrial septal defect allows excess blood to drain off into the right atrium and the regurgitation is often directly into the right atrium.

The x-ray features are similar to those of the usual type of atrial septal defect, except that in the ostium primum syndrome there may be evidence of left ventricular enlargement. The degree of left ventricular enlargement depends on the severity of the mitral regurgitation.

Electrocardiography

The typical electrocardiogram is quite characteristic and virtually pathognomonic (Figure 112). Superior axis deviation is invariably present, usually with a mean QRS frontal plane axis between $-30°$ and $-90°$. There is a prolonged P-R interval, perhaps because of atrial enlargement. Right ventricular hypertrophy is usually denoted by an rsR′ pattern in leads V_3R and V_1. Left ventricular hypertrophy indicates the presence of moderate or severe mitral insufficiency, although many patients with mild to moderate mitral insufficiency may not show left ventricular hypertrophy. The VCG typically demonstrates the following:

1. The frontal plane QRS loop is shifted leftward and superiorly and is inscribed in a counterclockwise direction. Occasionally this loop forms a figure eight or propellor loop along the superior-inferior axis.
2. The initial QRS forces are directed rightward and inferiorly, producing a q wave in leads I and aVL.
3. The horizontal plane QRS loop demonstrates increased rightward and terminal QRS forces.

Superior orientation of the QRS forces is characteristic of atrioventricular canal defects but may be seen in other defects, among which are:

1. A small percentage (approximately 7%) of secundum atrial septal defects, particularly those associated with mitral valve prolapse (see Chapter 29)
2. Origin of both great vessels from the right ventricle without pulmonic stenosis
3. Single ventricle
4. Post-rubella syndrome

The genesis of this electrocardiographic pattern is not fully established, but the weight of experimental evidence indicates that the anatomic abnormality is responsible. There is posterior displacement of the common bundle that courses along the rim of the defect, with displacement of the distal left bundle branches to the posterior aspect of the ventricular septum. The left bundle fibers emerge from the main bundle earlier than usual and thus cause early depolarization of the posterior aspect of the ventricular septum.

Superior orientation of the QRS forces is not affected by the type of atrioventricular canal defect nor the ventricular hypertrophy pattern. As right

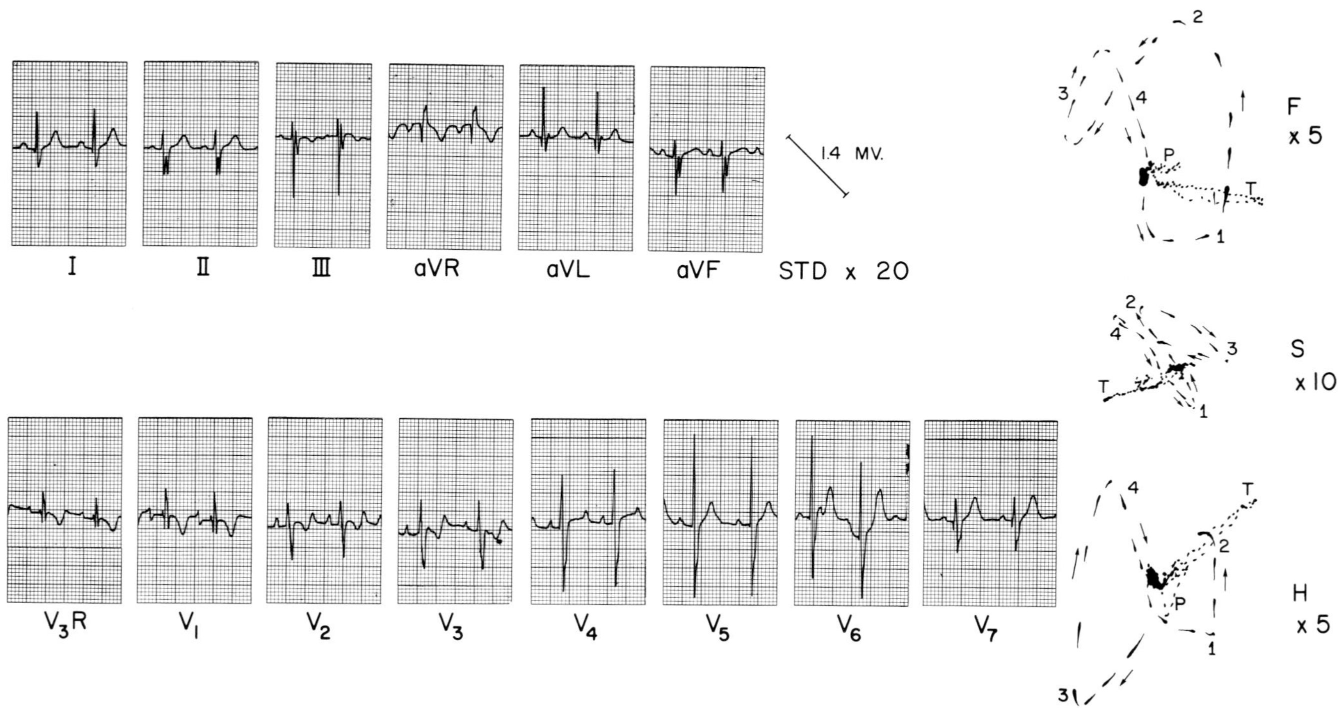

Figure 112. Electrocardiogram and vectorcardiogram of a 4-year-old child with an ostium primum and cleft mitral valve. Note the rsR′ in leads V_3R and V_1 and the superior orientation of the QRS loop, which is basically counterclockwise although forming a figure-eight loop. (From Elliott, L. P., and Schiebler, G. L. 1968. X-Ray Diagnosis of Congenital Cardiac Disease. Courtesy of Charles C Thomas, Publisher, Springfield, Ill.)

ventricular hypertrophy increases, the frontal QRS axis moves to the right but remains superior, with counterclockwise frontal plane rotation.

Echocardiography

The echocardiogram frequently demonstrates characteristic features. Paradoxical septal motion indicating right ventricular volume overload correlates with the size of the shunt. The mitral valve is displaced anteriorly and the anterior leaflet echo appears to move through the ventricular septum in diastole (Figure 113).

Prognosis

Mean age of death in these individuals is approximately the same as that of patients having simple atrial septal defects, unless there is significant mitral insufficiency.

Management

In the presence of a significant left-to-right shunt and/or significant mitral insufficiency, surgery is indicated. We presently favor 4 to 8 years as the

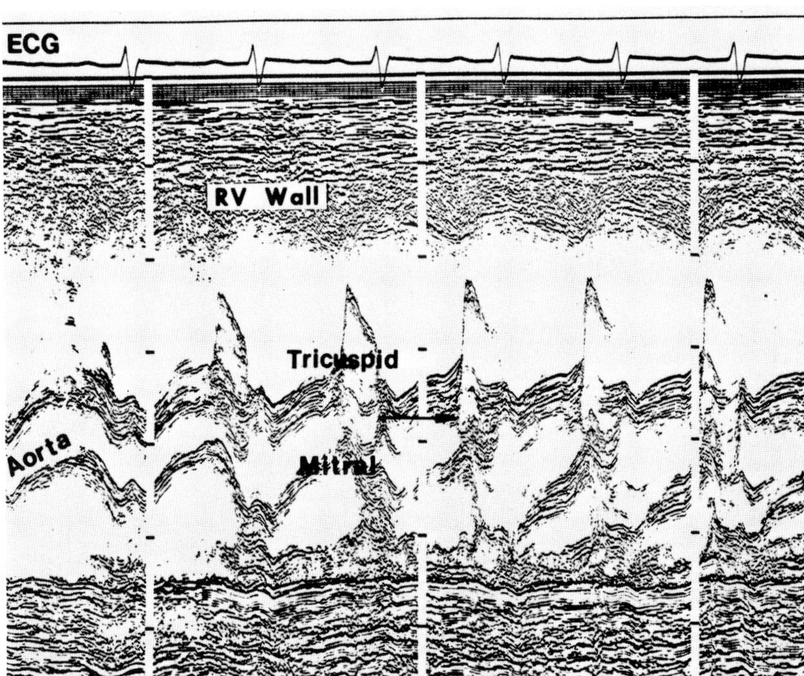

Figure 113. Echocardiogram of a 3-month-old child with a complete atrioventricular canal. Note that the tricuspid valve crosses the septum to meet the mitral valve at the arrow.

optimal age for surgery, although operation at an earlier age may be indicated when mitral insufficiency is significant. Surgical mortality is currently less than 2%.

COMPLETE ATRIOVENTRICULAR CANAL

Pathology

Failure of fusion of cardiac septa and lack of central fusion of atrioventricular valve tissue results in shunts at the atrial and ventricular levels, and incompetence of the common atrioventricular valve is frequent, although not invariable.

About one-third of these hearts have, in addition, a secundum atrial septal defect. The whole atrial septum may be absent, so that a single atrium exists. An associated patent ductus arteriosus is common, particularly in the infant.

Over one-third of all complete atrioventricular canals occur in the Down syndrome. They are also characteristically present in asplenia syndrome (Ivemark syndrome), in association with transposition of the great vessels, anomalies of systemic and pulmonary venous return, and pulmonary outflow tract obstruction.

Clinical Features

Affected infants are usually underweight, tachypneic, and in chronic congestive heart failure. The murmurs resemble those of a ventricular septal defect, with a pansystolic murmur and thrill along the lower left sternal border to the apex (Figure 114). Since there usually is associated pulmonary artery hypertension, the pulmonic component of the second sound is accentuated and may even be palpable. Furthermore, splitting of the two components is less marked or even absent. A mid-diastolic atrioventricular valve flow murmur is heard maximally at the lower left sternal border radiating toward the apex. As pulmonary resistance increases, pulmonary blood flow decreases, and cyanosis becomes apparent. The intensity of the murmurs and the size of the heart decrease, and the pulmonic valve closure sound becomes louder. A high-frequency early diastolic murmur of pulmonic insufficiency may be heard.

Roentgenographic Features

Diffuse enlargement of all four chambers produces a round globular heart (Figure 115). Increased pulmonary vasculature is invariably present and the lung fields are often plethoric in appearance because of an increase in both arterial and venous components. The pulmonary artery is enlarged and the aorta is small.

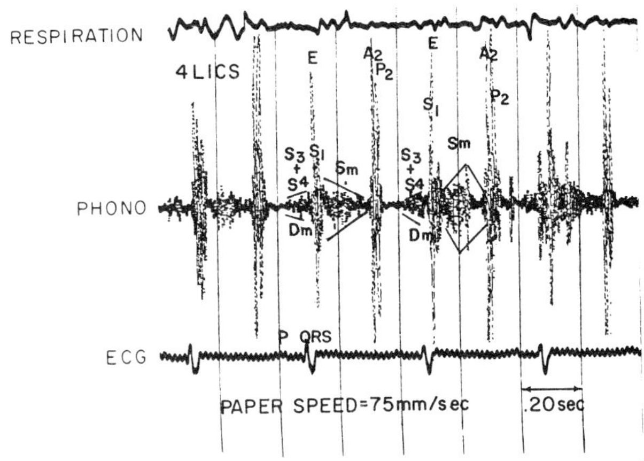

Figure 114. Phonocardiogram of a 14-day-old female infant with a complete atrioventricular canal and a patent ductus arteriosus. Note the prominent diastolic murmur, loud ejection click (E), and narrowly split second sound, with an accentuated pulmonic component.

Electrocardiography

The frontal plane QRS axis generally lies between −90° and −150°. The P-R interval is almost always prolonged, right atrial enlargement is common, and some cases also show left atrial enlargement. Right ventricular hypertrophy is invariable, with many patients also showing left ventricular hypertrophy (Figure 116).

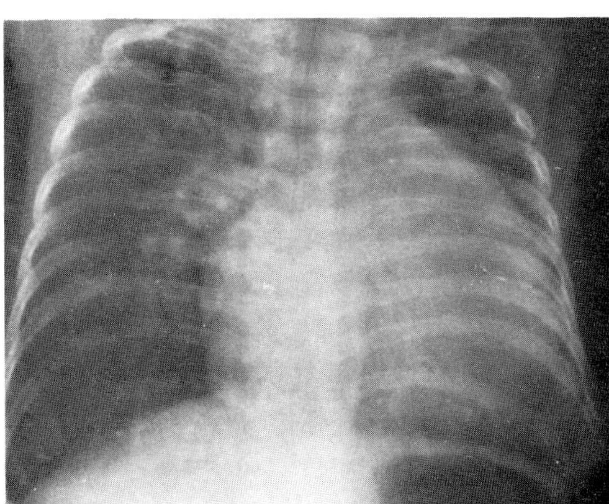

Figure 115. Chest film of the infant in Figure 114 with an atrioventricular canal at 6 months of age. Note the marked enlargement of the heart. On occasion, the cardiac enlargement may be so extreme that it is difficult to decide if the pulmonary vascular markings are increased or not.

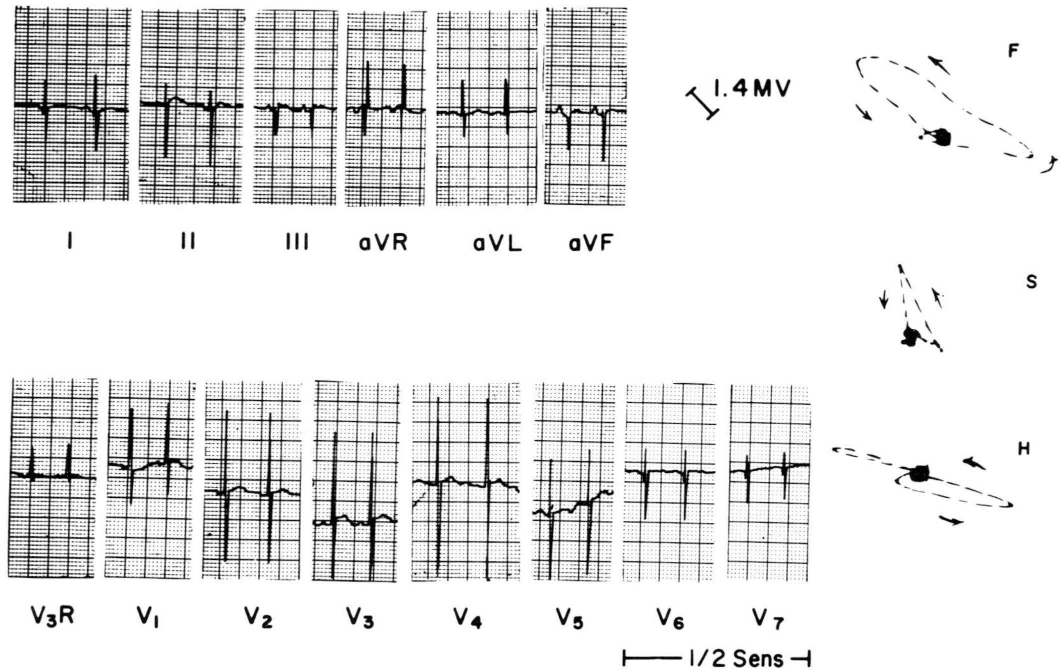

Figure 116. Typical electrocardiogram of a patient with a complete AV canal. Note the extreme left axis deviation and evidence of biventricular hypertrophy.

Echocardiography

Echocardiographic features are similar to those described in the partial form. It may be possible to demonstrate deficiency of the ventricular septum.

Prognosis

Affected children frequently die in the first year of life, and rarely live beyond the age of 4 years. With associated pulmonic stenosis, longer survival can be expected. Pulmonary vascular obstructive disease occurs more frequently in these patients than in patients with only large ventricular septal defects.

Management

Because of the high mortality rate in the first year of life, surgery should be performed during infancy. Mortality for complete correction of these defects in infancy is unfortunately still high at many centers. This is the result of a number of problems:

1. Residual mitral insufficiency
2. Complexity of the lesion, requiring a longer pump perfusion
3. Surgically induced heart block (the conduction system lies very close to the defect)
4. Early development of severe pulmonary vascular disease

Therefore, palliative surgery utilizing pulmonary artery banding has been advocated, but only about 60% of patients will show significant improvement. The remainder either do not survive surgery or show no improvement, because, although the cardiac work secondary to a large left-to-right shunt can be reduced, the work load caused by the incompetent atrioventricular valves has not been altered. Alternatively, referral to a cardiovascular center with acceptably low surgical mortality should be considered.

Corrective surgery can be performed later in life at a mortality rate of less than 10% if the infant responds well to medical treatment or pulmonary artery banding. Insertion of prosthetic material to close the septal defects and plastic repair of the valves are indicated.

BIBLIOGRAPHY

Baron, M. G. 1972. Abnormalities of the mitral valve in endocardial cushion defects. Circulation 45:672–680.

Borkon, A. M., Pieroni, D. R., Varghese, P. J., Ho, C. S., and Rowe, R. D. 1975. The superior QRS axis in ostium primum ASD: a proposed mechanism. Am. Heart J. 90:215–221.

Feldt, R. H. (ed.) 1976. Atrioventricular Canal Defects. W.B. Saunders Company, Philadelphia.

McGoon, D. C., McMullan, M. H., Mair, D. D., and Danielson, G. K. 1972. Correction of complete atrioventricular canal in infants. Mayo Clinic Proc. 48:769–772.

Newfeld, E. A., Sher, M., Paul, M. H., and Nikaidoh, H. 1977. Pulmonary vascular disease in complete atrioventricular canal defect. Am. J. Cardiol. 39:721–726.

Okamura, K., Kudo, T., Koyanagi, H., Imai, Y., and Konno, S. 1974. Evaluation of mitral regurgitation in endocardial cushion defect by selective left ventriculography with reference to surgical intervention on mitral valve cleft. Am. Heart. J. 88:579–587.

Pieroni, D. R., Homcy, E., and Freedom, R. M. 1975. Echocardiography in atrioventricular canal defect. Am. J. Cardiol. 35:54–58.

chapter 15

VENTRICULAR SEPTAL DEFECT

HISTORICAL NOTES

Decaisne published in 1877 a case report of a 26-month-old female with "an intense systolic murmur occupying the entire precordial region . . . maximum of this murmur was over the base and middle portion of the heart. There was considerable bulging with a purring thrill." The child died of "some pulmonary mishap" and at autopsy was found to have a ventricular septal defect.

An accurate description of the clinical manifestations of ventricular septal defects (VSD) was made by Henri Roger in 1879, when he published his observations of a small group of patients ranging in age from 6 months to 50 years. He described the characteristic murmur and noted that symptoms were rare after infancy.

Victor Eisenmenger, in 1897, described a young cyanotic male who at autopsy proved to have a large ventricular septal defect. Eisenmenger correctly deduced that the overriding of the aorta was more apparent than real and that the cyanosis was most likely due to changes in the lungs. Nearly half a century passed before adequate confirmation of his views was obtained. The association of a large ventricular septal defect and severe pulmonary arteriolar damage is called the Eisenmenger complex, and a similar physiologic picture associated with other shunt defects is called the Eisenmenger reaction or syndrome.

Credit for the first successful closure of a series of ventricular septal defects goes to Lillehei and his colleagues, in 1955, who also developed one of the first adequate heart-lung machines.

INCIDENCE

This is a common congenital heart defect. One out of every four children with congenital heart anomalies will have an isolated ventricular septal defect. If we include patients in whom a ventricular septal defect is but one component of the clinical picture, it is found in two out of every five congenital heart patients. There are no known sex or racial differences in incidence rates.

ETIOLOGY

Although cases of several afflicted members of a family are known, there is little concrete evidence that this defect is inherited. It has been noted to follow maternal rubella during early pregnancy and has also been found in children born of mothers who had taken thalidomide during pregnancy. VSD is also commonly found in the autosomal trisomic syndromes.

HEMODYNAMICS

The hemodynamics, as well as clinical features and prognosis, are largely dependent on the size of the defect (Table 16). VSD in combination with obstruction of right ventricular outflow is discussed in Chapter 23.

Large-sized defects are those that are nearly equal in cross-sectional area to the area of the aortic annulus, thereby allowing free communication between the two ventricles (Figure 117). Pressures are equal in the right and left ventricles. Since pulmonary vascular resistance is ordinarily about one-sixth of systemic resistance, it is easier for blood to flow out the pulmonary artery than out the aorta. Pulmonary blood flow is therefore greater than systemic

Table 16. Classification of ventricular septal defects[a]

Type of defect	Size of defect (cm)	Percentage of total after age 3 years	Right ventricular systolic pressure (mm Hg)	Left-to-right shunt
Small	0.1–0.6	41	12–30	Less than 40% of PBF[b]
Moderate	0.8–1.5	23	15–40	40 to 65% of PBF
Large—no pulmonary hypertension	1.5–2.4	4	20–70	Over 65% of PBF
Large—with pulmonary hypertension	1.5–3.0	15	60 to systemic	30 to 70% of PBF
Eisenmenger complex	1.5–3.0	17	Systemic	Predominantly right-to-left

[a] Adapted from Bloomfield, D. K. 1964. The natural history of ventricular septal defect in patients surviving infancy. Circulation 29:914. By permission of the American Heart Association, Inc.

[b] PBF = pulmonary blood flow.

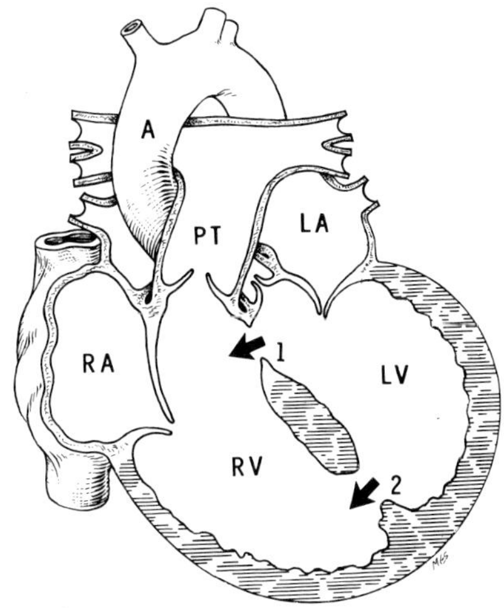

Figure 117. Schematic intracardiac circulation with ventricular septal defects. The more common location is in the membranous portion of the septum (1), but occasionally the defect may occur in the muscular portion of the septum (2). (From Elliott, L. P., and Schiebler, G. L. 1968. X-Ray Diagnosis of Congenital Cardiac Disease. Courtesy of Charles C Thomas, Publisher, Springfield, Ill.)

blood flow. This excess pulmonary flow causes enlargement of the left atrium, the left ventricle, and, unless the VSD is located just below the pulmonary artery, the right ventricle. The more blood that enters the right ventricle and the pulmonary artery through the shunt, the more blood must exit from the pulmonary veins into the left atrium and across the mitral valve into the left ventricle. Although the mitral valve orifice is adequate for normal flow, when the pulmonary flow is approximately doubled, the valve restricts flow. This in turn produces a pressure drop across the valve and a murmur, sometimes referred to as "relative mitral stenosis."

Moderate-sized defects are those in which the size of the defects restricts flow and pressure across them. The pressure in the right ventricle ranges from slightly above normal to nearly equal to that found in the left ventricle. Pulmonary blood flows may be almost as great as with a large VSD. Similarly, enlargement of the left atrium, the left ventricle, and the right ventricle and a diastolic apical flow murmur may be present. Moderate-sized defects probably represent a transitional stage, as larger defects become relatively smaller as a result of growth of the child or absolutely smaller as cardiac muscle or tricuspid valve tissue narrows the orifice.

Small-sized defects are those with further restriction to pressure and flow. By definition, the right ventricular pressure is normal and the pulmonary-to-systemic flow ratio less than 1.5:1. The left atrial pressure is normal or only slightly elevated.

CLINICAL FEATURES

As one would expect from the hemodynamics, the clinical features depend on the size of the VSD. On physical examination, all three groups are acyanotic except when they have a pulmonary diffusion problem secondary to pneumonia or congestive heart failure.

Children with *large ventricular septal defects* commonly present in congestive heart failure between 1 and 3 months of age. They are subject to frequent bouts of pneumonia. They often gain weight slowly, with growth in length being only slightly faster. They occasionally present with mild cyanosis, secondary to pulmonary infections or congestive heart failure, which can be relieved by oxygen. These infants have increased precordial activity, and commonly have both a left ventricular heave and a right ventricular lift.

Children with *moderate ventricular septal defects* are typically asymptomatic, although they may tire more easily than their contemporaries. They may have more frequent bouts of pneumonia and other lower respiratory tract infections. (Although they are also said to have more *upper* respiratory tract infections, this has not been borne out in our experience.) They do not develop congestive heart failure, unless some complication such as infective endocarditis or marked anemia occurs. Physical and laboratory findings may be so similar to those of a large VSD that cardiac catheterization is needed to separate them clearly.

Large- and moderate-sized ventricular septal defects produce very loud murmurs, at least grade 3 in amplitude. The murmurs are pansystolic in timing, loudest at the fourth left intercostal space, and usually accompanied by a thrill. The typical murmur is harsh and the frequency content varies from one beat to the next (Figure 118). Since very large defects may cause increased pulmonary resistance, such patients may have lower pulmonary blood flows and hence softer murmurs.

Almost by definition, children with *small ventricular septal defects* are asymptomatic. The murmur of a tiny VSD often is not pansystolic but instead ends a short time prior to S_2. Small defects, sometimes referred to as *maladie de Roger,* appear to be compatible with an active and long life. Many of these small defects will close spontaneously. The murmur of small ventricular septal defects is sometimes said to sound much like an innocent murmur. In our experience, even the smallest defects detectable at catheterization have had a characteristically harsh systolic murmur, but one that may end before the second heart sound rather than being pansystolic. Diastolic flow murmurs are not heard in small VSDs.

In the *newborn,* one may hear a moderately loud early systolic murmur along the lower left sternal border. These murmurs are most common about the second or third day of life. A few days later, these murmurs may become louder and longer in duration, but they tend to shorten again between the age

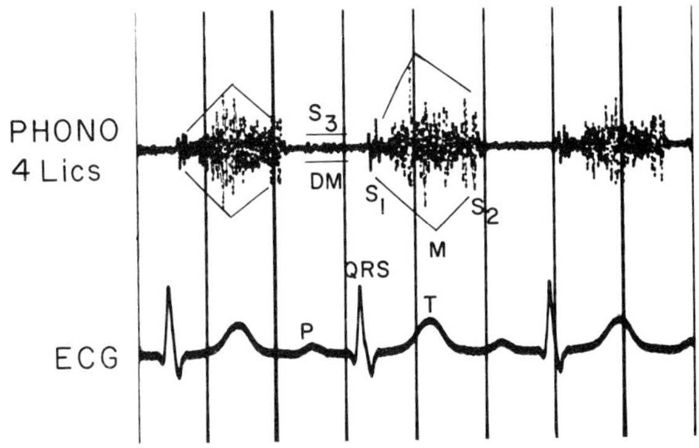

Figure 118. Phonocardiogram of a 5-year-old child with a ventricular septal defect. Note that the murmur begins shortly after the first heart sound and lasts throughout systole, obscuring the aortic component of the second sound. The murmur is almost totally irregular in amplitude, although there is a slight suggestion of an increase near midsystole. The components of the second sound are often difficult to distinguish due to the extent of the murmur. There is a low-amplitude, low-frequency diastolic murmur beginning with S_3 that actually is heard better than it is reproduced on the phonocardiogram.

of 3 to 6 weeks. Rowe thinks that these murmurs are usually due to small muscular ventricular septal defects that are particularly likely to close spontaneously in early infancy.

In *infants* the murmur may be loudest near the base of the heart and suggest pulmonic stenosis.

The intensity of the *diastolic murmur* at the apex is roughly proportional to the left-to-right shunt. This rumbling mid- to late diastolic murmur begins with the third heart sound and, in infants with a fast heart rate, may encompass S_3 or S_4. Diminution or disappearance of this murmur suggests a decrease of pulmonary blood flow resulting from creation of infundibular stenosis, pulmonary vascular bed damage, or a decrease in size of the VSD.

Another important physical finding is the intensity of the pulmonic component of the second sound (P_2). When the pulmonary artery pressure is normal, P_2 is as loud as or slightly louder than the aortic component in the second and third left intercostal spaces. If the pulmonary artery pressure is increased, P_2 is louder and closer in time to the aortic component (A_2) and may even be superimposed on A_2. With severe pulmonary hypertension, P_2 may be palpable and even visible on inspection. P_2 will then have a loud tambour quality and is often followed by a short diastolic murmur of pulmonic insufficiency. The second sound is often the most striking finding on physical examination in patients with Eisenmenger complex.

Elevated pulmonary resistance manifests itself on auscultation by a loud, banging pulmonic component of the second sound. There may be a right ventricular lift and an easily palpable pulmonary artery impulse. The characteristic systolic murmur is still present, but the diastolic flow murmur may be difficult to hear. Patients often complain of breathlessness on exertion, which is thought to be due to stiffening of the lungs by pulmonary vascular bed changes. The vast majority, or perhaps even all, of these patients will ultimately develop a predominant right-to-left shunt (Eisenmenger complex).

The Eisenmenger complex is the terminal stage of this spectrum (Figure 119). In the large VSD, the prime determinant of direction of blood flow is the ratio of resistances of the pulmonary and systemic vascular beds. The degree of "aortic overriding" is relatively unimportant. Average age of death is about 30 years, most commonly due to hemoptysis from enlarged bronchial arteries or to ill-advised surgery. Surgical closure of the defect is definitely contraindicated. There appears to be little risk of bacterial endocarditis in this group.

ROENTGENOGRAPHIC FEATURES

Patients with a small VSD have a normal chest x-ray or only equivocally increased pulmonary arterial markings. Patients with a moderate to large VSD will exhibit varying degrees of biventricular hypertrophy, left atrial enlargement, pulmonary artery enlargement, and increase in pulmonary arterial markings (Figure 120). This particular combination of findings is characteristic of a left-to-right shunt at the ventricular level.

The Eisenmenger complex produces an x-ray picture of a large main pulmonary artery and a paucity of small- and medium-sized pulmonary arteries distally (peripheral cutoff). However, the chest x-ray is notoriously unreliable for detection of the Eisenmenger syndrome.

ELECTROCARDIOGRAPHY

The ECG is usually normal in patients with small defects (Figure 121). The most common electrocardiographic pattern in moderate and large VSDs is that of biventricular hypertrophy with left atrial enlargement (Figure 122). Children with severe pulmonary hypertension may show a pattern of pure right ventricular hypertrophy.

PROGNOSIS

The infant with a large VSD in congestive heart failure may follow one of several courses. The baby may be unable to produce enough systemic blood flow for vital body functions, particularly growth. Pulmonary vascular resistance is normally one-sixth of systemic vascular resistance; thus it is far easier for blood to enter the pulmonary artery than the aorta. These infants present

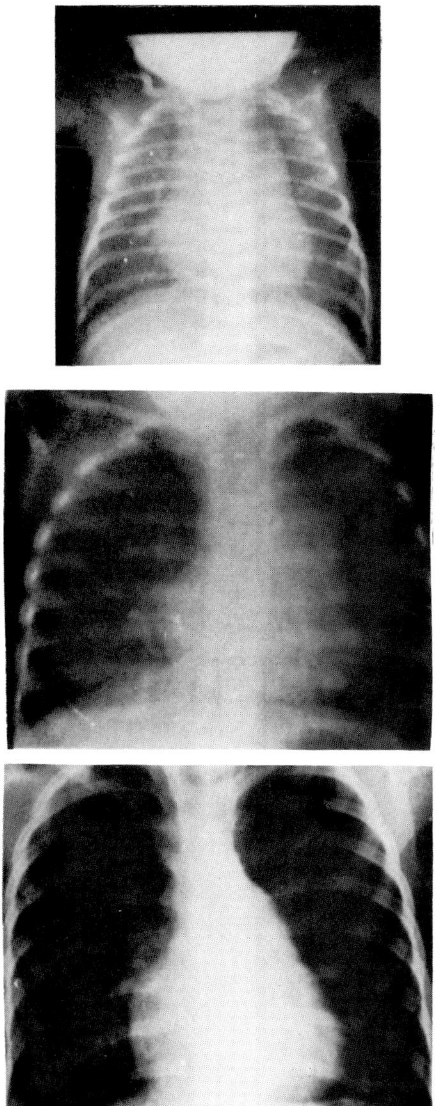

Figure 119. Development of the Eisenmenger syndrome in a child with a large ventricular septal defect. The figure at the top is the child at the age of 3 months, showing markedly increased pulmonary vascularity. The middle panel, at 1 year of age, shows diminished vascularity. Shortly after this x-ray was taken, the diastolic flow murmur previously heard at the apex had disappeared. The bottom panel shows this child at age 4, when initially seen in our center. He is now clinically cyanotic and has all the classical features of the Eisenmenger complex.

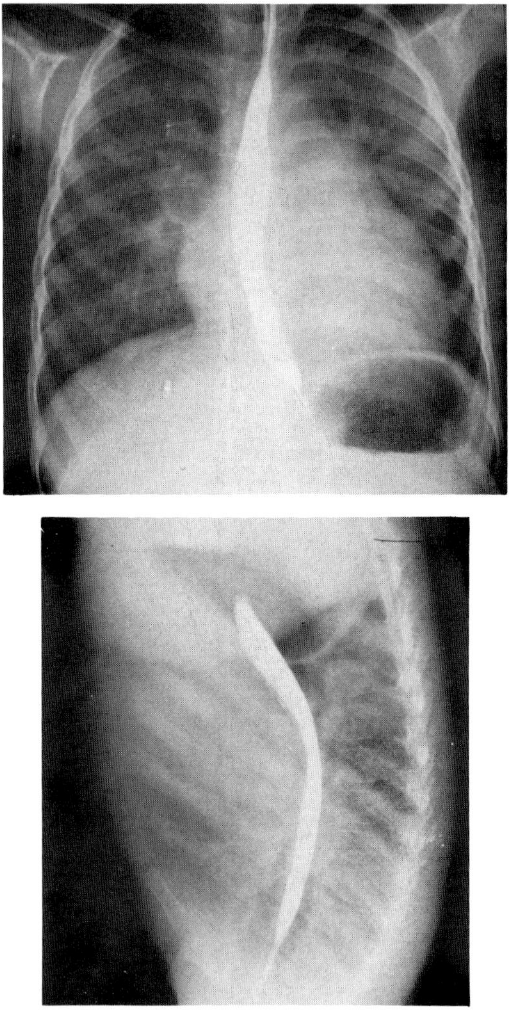

Figure 120. AP (top) and lateral (bottom) chest x-ray of a 5-year-old male with a ventricular septal defect. Note the moderate cardiomegaly, the increased pulmonary vascular markings, and the left atrial enlargement.

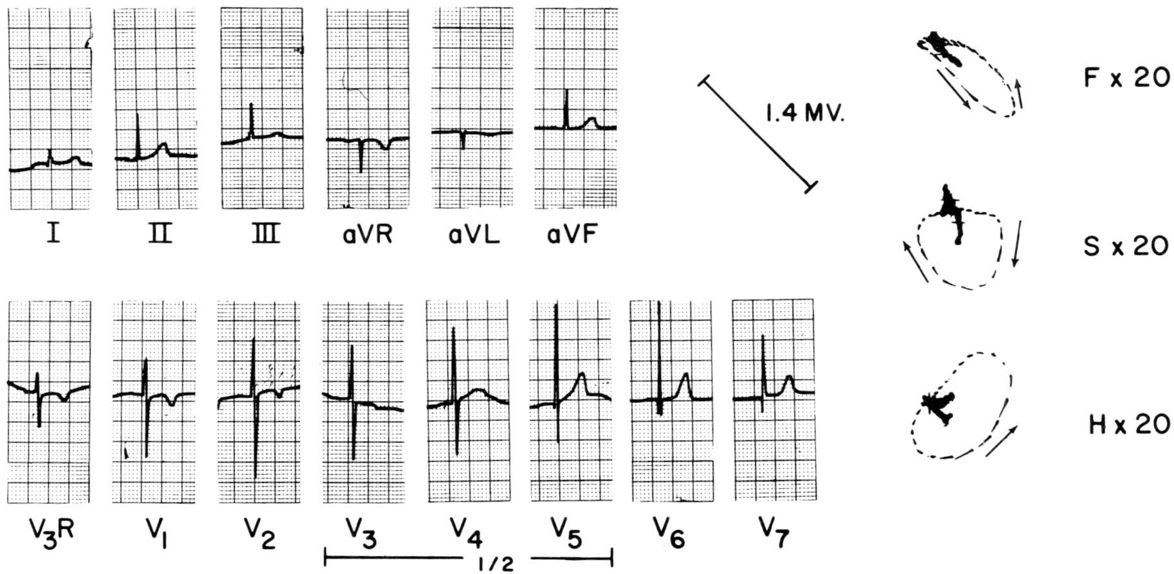

Figure 121. Patients with small ventricular septal defects may have normal electrocardiograms. Here, absence of terminal R in lead aVR, a 50-mm R wave in lead V_5, and a 3-mm q wave in lead V_6 with peaked T waves suggest left ventricular volume overloading. The counterclockwise rotation in the frontal plane, as well as the predominantly posterior forces, also suggests left ventricular hypertrophy.

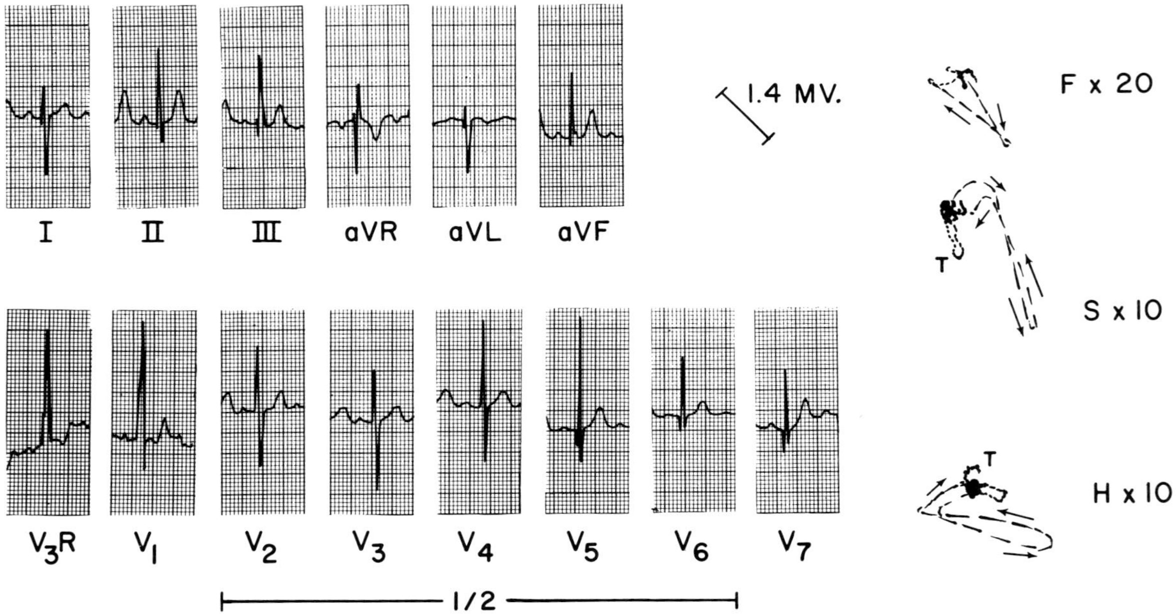

Figure 122. Electrocardiogram of a patient with a moderate-sized ventricular septal defect. Note the biphasic P wave in V_3R, indicating left atrial enlargement. Tall R waves over the right precordium indicate right ventricular systolic overloading, and the large isodiphasic QRS complexes over the mid-precordium indicate biventricular enlargement. The tall T waves in leads II, III, and aVF and the deep q wave in lead V_7 suggest left ventricular diastolic overloading.

with severe congestive heart failure manifested by such signs as hepatomegaly, splenomegaly, tachypnea, labored respirations, and excessive sweating. One hopes, of course, that these patients will gain weight so that, with growth, the size of the ventricular septal defect will become relatively smaller, making clinical management easier. If after an adequate trial this has not occurred, surgical intervention is in order.

In a few infants, pulmonary vascular resistance increases with thickening of the intima and media of the smaller pulmonary arteries and a corresponding reduction in the average cross-sectional area. This results in clinical improvement, but, if allowed to persist beyond approximately 2 years of age, irreversible damage to the pulmonary vascular bed may preclude corrective surgery.

A third possibility is that the infant will develop hypertrophy of the right ventricular infundibulum. We estimate that 5% to 15% of infants with large ventricular defects will develop "protective" *infundibular stenosis*. This decreases the risk of congestive heart failure and of pulmonary vascular changes, but may increase the risk of bacterial endocarditis. Some so-called acyanotic tetralogies of Fallot demonstrate this type of transformation (see Chapter 23). While there is an increase in resistance to blood flowing out the right ventricle, the pulmonary vascular resistance remains normal. Progressive narrowing may occur and become the major cardiac anomaly, and the infant may develop cyanosis and a clinical picture indistinguishable from tetralogy of Fallot. In such cases, the anatomy of the right ventricle differs from that seen in the cyanotic tetralogy of Fallot. Rare instances have been reported in which the VSD has closed spontaneously, but the infundibular stenosis required surgical resection.

Finally, the most favorable course is an absolute or relative reduction in size of the ventricular septal defect. If the infant manages to grow, the size of the defect will become less important with increasing body and cardiac size. It is not uncommon for the VSD to close spontaneously either through apposition of adjacent musculature or by being sealed off by part of the tricuspid valve apparatus. Spontaneous closure of a VSD is most common during the first few months of postnatal life and with small-sized defects. Estimates of spontaneous closure range from 21% to 90%, depending on the age of the population studied, the follow-up period, and the criteria for inclusion. Spontaneous closure becomes less common with increasing age (Table 17). However, the rarity of VSD in adults would suggest that closure must continue to occur throughout life.

Risk of Infective Endocarditis (see also Chapter 37)

The hospital incidence of infective endocarditis is not decreasing, and, after spectacular gains in the early antibiotic era, the hospital mortality rate seems to have stabilized at 20% to 25%. The relative incidence of infective endocar-

Table 17. Spontaneous closure of ventricular septal defects[a]

Age defect was last open (years)	Small sized	Large sized	Large sized with pulmonary vascular disease
0–4	29 of 86 (34%)	7 of 88 (8%)	1 of 44 (2%)
5–9	16 of 91 (18%)	1 of 77 (1%)	0 of 47
10–14	11 of 97 (11%)	2 of 39 (5%)	0 of 34
15–19	2 of 97 (4%)	0 of 18	0 of 10
20	0 of 47	0 of 14	0 of 13

[a] Modified from Corone, P., Doyon, F., Gaudeau, S., Guerin, F., Vernant, P., Ducam, H., Rumeau-Roquette, C., and Gaudeul, P. 1977. Natural history of ventricular septal defect. Circulation 55: 908. By permission of the American Heart Association, Inc.

ditis superimposed on a congenital heart lesion is increasing, and VSD is the most common congenital heart lesion associated with it, reflecting the high prevalence of VSD in the population. Infective endocarditis most commonly occurs during the fourth and fifth decades. Estimates of the lifetime risk of contracting it range from 10% to 30%, with an estimated lifetime mortality of 2% to 5%.

MANAGEMENT

Initial treatment of the patient in congestive heart failure consists of digitalis, diuretics, and usually antibiotics (since infants in failure commonly have pneumonia) for a period of some 24–48 hr. It is our policy to catheterize all infants with congestive heart failure as soon as they have stabilized. After 3–6 months, if the infant appears to be improving but still has manifestations of a large ventricular septal defect, we recatheterize the infant. If pulmonary vascular resistance has increased or is unchanged at the time of the second catheterization, we recommend early surgical intervention.

For the infant whose congestive heart failure cannot be managed by medical means alone or who appears to be developing severe pulmonary vascular bed changes, *pulmonary artery banding* was formerly the procedure of choice. This is an attempt to imitate the natural development of infundibular stenosis that occurs spontaneously in some infants with large VSDs. When properly performed, it results in a decrease in pulmonary blood flow, but not to the extent of producing a right-to-left shunt. However, the hemodynamics of banding are not well understood, and there is no reliable method of determining how much banding is adequate. Furthermore, a band that is adequate in infancy is apt to become too tight with subsequent growth; it is not uncommon for these children to be cyanotic in later childhood. The bands tend to become incorporated into the pulmonary artery wall and subsequent repair of the stenosis may be a problem at the time of open heart repair. Pulmonary artery banding duplicates the body's natural way of protecting the lungs and may be helpful; a 25% mortality rate and a 25% failure rate are seen in most series. However, as a result of the recent success of open heart repair even in small infants, many centers have abandoned this procedure in favor of a one-stage repair.

Open heart surgery has been remarkably successful in this defect. Many surgeons prefer to wait until the infant weights at least 12 kg. For elective procedures in the absence of pulmonary vascular disease, we prefer to operate at age 4 to 6 years. Our criteria for surgery are: 1) significant pulmonary hypertension; 2) cardiomegaly, either on physical or roentgenographic examination; and 3) a predominant left-to-right shunt in excess of 50% of the pulmonary blood flow.

Operative mortality rates for closure of ventricular septal defects should be less than 2% in the absence of severe pulmonary hypertension. With severe pulmonary hypertension (pulmonary artery pressure in excess of two-thirds of systemic pressure), the operative mortality rate is about 10%.

Postoperative catheterizations have demonstrated the absence of a significant shunt in the absence of a significant murmur. However, patients with severe pulmonary hypertension should be restudied to ascertain prognosis, and children with murmurs suggesting residual defects should be recatheterized to assess the degree and location of the shunt and the advisability of repeat surgery.

CONCLUSIONS AND RECOMMENDATIONS

1. Patients with small ventricular septal defects need not undergo surgery, since the development of proven pulmonary hypertension and vascular bed damage is unknown. Infective endocarditis is rarely associated with small defects, but when it does occur we recommend closure of the VSD 1 year later, since the risk of recurrence is increased significantly.
2. Patients with increased pulmonary vascular resistance need early surgery. If not operated by 2 years of age, most, if not all, of these patients will develop irreversible pulmonary bed changes.
3. Patients with Eisenmenger complex do not benefit from surgical closure and usually die as a result. Since these patients may enjoy relatively good health for many years, surgery is contraindicated.
4. Infants with congestive heart failure and ventricular septal defect should be initially managed medically and catheterized as soon as they are stable and free of infections or after an adequate trial of unsuccessful therapy. If congestive heart failure cannot be managed by medical means alone, or if repeat catheterization 3–6 months later shows evidence of increasing pulmonary vascular resistance, surgical intervention should be considered.
5. There is often amelioration of symptoms secondary to reduction in size of the VSD or development of pulmonary stenosis.

BIBLIOGRAPHY

Campbell, M. 1971. Natural history of ventricular septal defect. Br. Heart J. 33:246–257.

Ching, E., DuShane, J. W., McGoon, D. C., and Danielson, G. K. 1971. Total correction of ventricular septal defect in infancy using extracorporeal circulation. Ann. Thorac. Surg. 12:1–10.

Collins, G., Calder, L., Rose, V., Kidd, L., and Keith, J. 1972. Ventricular septal defect: Clinical and hemodynamic changes in the first five years of life. Am. Heart J. 84:695–705.

Corone, P., Doyon, F., Gaudeau, S., Guerin, F., Vernant, P., Ducam, H., Rumeau-Rouquette, C., and Gaudeul, P. 1977. Natural history of ventricular septal defect. Circulation 55:908–915.

Evans, J. R., Rowe, R. D., and Keith, J. D. 1960. Spontaneous closure of ventricular septal defects. Circulation 22:1044–1054.

Friedli, B., Kidd, B. S., Mustard, W. T., and Keith, J. D. 1974. Ventricular septal defect with increased pulmonary vascular resistance. Am. J. Cardiol. 33:403–409.

Ho, C. S., Krovetz, L. J., Strife, J. L., Brawley, R. K., and Rowe, R. D. 1973. Postoperative assessment of residual defects following cardiac surgery in infants and children. II. Ventricular septal defects. Johns Hopkins Med. J. 133:270–294.

Hoffman, J. E. E., and Rudolph, A. M. 1965. The natural history of ventricular septal defects in infancy. Am. J. Cardiol. 16:634–653.

Jarmakani, J. M., Graham, T. P., Jr., Canent, R. V., Jr., and Capp, M. P. 1971. The effect of corrective surgery of left heart volume and mass in children with ventricular septal defect. Am. J. Card. 27:254–258.

Kidd, L., Rose, V., Collins, G., and Keith, J. 1965. Ventricular septal defect in infancy. A hemodynamic study. Am. Heart J. 69:4–10.

Levin, A. R., Spach, M. S., Canent, R. V., Boineau, J. P., Capp, M. P., Jain, V., and Barr, R. C. 1967. Intracardiac pressure-flow dynamics in isolated ventricular septal defects. Circulation 35:430–441.

Naeye, R. L. 1966. The pulmonary arterial bed in ventricular septal defect. Circulation 34:962–970.

Park, C. D., Nicodemus, H., Downes, J. J., Miller, W. W., and Waldhausen, J. A. 1969. Changes in pulmonary vascular resistance following closure of ventricular septal defects. Circulation 39/40:Suppl. I:193–200.

Pieroni, D. R., Bell, B. B., Krovetz, L. J., Varghese, P. J., and Rowe, R. D. 1971. Auscultatory recognition of aneurysm of the membranous ventricular septum associated with small ventricular septal defect. Circulation 44:733–739.

Sigmann, J. M., Perry, B. L., Behrendt, D. M., Stern, A. M., Kirsh, M. M., and Sloan, H. E. 1977. Ventricular septal defect: results after repair in infancy. Am. J. Cardiol. 39:66–71.

Stanton, R. E., and Fyler, D. C. 1961. The natural history of pulmonary hypertension in children with ventricular septal defects assessed by serial hemodynamic studies. Pediatrics 27:621–626.

chapter 16

PATENT DUCTUS ARTERIOSUS

HISTORICAL NOTES

The ductus arteriosus was known to Galen, although its function was not clearly understood until depicted by Harvey in 1628.* In *De motu cordis,* Harvey described with remarkable accuracy the function of both the foramen ovale and the ductus arteriosus and how they close after birth.

Failure of the ductus to close and the resultant clinical picture were first described by Gibson in 1900. The first systematic experimental studies to determine why the ductus constricts at birth were undertaken by Barcroft in 1938.

In August, 1938, Gross and Hubbard successfully ligated a persistently patent ductus. This first surgical correction of a cardiovascular anomaly was the major impetus in the rapid development of both cardiac surgery and pediatric cardiology.

INCIDENCE

Persistent patency of the ductus arteriosus is the fourth most common congenital heart defect, accounting for one out of every nine congenital heart anomalies. Approximately 15% of patients with a patent ductus arteriosus (PDA) have additional cardiac anomalies, particularly a ventricular septal defect, coarctation of the aorta, and atrioventricular canals. There is a striking difference in sex incidence—patent ductus arteriosus is found three times as often in females as in males. In some types of cyanotic congenital heart disease, e.g., pulmonic atresia or tricuspid atresia, the ductus is the primary

---

*In 1564, Leonardo Botallo published a short description of part of the heart. According to Franklin (Ann. Sci. 5:57, 1944), "Through strange turn of events and the carelessness of many writers in checking their references," it became known as the *ductus arteriosus Botalli.* Unfortunately Botallo never described the ductus arteriosus in his paper.

conduit carrying blood to the lungs and acts to compensate for a reduced pulmonary blood flow. These forms are not considered further in this chapter.

Pediatric cardiologists and neonatologists have come to recognize that the incidence of patent ductus arteriosus in small premature infants has recently increased dramatically. Survival of premature infants with severe respiratory distress syndrome (RDS) has increased from less than 20% a decade ago to over 80% today. During this time interval, the use of respirators, continuous distending airway pressure, blood transfusions, and hyperalimentation have all become more frequent. Improvement in neonatal care has resulted not only in an increasing survival of premature infants but also an increase in disorders associated with prematurity, such as retrolental fibroplasia, necrotizing entercolitis, and patent ductus arteriosus. The Communicable Disease Center has reported that the incidence of PDA has more than doubled during the last decade.

ETIOLOGY

The major factor in the incidence of patent ductus arteriosus is *prematurity*. Premature infants with PDA tend to be symptomatic earlier in life, especially if they also have RDS (Table 18). Patent ductus arteriosus is also more common among children born in high altitudes. Both of these factors point to a hypoxic stimulus as one cause of failure of the ductus arteriosus to close. Recent evidence suggests that these effects are mediated via the prostaglandin system.

The occurrence of *maternal rubella* in the first 3 or 4 months of pregnancy is also associated with a high incidence of patent ductus arteriosus (Table 19). These infants may also have cataracts, deafness, and microcephaly. Apparent mental retardation is almost always secondary to sensory deprivation, and learning potential may not be impaired. Thrombocytopenic purpura and hepatosplenomegaly have also been reported in the neonatal period. When congenital heart disease is present, it is usually a PDA or

Table 18. Etiological factors in patent ductus arteriosus[a]

	Infants (under 1 year)	Older children (1–16 years)
Number of patients	39	309
Maternal rubella	18%	2%
Prematurity	41%	11%
Family history of congenital heart disease	0%	4%

[a] Adapted from Krovetz, L. J., Lester, R. G., and Warden, H. E. 1962. The diagnosis of patent ductus arteriosus in infancy. Dis. Chest 42: 241.

Table 19. Cardiac Findings in 60 children with post-rubella syndrome[a]

Finding	Incidence
Patent ductus arteriosus	26
Pulmonary artery coarctations	13
Pulmonic stenosis, valvar	10
PDA and VSD	6
Ventricular septal defect	4
PDA and PSV	3
Aortic stenosis, valvar	1
Idiopathic myocardial hypertrophy	1
No significant heart disease	5
PDA and Coarctation	1
Transposition of great arteries and VSD	1

[a] This table includes only children seen on our service. It does not reflect the incidence of congenital heart disease, but only the relative importance of the various lesions.

multiple pulmonary artery coarctations. Post-rubella patients with PDA tend to develop symptoms during infancy.

There is a moderately high incidence of more than one case occurring in a family, and 4% of our patients with PDA had other first degree family members with congenital heart disease. Families with three or more instances of patent ductus arteriosus have been reported.

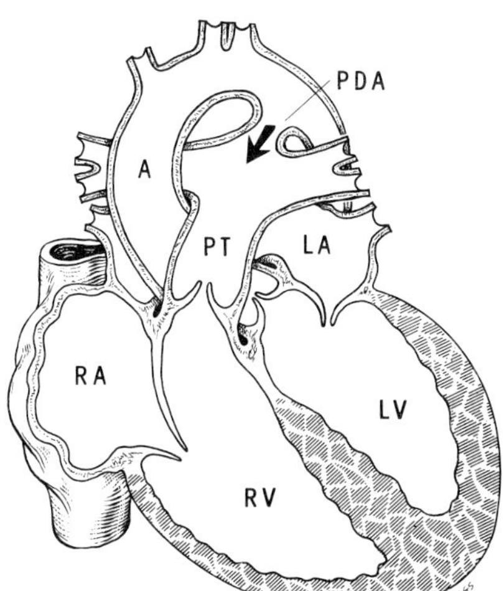

Figure 123. Schematic drawing of a circulation with a patent ductus arteriosus. In the usual postnatal situation, the pressure in the aorta (A) is higher than the pressure in the pulmonary trunk (PT), and there is a left-to-right shunt. (From Elliott, L. P., and Schiebler, G. L. 1968. X-Ray Diagnosis of Congenital Cardiac Disease. Courtesy of Charles C Thomas, Publisher, Springfield, Ill.)

HEMODYNAMICS

Patients having the most hemodynamically significant lesions will exhibit the highest pulmonary blood flows and pressures (Figure 123). The runoff from the aorta during diastole decreases arterial diastolic pressure and widens the pulse pressure, producing prominent arterial pulses. When the shunt is large enough to increase mitral valve flow substantially, a rumbling diastolic murmur will be heard at the apex, and left atrial enlargement occurs.

Excess pulmonary blood flow may produce congestive heart failure in the infant. Initially, the left-to-right shunt places the extra burden solely on the left ventricle. If the shunt is quite large, pulmonary artery pressure increases, and evidence of right ventricular pressure overloading develops.

CLINICAL FEATURES

The more hemodynamically significant the lesion, the earlier the patient develops symptoms and comes to the attention of the physician. Infants with a large patent ductus arteriosus usually present with tachypnea, slow motor development, congestive heart failure, and failure to thrive. Occasionally hoarseness or a chronic nonproductive cough, due to irritation of the left recurrent laryngeal nerve as it courses around the ductus, may be present. The PDA may be large enough to compress the left bronchus, producing ''asthma'' or even atalectasis.

It is uncommon for an asymptomatic infant with a PDA to be brought to our attention. Whether this is due to the referral nature of our practice, the greater difficulty in identifying murmurs during infancy, or the possibility that

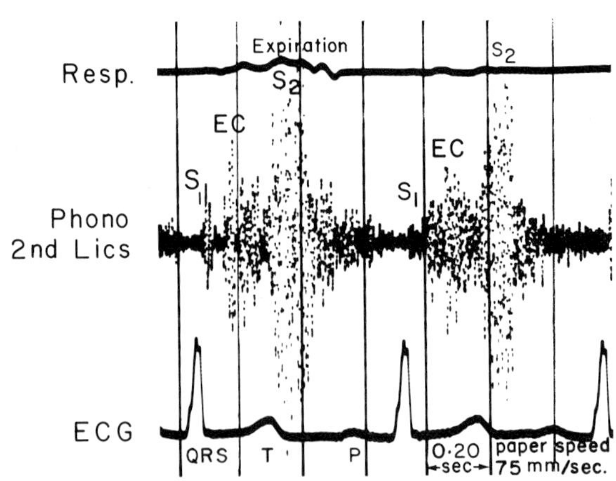

Figure 124. The phonocardiogram of a 5-year-old patient with a patent ductus arteriosus secondary to post-rubella syndrome. Note that peak accentuation of the continuous murmur centers around the second heart sound.

the murmur becomes more obvious with time cannot be stated on the basis of our evidence.

Older children rarely have significant symptoms. Forty-four percent of the children in one series were discovered on routine physical examination. This certainly must be considered a plus for routine examinations of apparently normal children!

A continuous machinery-like murmur, loudest in the second left intercostal space at the sternal margin and under the left clavicle, is heard in about 85% of children (Figure 124). Peak accentuation of the murmur centers around the second sound and often obscures it. There is usually a diastolic flow murmur at the apex, secondary to increased flow through the left heart. Neonates with patent ductus arteriosus have a variety of murmurs (Table 20). We have seen neonates with systolic murmurs alone, only a diastolic murmur, a murmur of mitral insufficiency, and even infants with no murmur at all (Figure 125). Thus a high index of suspicion is warranted, especially if the peripheral arterial pulses are easily palpable.

A widened pulse pressure is a frequent and valuable finding. This is due to flow of blood from aorta to pulmonary artery, hemodynamically similar to cases of aortic regurgitation, large systemic AV fistulas, or truncus arteriosus.

Extracardiac anomalies are found frequently in infants, especially those with post-rubella syndrome. They are found in only 5% of older children.

ROENTGENOGRAPHIC FEATURES

During infancy, chest x-rays almost invariably reveal increased pulmonary vasculature, gross cardiomegaly, and enlargement of the left atrium. In con-

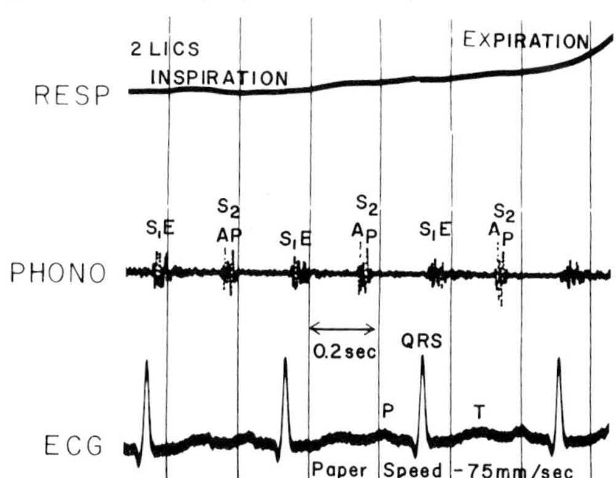

Figure 125. Phonocardiogram of an 8-month-old girl with a large surgically proven patent ductus arteriosus. When the pulmonary artery pressure approximates the pressure in the aorta, the murmur may be unimpressive or even absent, as in this child. (From Cruze, K., Elliott, L. P., Schiebler, G. L., and Wheat, M. W., Jr. 1963. Unusual manifestations of patent ductus arteriosus in infancy. Dis. Chest. 43:563.

trast, x-rays of older children usually show a normal or slightly enlarged heart with normal or slightly increased pulmonary arterial markings (Figure 126).

An increase in the size of the ascending aorta is produced by the increased flow traversing this portion of the aorta. The aorta may be slightly to markedly enlarged. At times, the ductus arteriosus itself may be visible as an extra bump between the aortic knob and the pulmonic trunk at the left upper mediastinal border.

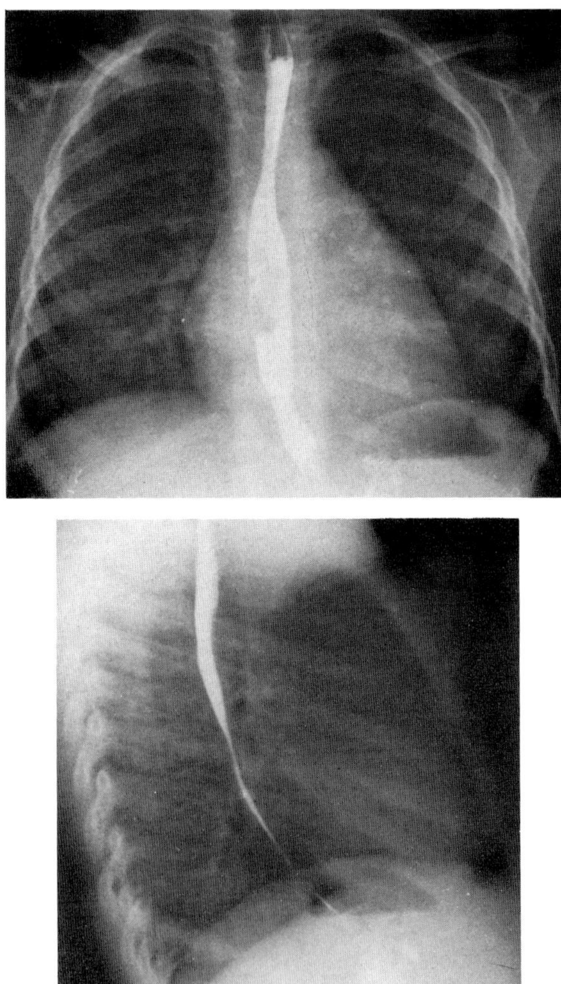

Figure 126. Chest x-ray of a 4-year-old male with patent ductus arteriosus. These x-rays show minimal cardiomegaly, a suggestive left ventricular contour, and perhaps increased pulmonary vascularity. A casual observer might pass these by as within normal limits.

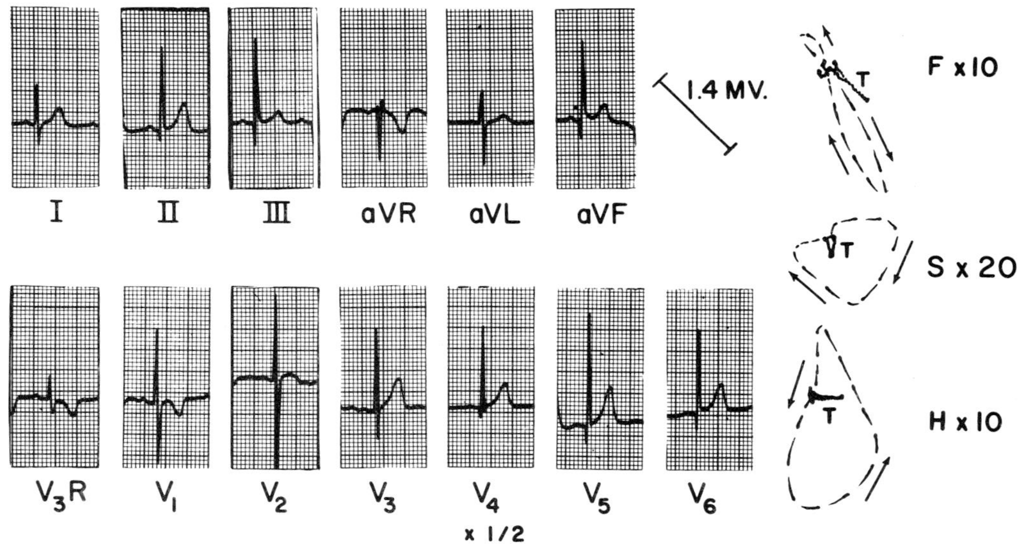

Figure 127. Electrocardiogram and vectorcardiogram of a 4-year-old patient with a patent ductus arteriosus. The rounding of the RS-T segment seen in leads II, III, aVF, and V_6 is common in patients with patent ductus arteriosus. The contour of the T waves in leads V_5 and V_6 suggests left ventricular volume overloading, and the entire pattern suggests mild biventricular hypertrophy.

Table 20. Physical findings in patent ductus arteriosus[a]

Murmur	Under 1 year (percentage)	Over 1 year (percentage)
Machinery-like	26	90
Systolic and diastolic	15	5
Systolic only	59	5
Thrill	52	17
Pulse pressure		
under 40 mm Hg	0	8
40–49 mm Hg	21	19
50–59 mm Hg	7	24
60 mm Hg and over	72	49

[a] Adapted from Krovetz, L. J., and Warden, H. E. 1962. Patent ductus arteriosus. An analysis of 515 surgically proven cases. Dis. Chest 42:46.

ELECTROCARDIOGRAPHY

In infancy, the most common electrographic pattern is that of biventricular hypertrophy, similar to that seen with a ventricular septal defect. In older children, the electrocardiogram is normal in approximately 60% of cases and shows left ventricular hypertrophy in an additional 25%.

A coved RS-T segment is found in nearly two-thirds of older children (Figure 127). This coving is far less frequent in other forms of congenital heart disease. When the differential diagnosis is either a ventricular septal defect or a patent ductus arteriosus, the presence of a coved RS-T segment would suggest a patent ductus arteriosus.

DIFFERENTIAL DIAGNOSIS

A large ventricular septal defect may be difficult to differentiate from a PDA when the PDA is manifested by a loud systolic murmur only, as often occurs in infancy. In both, the pulmonic component of S_2 may be increased and a mitral flow murmur may be present. Persistent careful auscultation at the left base, especially with the infant quiet or asleep, may reward the listener with recognition that the murmur extends slightly into diastole, confirming the diagnosis of PDA. In both anomalies the peripheral pulses may be increased, but the increase with a PDA is far more striking. Frequently, however, cardiac catheterization will be required to establish the diagnosis unequivocally.

Ventricular septal defect with aortic insufficiency has a murmur that superficially mimics that of patent ductus arteriosus; however, the diastolic component is higher pitched than in PDA. The murmur also does not have the crescendo type of accentuation surrounding S_2 that is usually found in patent ductus arteriosus.

A ruptured aortic sinus of Valsalva or a *coronary-cardiac fistula* may also mimic a PDA. However, in these anomalies the diastolic component of the murmur is at least as loud as if not louder than the systolic component.

Truncus arteriosus is sometimes difficult to differentiate from PDA. If the clinical findings are not completely typical for a PDA, cardiac catheterization and angiocardiography are warranted.

PROGNOSIS

The vast majority of children are asymptomatic and have an excellent prognosis, except for the risks of infective endocarditis and congestive heart failure later in life. Infective endocarditis rarely occurs before age 5. In one series, 13% of patients over 20 years of age had congestive heart failure.

Since transient patency of the ductus arteriosus may occur in normal newborns, there may be some question as to when a ductus that is patent in early infancy is abnormal. When symptoms can be attributed to its presence, however, there can be little doubt that it is abnormal. Even then, it is still possible for a ductus to close spontaneously. Small premature infants may develop congestive heart failure secondary to a patent ductus arteriosus, especially in the presence of severe respiratory distress syndrome. With digitalization, diuretics, and restriction of fluids, the murmurs and wide pulse pressures have disappeared with closure of the PDA.

In full-term patients with patent ductus arteriosus, spontaneous closure rarely occurs. This is particularly true of children who have a large symptomatic PDA during the first year of life. Cosh reported four patients with typical murmurs of PDA in whom the murmur spontaneously disappeared. Unfortunately, none of these was catheterized either before or after the "closure" of the patent ductus arteriosus.

MANAGEMENT

Surgical results for this lesion are among the best for any cardiac defect. Overall mortality rate is less than 2%, even though the patients operated on range in age from a few months to over 60 years. The results of surgery are so gratifying that we recommend prompt surgery for a symptomatic patient unless there is some other problem that needs prior attention. Although a few of these ducti *might* close spontaneously later in life, the risk of waiting is greater than the risk of surgery. For the usual asymptomatic child, timing of surgery should depend first on local surgical results and second on the desires of the parents.

Obviously, children with pneumonia or congestive heart failure should be treated prior to surgery. However, prolonged procrastination is unwise. If the infant does not respond to medical management with clearing of congestive heart failure and pneumonia within 2 days, surgery should not be further postponed. We have seen several dramatic instances of clearing of chronic pneumonia following surgical closure of a large PDA.

In *premature infants* without RDS, an attempt should be made to control congestive heart failure by use of digitalis, diuretics, and limitation of fluid intake. If this is successful, surgery may be postponed for 3 months or longer, since many of these ducti will close spontaneously. For those premature infants whose congestive heart failure cannot be controlled medically within 48 hr, closure is indicated, either surgically or pharmacologically (see below).

In the *infant with RDS and PDA,* the management problem becomes much more complex. It is often difficult to tell which part of the clinical picture is due to respiratory disease and which part is cardiac in nature. Demonstration by echocardiography that the left atrium is considerably larger than normal may be helpful in documenting significant left atrial overloading secondary to a large left-to-right shunt and may warrant concentration on the PDA. Early evidence would indicate that the closure of a PDA in a premature infant with respiratory distress syndrome will reduce the amount or need for respirators and even shorten the length of time needed in the intensive care unit, but may not prevent the development of chronic lung disease, such as bronchopulmonary dysplasia.

Recently, indomethacin, a prostaglandin antagonist, has been demonstrated to cause pharmacological closure of the ductus. Prostaglandin administration can maintain patency of the ductus, benefiting infants with ductus-dependent cyanotic heart disease. These techniques are potentially valuable, particularly for tiny prematures with respiratory distress syndrome or other complicating lesions that would tend to increase the hazard of surgery. The long-term hazards of indomethacin and prostaglandins are still unknown. Obviously these drugs have the potential for affecting arterial musculature in many blood vessels. Our suggestion at the present time is that their use be restricted to major centers that are involved in clinical research of those potent drugs and that have the capacity (and obligation) to conduct appropriate long-term follow-up studies.

BIBLIOGRAPHY

Cosh, J. A. 1957. Patent ductus arteriosus: A follow-up study of 73 cases. Br. Heart J. 19:13–22.

Cruze, K., Elliott, L. P., Schiebler, G. L., and Wheat, M. W., Jr. 1963. Unusual manifestations of patent ductus arteriosus in infancy. Dis. Chest 43:563–571.

Friedman, W. F., Hirschklau, M. J., Printz, M. P., Pitlick, P. T., and Kirkpatrick, S. E. 1976. Pharmacologic closure of patent ductus arteriosus in the premature infant. N. Engl. J. Med. 295:526–529.

Kilman, J. W., Sirak, H. D., Clatworthy, H. W., Jr., Craenen, J., and Hosier, D. M. 1970. The case for the early closure of a patent ductus arteriosus. Surgery 67:197–203.

Krovetz, L. J. 1963. Weight gain in children with patent ductus arteriosus. Dis. Chest 44:274–283.

Krovetz, L. J., Lester, R. G., and Warden, H. E. The diagnosis of patent ductus arteriosus in infancy. Dis. Chest 42:241–250.

Krovetz, L. J., and Warden, H. E. 1962. Patent ductus arteriosus. An analysis of 515 surgically proven cases. Dis. Chest 42:46–57.

Oberhansli-Weiss, Haymann, M. A., Rudolph, A. M., and Melon, K. L. 1972. The pattern and mechanisms of response to oxygen by the ductus arteriosus and umbilical artery. Pediat. Res. 6:693–700.

Rudolph, A. M., Scarpelli, E. M., Golinko, R. J., and Gootman, N. L. 1964. Hemodynamic basis for clinical manifestations of patent ductus arteriosus. Am. Heart J. 68:447–458.

Zachman, R. D., Steinmetz, G. P., Botham, R. J., Graven, S. N., and Ledbetter, M. K. 1974. Incidence and treatment of the patent ductus arteriosus in the ill premature neonate. Am. Heart J. 87:697–703.

chapter 17

TOTAL ANOMALOUS PULMONARY VENOUS CONNECTION

HISTORICAL NOTES

Total anomalous pulmonary venous connection (TAPVC) was first described by Wilson in 1798. By 1942, Brody was able to locate only 38 cases in the medical literature. In the next two decades Gott et al. reported 30 personal cases and Darling et al. reported an additional 17 personal cases, clarifying the classification and clinical features of TAPVC. Kauffman et al. in 1962 first clearly described those cases of TAPVC to the left superior vena cava, in which obstruction occurs, a point also emphasized by Elliott and Edwards that same year. Reports of successful surgical repair by Burroughs and Kirklin and by Lewis et al. appeared in 1956.

INCIDENCE

This defect occurs with equal frequency in both sexes and accounts for approximately 1% of all congenital heart anomalies.

EMBRYOLOGY

The basic malformation is considered to be a failure of development of the common pulmonary vein from the left atrium. The pulmonary venous system is forced to develop an alternate drainage pathway. Because of its intimate connection with other developing venous systems (see Chapter 2), this alternate drainage can be via several routes.

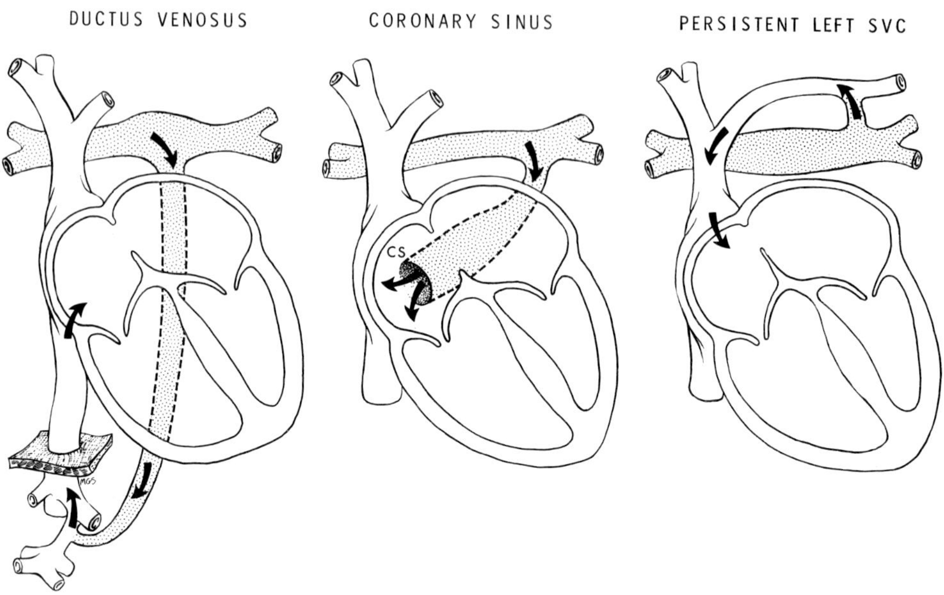

Figure 128. Schema of the venous circulation in total anomalous pulmonary venous connection. Shown are examples of infracardiac, cardiac, and supracardiac drainage. Regardless of the site of connection, there is an obligatory shunt at the atrial level.

PATHOLOGY

Many combinations of anomalous pulmonary venous connection may occur. Partial anomalous venous connection, in which some pulmonary veins connect normally to the left atrium and some abnormally, is rather common, particularly in association with atrial septal defects of the sinus venosus type.

Table 21. Occurrence of drainage site in total anomalous pulmonary venous connection (composite of reported literature)

Type of TAPVC	Cases (N = 513)	Incidence (percentage)
Supracardiac		
Left superior vena cava	203	40
Right superior vena cava	63	12
Cardiac		
Coronary sinus	83	16
Right atrium	65	13
Infracardiac	65	13
(Portal veins, ductus venosus, hepatic veins, or inferior vena cava)		
Mixed drainage sites	34	7

Table 22. Pulmonary venous obstruction in TAPVC (excluding complex varieties)

Author	Year	Age (years)	Total	Obstructed
Behrendt	1972	< 1	37	9 (24%)
Carter	1969	0–12	58	11 (19%)
El-Said	1972	< 2	35	16 (46%)
Gathman	1970	0–16	75	40 (53%)
Totals			205	76 (37%)

Total anomalous pulmonary venous connection is complicated by the presence of other cardiac anomalies in about one-fourth of cases. However, this discussion is limited to the more common form, unassociated with any other major cardiovascular anomaly.

In TAPVC, all four pulmonary veins are connected either directly or indirectly to the right atrium. An interatrial communication is the only route by which pulmonary venous blood enters the left atrium and thence the left ventricle and aorta (Figure 128). This opening may range from a 3–4 mm patent foramen ovale to a large secundum atrial septal defect, or (rarely) an ostium primum defect.

TAPVC can be divided into four major groups based on the level of entrance of the pulmonary venous return (Table 21). Of more importance from a clinical point of view is the presence of obstructed pulmonary venous drainage.

Some degree of obstruction of the pulmonary venous pathway is seen in nearly 40% of TAPVC (Table 22). In the infracardiac type, once the ductus venosus closes, pulmonary venous blood must traverse the hepatic portal capillary system before reaching the heart. Obstruction may also occur with supracardiac drainage, when, for example, the left superior vena cava is compressed between the left pulmonary artery and the left main stem bronchus. Internal anatomic stenosis of the individual pulmonary veins may also occur, but fortunately is rare, since this makes surgical repair more difficult.

In unobstructed forms of TAPVC, the right atrium, right ventricle, and pulmonary artery are hypertrophied and dilated. In all forms, because the common pulmonary vein is not incorporated, the left atrium is reduced in size. Its subsequent development, as well as that of the left ventricle, depends on the amount of blood flow reaching the left heart.

HEMODYNAMICS

Pulmonary hypertension is nearly always seen in those cases presenting in infancy. In contrast, cases first detected at an older age have normal or only slightly elevated pulmonary artery pressures. Obstruction to pulmonary venous drainage may result in pressure differences of 30 mm Hg or more across the site of obstruction.

There is marked volume overloading of the right heart, since both systemic and pulmonary venous blood return to the right atrium. Because all oxygenated blood entering the left heart must first pass through the right heart, oxygen saturations in the right heart are equal to or greater than those in the systemic circulation. An increase in oxygen saturation occurs at the site of insertion of the anomalous pulmonary veins. This is particularly helpful at cardiac catheterization if the increase occurs in either the inferior or superior vena cava.

CLINICAL FEATURES

Over 80% of TAPVC patients are asymptomatic in infancy. Tachypnea, poor feeding, and failure to gain weight are common early symptoms. Frank congestive failure is seen in about one-half of affected patients, usually prior to 3 months of age.

Mild cyanosis, which may not be easily appreciated, is seen in nearly all cases. A widely split second sound with accentuation of the pulmonic component is a valuable sign, but may be difficult to appreciate in an infant with a rapid heart rate. A right ventricular parasternal lift and a systolic thrill occasionally are present. A pulmonary systolic ejection murmur is almost invariably present, and a tricuspid diastolic flow murmur may be heard. Continuous murmurs may be audible over the sites of drainage of the anomalous veins.

With obstruction to pulmonary venous drainage or when pulmonary resistance is elevated, the clinical findings will be appropriately modified. The patient is more cyanotic, and usually in distress shortly after birth. These infants demonstrate pulmonary edema, tachycardia, and marked tachypnea. Since pulmonary blood flow is reduced, the murmurs are either absent or unimpressive. The systolic ejection murmur is softer, and the tricuspid flow murmur is often absent. The second sound will not be widely split, whereas the pulmonic component may be quite loud. A loud fourth heart sound is common.

ROENTGENOGRAPHIC FEATURES

The right atrium, the right ventricle, and the main pulmonary artery are enlarged and the pulmonary markings are increased. Most patients with pulmonary venous obstruction have normal-sized hearts, with a vascular pattern of pulmonary venous engorgement (Figure 129). With TAPVC to the left superior vena cava, the cardiac shadow may resemble a snowman or a figure eight, establishing the diagnosis as well as the drainage site (Figures 130 and 131).

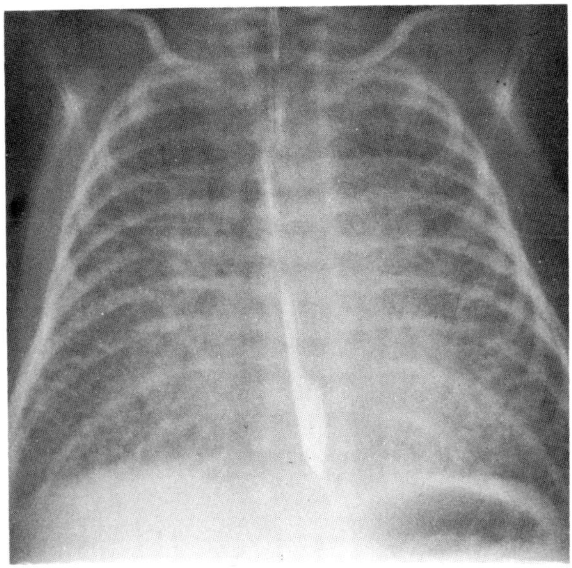

Figure 129. X-ray of a 10-day-old child showing a diffuse mottled appearance of entire lung fields, characteristic of severe pulmonary venous obstruction. In this instance, the pulmonary venous return was obstructed at the junction with the innominate vein. A similar picture is seen in infracardiac return.

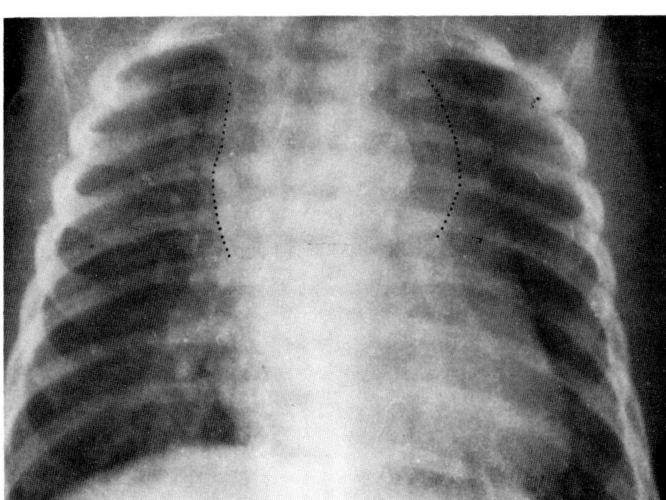

Figure 130. Total anomalous pulmonary return illustrating the "snowman" contour, which is partially obscured by the thymus. The great vessels (persistent left superior vena cava) and the heart form the outline of the snowman or figure eight. These x-rays were taken at 2 days of age. The angiocardiogram of the same patient appears in Figure 131.

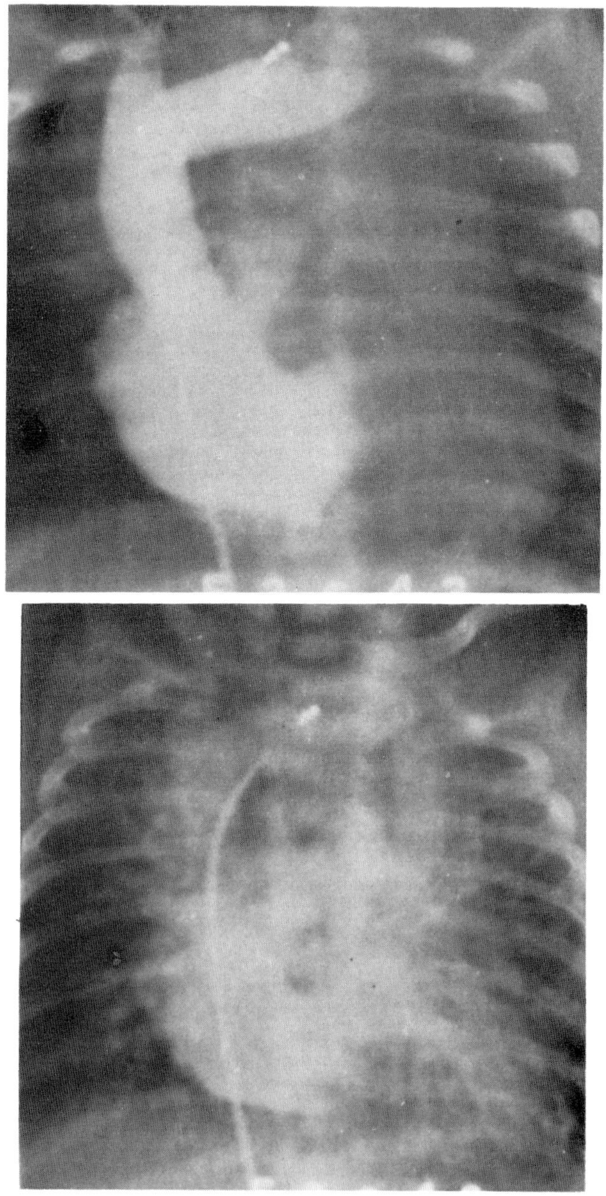

Figure 131. (Top) The catheter is in the innominate vein and contrast media may be seen to fill a large distended innominate vein, the right superior vena cava, and the right atrium. (Bottom) The contrast media has now recirculated through the lungs and outlines the persistent left superior vena cava. This illustrates how the top part of the snowman is formed.

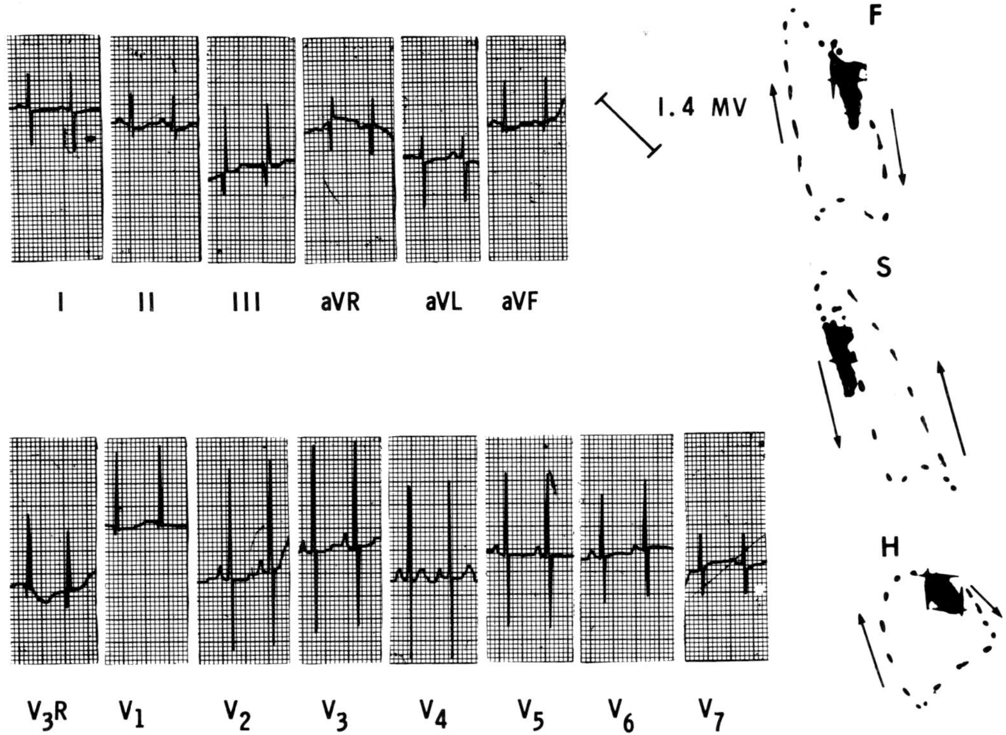

Figure 132. Electrocardiogram of a 30-day-old child with total anomalous return. Note particularly the q in lead V_3R and tne absence of a q in left precordial leads. This is indicative of marked right ventricular hypertrophy.

It is occasionally possible to detect a dilated coronary sinus on a lateral chest roentgenogram as a small, discrete indentation on the barium-filled esophagus at approximately the same level as one would expect to find an impression caused by the left atrium. However, the size of the impression is significantly smaller than would be caused by true left atrial enlargement. Similarly, infracardiac total anomalous pulmonary venous return may be marked by a small impression on the barium-filled esophagus, seen in the lateral view, as the common pulmonary vein passes through the diaphragm. This small impression just above the diaphragm, if detected with other evidence of pulmonary venous obstruction, is virtually diagnostic.

ELECTROCARDIOGRAPHY

Right axis deviation is usually found, but (rarely) there may be superior axis deviation due to a complicating ostium primum defect or an abnormality of atrial conduction. Right ventricular hypertrophy and right atrial enlargement are always present. A qR pattern in lead V_1 is seen in approximately 35% of patients (Figure 132). Patients with lower right ventricular pressures and higher pulmonary:systemic flow ratios show more leftward QRS forces. A small q wave in lead V_6 may be seen, indicating the presence of a ventricular septum, but left ventricular hypertrophy is not consistent with TAPVC.

DIFFERENTIAL DIAGNOSIS

Hypoplastic left heart syndrome need be considered only during the first month.

Common atrium frequently will show left axis deviation, whereas this is rare in total anomalous pulmonary venous connection.

Atrial septal defect, with or without partial anomalous return, will not cause cyanosis or pulmonary hypertension in childhood. Atrial septal defect in association with primary pulmonary hypertension can usually be differentiated only by catheterization.

Cor triatriatum and *mitral stenosis* may be indistinguishable from obstructive total anomalous pulmonary venous return without catheterization.

Respiratory distress syndrome is more likely in premature infants with labored respiration within a few hours after birth.

PROGNOSIS

With medical management alone, 70% of patients will die prior to their first birthday and less than 5% survive past their tenth year. Survival is closely related to the degree of pulmonary hypertension, which in turn depends largely on the type of anomalous venous drainage and the presence of pulmonary venous obstruction. Survival is longest in patients without obstruction to pulmonary venous return and in whom a large interatrial communication exists. Average life span is poorest in TAPVC with pulmonary venous obstruction, usually being less than 1 month. Early onset of severe cyanosis usually means an early death. Rarely, a patient may be asymptomatic and reach adult life before this cardiac anomaly is diagnosed.

MANAGEMENT

Patients presenting with congestive heart failure should be appropriately treated with digoxin and diuretics as well as other supportive measures. After stabilization or if no improvement is evident, cardiac catheterization should be carried out promptly. On confirmation of the diagnosis of unobstructed total anomalous pulmonary venous return, balloon atrial septostomy should be done to allow freer communication between the atria. Because of the small left atrial size and the fact that many patients are 2 to 3 months old when first seen, this procedure is more difficult to accomplish than in neonates with complete transposition of the great arteries. However, if successful, balloon atrial septostomy may permit delaying definitive surgery for several months. Patients with severe pulmonary venous obstruction will not benefit from balloon septostomy and must be operated on without delay.

Complete repair must usually be accomplished in infancy. Although previously published figures indicated an overall operative mortality of 40% or more, recent surgical results have been more encouraging. After 3 months of age, operative mortality should be 20% or less and, after 1 year of age, under 5%. Of 14 consecutive patients less than 1 year of age operated on at the University of Florida from 1968 to 1978, 12 are now alive and well. Sporadic reports of successful repair on infracardiac total anomalous pulmonary venous return have also appeared in recent years.

Since the heart itself is usually anatomically normal, there is at least a theoretical basis for surgical cure in all of these patients. Thus each patient deserves rapid and vigorous diagnosis and treatment. Prompt, accurate diagnosis, palliative balloon atrial septostomy, and early referral to a cardiovascular center with acceptably low operative mortality are the best ways to increase survival.

BIBLIOGRAPHY

Behrendt, D. M., Aberdeen, E., Waterson, D. J., and Bonham-Carter, R. E. 1972. Total anomalous pulmonary venous drainage in infants. I. Clinical and hemodynamic findings, methods and results of operation in 37 cases. Circulation 46:347–356.

Bonham-Carter, R. E., Capriles, M., and Noe, Y. 1969. Total anomalous pulmonary venous drainage. Br. Heart J. 31:45–51.

El-Said, G., Mullins, C. E., and McNamara, D. G. 1972. Management of total anomalous pulmonary venous return. Circulation 45:1240–1250.

Gathman, G. E., and Nadas, A. S. 1970. Total anomalous pulmonary venous connection. Circulation 42:142–154.

Haworth, S. G., and Reid, L. 1977. Structural study of pulmonary circulation and of heart in total anomalous pulmonary venous return in early infancy. Br. Heart J. 39:80–92.

Jensen, J. B., and Blount, S. G., Jr. 1971. Total anomalous pulmonary venous return. Am. Heart J. 82:387–407.

Mathew, R., Thilenius, O. G., Replogle, R. L., and Arcilla, R. A. 1977. Cardiac function in total anomalous pulmonary venous return before and after surgery. Circulation 55:361–370.

Nakazawa, M., Jarmakani, J. M., Gyepes, M. T., Prochazka, J. V., Yabek, S. M., and Marks, R. A. 1977. Pre- and postoperative ventricular function in infants and children with right ventricular volume overload. Circulation 55:479–484.

chapter 18

COMPLETE TRANSPOSITION OF THE GREAT ARTERIES

HISTORICAL NOTES

After recorded observations by Steno (1672), Baillie (1797), Langstaff (1811), and Farre (1814), von Rokitansky, in 1875, presented a systematic classification of transposition of the great arteries (TGA). Spitzer, in 1923, described four degrees of transposition and offered a phylogenetic theory of origin. Antemortem recognition on clinical grounds was shown to be possible by Fanconi in 1930, who recognized that a narrow vascular pedicle on x-ray was characteristic. Castellanos demonstrated in 1937 that the diagnosis could be established by the injection of radiopaque material into the heart.

Blalock and Hanlon, in 1948, created an artificial atrial septal defect to increase the degree of mixing. Lillehei and Varco (1953), Baffes (1956), and Edwards (1964) tried to reroute the great veins, and Mustard (1954), Bailey (1954), and Kay (1955) attempted to transpose the great vessels. However, in this latter operation the coronary arteries now arose from the venous trunk, and attempts to transpose them were generally unsuccessful. The operation currently in use was developed in 1964 by Mustard, who devised an ingenious technique of rerouting the venous inflows using a pericardial tunnel. In 1966, Raskind developed a technique for creating atrial septal defects at the time of catheterization.

INCIDENCE

TGA is the most common severe congenital cardiac anomaly, especially during infancy, comprising 12% of all autopsied cases of congenital heart lesions. Males predominate by a ratio of almost three to one.

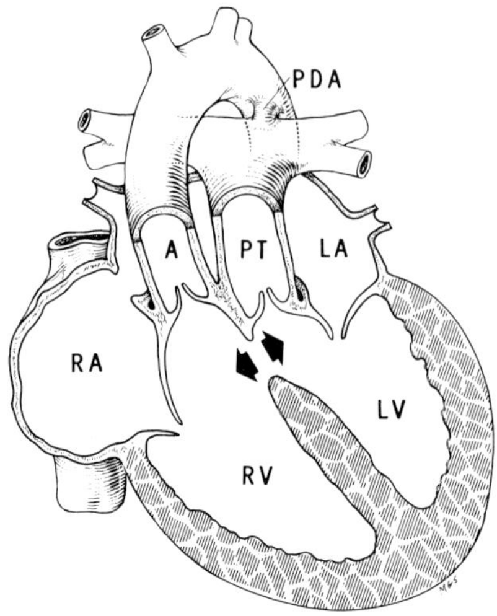

Figure 133. Schema of the intracardiac circulation in complete transposition of the great vessels. Although mixing is shown at the ventricular as well as the atrial level, mixing only at the atrial level is more common. (From Elliott, L. P., and Schiebler, G. L. 1968. X-Ray Diagnosis of Congenital Cardiac Disease. Courtesy of Charles C Thomas, Publisher, Springfield, Ill.)

PATHOLOGY

Complete transposition of the great arteries with an intact ventricular septum is the most common type, accounting for one-half of our cases (Table 23). The architecture of the ventricles is essentially normal, but usually the right and left ventricular walls are of equal thickness. The aorta emerges from the right ventricle and the pulmonary artery emerges from the left ventricle. The aorta is situated anteriorly and to the right and the pulmonary artery posteriorly and to the left (Figure 133). The pulmonary artery may be larger than or equal to the aorta. The coronary arteries always arise from the aorta. Additional cardiac or noncardiac anomalies are rare, and this is an important point in differential diagnosis.

Table 23. Autopsy findings in cases of TGA[a]

Group	Total cases	Autopsied cases	PFO	PDA	VSD	Single ventricle	Pulmonic stenosis
1	37	20	19	14	3	0	0
2	11	5	4	0	5	0	0
3	10	4	2	0	3	1	3
4	8	7	5	4	3	3	0
5	10	5	2	1	3	1	3

[a] Conducted at the J. Hillis Miller Health Center, Gainesville, Florida.

Complete transposition with ventricular septal defect is next in frequency, accounting for one-fifth of our total cases. The position of the arterial trunks is essentially the same as in the previous type, but the pulmonary artery is usually larger than in those cases with an intact septum. The ventricular septal defect may be in almost any area of the septum, but is most commonly posterior and inferior to the crista supraventricularis. The VSD is usually large and the architecture of the right ventricle may be abnormal.

Complete transposition with pulmonic stenosis accounts for 5% of our series of complete TGAs. These patients nearly always have an additional ventricular septal defect. Either the pulmonic orifice or the subpulmonic area may be narrow. A bicuspid pulmonic valve is a common finding, and the pulmonary artery is smaller than the aorta. The ductus arteriosus is usually closed. A right aortic arch is sometimes seen with this grouping.

In *complete transposition with a single ventricle,* there is usually a hypoplastic outlet chamber, which may give rise to either the pulmonary artery or the aorta. These vessels may be arranged in the configuration of either d-loop or l-loop transposition (see Chapter 19). The main ventricular chamber, which is usually the left ventricle, receives both mitral and tricuspid valve orifices.

Of our 14 patients with *complete transposition with obstruction to systemic arterial flow,* 13 had coarctation of the aorta and one had complete interruption of the aortic arch. Seven of these patients had an associated ventricular septal defect, five a single ventricle, and two an intact ventricular septum with a patent ductus arteriosus.

Complete transposition may also be associated with *complex lesions* such as dextroversion and absent spleen syndrome (asplenia). Associated lesions include single atrium, single ventricle, pulmonic atresia, absence of the hepatic portion of the inferior vena cava, total anomalous pulmonary venous connection, vascular ring, and right aortic arch. As if this weren't enough, there are often extracardiac anomalies as well.

HEMODYNAMICS

Patients with complete transposition of the great vessels can be divided into five main functional groups:

1. Patients with *inadequate mixing* of pulmonary and systemic venous blood, either intra- or extracardiac. These patients usually have an intact ventricular system, but may have a small VSD. The only opportunity for mixing of systemic return and pulmonary return is through a small foramen ovale or a patent ductus arteriosus. In these cases left atrial pressure becomes elevated and some degree of pulmonary venous congestion is present.

2. Patients with *adequate mixing* usually have large ventricular septal defects or even a single ventricle. These patients generally have higher pulmonary blood flows and left atrial pressures than those found in Group 1. The degree of cyanosis is less than seen in Group 1 patients.
3. Patients with *adequate mixing and obstruction to pulmonary flow* have varying pulmonary blood flow, ranging from slightly high to grossly inadequate, and the flow is lower than in either Group 1 or Group 2 patients. Left atrial pressures are usually normal and there is no pulmonary venous hypertension. There is usually more cyanosis than in Group 2 patients.
4. Patients with *associated aortic anomalies* causing obstruction to systemic arterial flow may have either the obstruction or the transposition as the dominant hemodynamic feature.
5. Patients with *complex lesions* (these are not discussed further in this chapter).

CLINICAL FEATURES

Infants with complete transposition of the great arteries usually have normal birth weights, since the anomaly is of little hemodynamic consequence prior to birth. Cyanosis is noted at birth or within 3 days in the vast majority of patients. Cyanosis tends to be most severe in patients with inadequate mixing or with inadequate pulmonary blood flow. However, the purplish appearance of intense cyanosis that is seen in tricuspid atresia or pulmonic atresia is rarely seen with complete TGA. Hypercyanotic spells are seen only with Group 3 patients. Clubbing may be seen as early as 5 months. Clubbing and cyanosis are constant and severe in older children in all groups.

Congestive heart failure, with its triad of tachypnea, cardiomegaly, and hepatomegaly, usually occurs within the first month of life. It is less commonly seen in TGA with adequate mixing, and rare in TGA with pulmonary obstruction (Table 24).

Table 24. Clinical findings of complete transposition of the great arteries, grouped according to hemodynamic status[a]

Group	Number of cases	Sex M	Sex F	CHF within first month	Murmurs: Systolic grade 0–2	Murmurs: Grade 3–4	Murmurs: Apical diastolic
1	37	28	9	78%	33	4	2
2	11	7	4	18%	3	8	7
3	10	7	3	10%	2	4	0
4	8	5	3	87%	2	6	4
5	10	7	3	60%	1	7	4

[a] Data collected at the J. Hillis Miller Health Center, Gainesville, Florida.

In patients with inadequate mixing (Group 1), the systolic murmur is usually short, decrescendo, and of only grade 1 or 2 intensity on a scale of 6 (Figure 134). Apical mid-diastolic flow murmurs are uncommon, but summation sounds (S_3 and S_4) are heard in 80% of patients. In patients with a VSD, the systolic murmur is usually of grade 3 to 4 intensity and apical mid- and late diastolic flow murmurs are common, except for those with inadequate pulmonary blood flow (Group 3). The second heart sound is usually single. Although a patent ductus arteriosus is commonly present, the elevated pulmonary artery pressure precludes the usual continuous murmur. Patients with TGA and obstruction to systemic arterial blood flow may present with either the symptoms of TGA or coarctation predominating.

ROENTGENOGRAPHIC FEATURES

In infants under 2 weeks of age, both cardiac size and pulmonary vascularity may be normal. After 2 weeks of age, the cardiac configuration is typically egg-shaped, with a narrow base and apparent diminution of the thymic shadow and the pulmonary artery segment (Figure 135). Pulmonary arterial and venous marking may both be increased. Pulmonary vascularity is decreased only in patients with inadequate blood flow (Group 3).

Patients with adequate mixing and excessive pulmonary blood flow usually show enlargement of both ventricles, whereas only right heart enlarge-

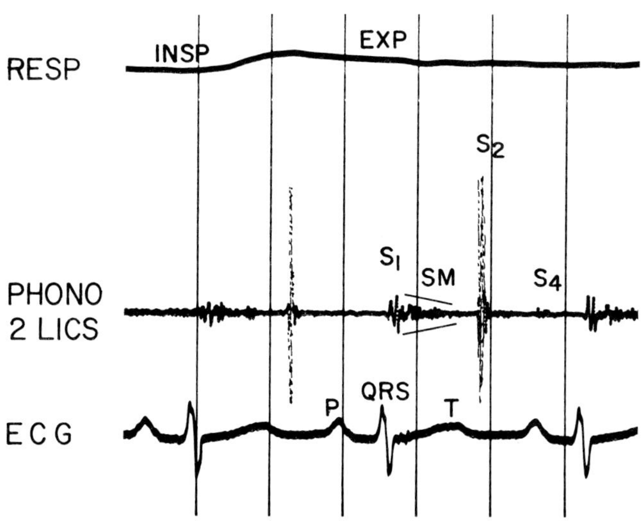

Figure 134. Phonocardiogram of a 15-month child with complete transposition of the great vessels with intact ventricular septum. In the common case, with intact ventricular septum and no pulmonic stenosis, the murmurs are quite innocuous. Note the loud single second sound caused by prominent closure of the anteriorly placed aorta. (From Elliott, L. P., and Schiebler, G. L. 1968. X-Ray Diagnosis of Congenital Cardiac Disease. Courtesy of Charles C Thomas, Publisher, Springfield, Ill.)

ment is evident in patients with inadequate mixing (Group 1) or with decreased pulmonary blood flow (Group 3).

Right atrial enlargement is seen most commonly when inadequate mixing is present. Patients with adequate mixing and excess pulmonary blood flow or associated aortic arch obstruction usually have evidence of left atrial enlargement.

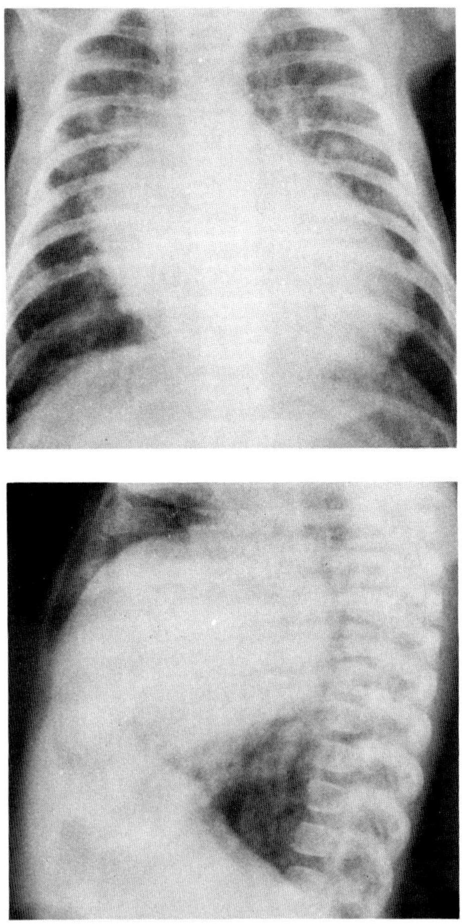

Figure 135. Chest x-ray of a patient with complete transposition of the great vessels. The narrow upper mediastinum and massive cardiomegaly cause the heart to look like a tilted hen's egg. The plethoric lung fields are probably due to both pulmonary arterial and pulmonary venous components, indicating congestive heart failure as well as increased flow. In the lateral view, there is a clear space behind the sternum, which in the presence of right ventricular hypertrophy indicates that the pulmonary artery is either absent or not in the normal location. (From Morgan, A. D., Krovetz, L. J., Schiebler, G. L., Shanklin, D. R., Wheat, M. W., Jr., and Bartley, T. D. 1965. Diagnosis and palliative surgery in complete transposition of the great vessels. Ann. Thorac. Surg. 1:711.)

ELECTROCARDIOGRAPHY

Patients with inadequate mixing usually have right axis deviation, right atrial enlargement, and right ventricular hypertrophy (Figure 136 and Table 25). Obviously, this pattern may be difficult to differentiate from normal right ventricular preponderance during the first few days of life.

Patients with adequate mixing usually exhibit a biventricular hypertrophy pattern (Figure 137), although those with decreased pulmonary blood flow usually have isolated right ventricular hypertrophy. In infants with single ventricles or aortic arch obstruction, there are often left axis deviation and left ventricular hypertrophy (Figure 138).

Isolated right atrial enlargement is seen with inadequate mixing or obstruction to pulmonary flow, whereas both left and right atrial enlargement is seen in patients with excessive pulmonary blood flow (Group 2).

DIFFERENTIAL DIAGNOSIS

Aortic atresia usually presents with fulminating congestive heart failure, weak peripheral pulses, and varying degrees of cyanosis during the first week of life, whereas the pulses are usually normal in TGA.

Respiratory distress syndrome has its initial onset within hours after birth, a time when complete transposition cases are asymptomatic.

Pulmonary atresia and *tricuspid atresia* usually have more profound cyanosis.

Ebstein's anomaly of the tricuspid valve may present with cyanosis, massive cardiomegaly, and profound failure during the first week. Patients who survive the first week improve markedly with time. In Ebstein's anomaly, electrocardiograms rarely reveal right ventricular hypertrophy, but may show WPW, 1° AV block, or right bundle branch block.

Hyperviscosity syndrome is manifested by a high hematocrit (greater than 60%), irritability, and cyanosis, with congestive heart failure occurring

Table 25. Electrocardiographic findings in TGA patients[a]

		Atrial enlargement			Ventricular hypertrophy[b]		
Group	Number of cases	Right	Left	Both	Right	Left	Both
1	37	20	0	9	34	0	3
2	11	2	1	8	5	2	4
3	10	3	0	1	4	2	0
4	8	0	1	7	0	5	3
5	10	5	0	0	4	2	0

[a] Seen at the J. Hillis Miller Health Center, Gainesville, Florida.

[b] In some cases, the precordial QRS complexes were normal or the pattern was indeterminate.

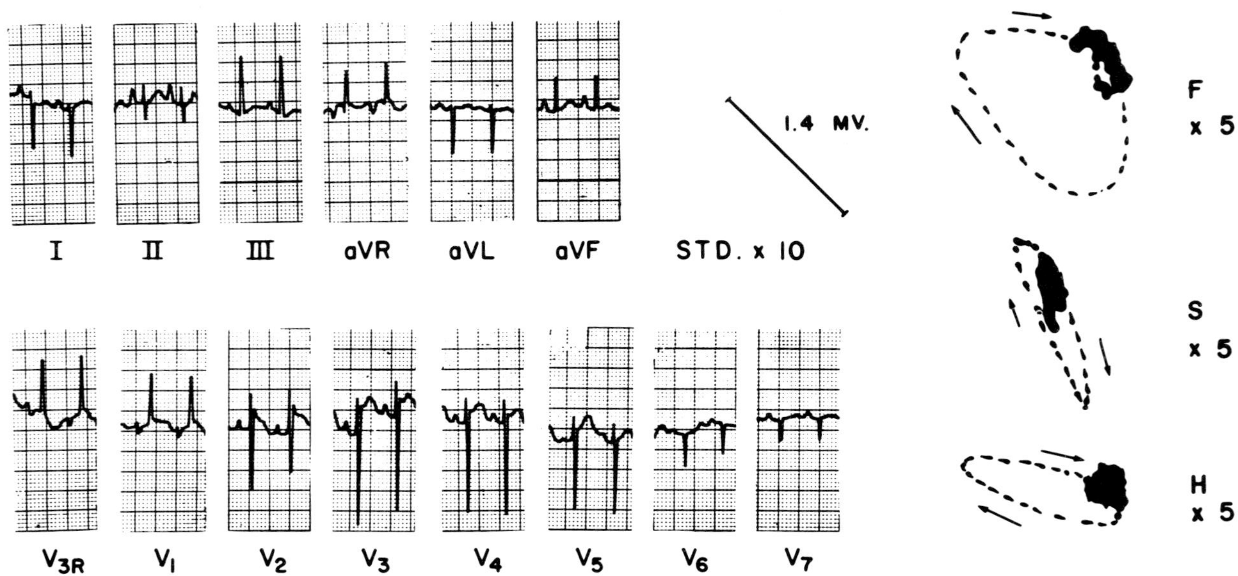

Figure 136. Electrocardiogram of patient with complete transposition of the great vessels with intact ventricular septum and inadequate mixing, indicating right atrial enlargement (lead II) and right ventricular hypertrophy. (From Morgan, A. D., Krovetz, L. J., Schiebler, G. L., Shanklin, D. R., Wheat, M. W., Jr., and Bartley, T. D. 1965. Diagnosis and palliative surgery in complete transposition of the great vessels. Ann. Thorac. Surg. 1:711.)

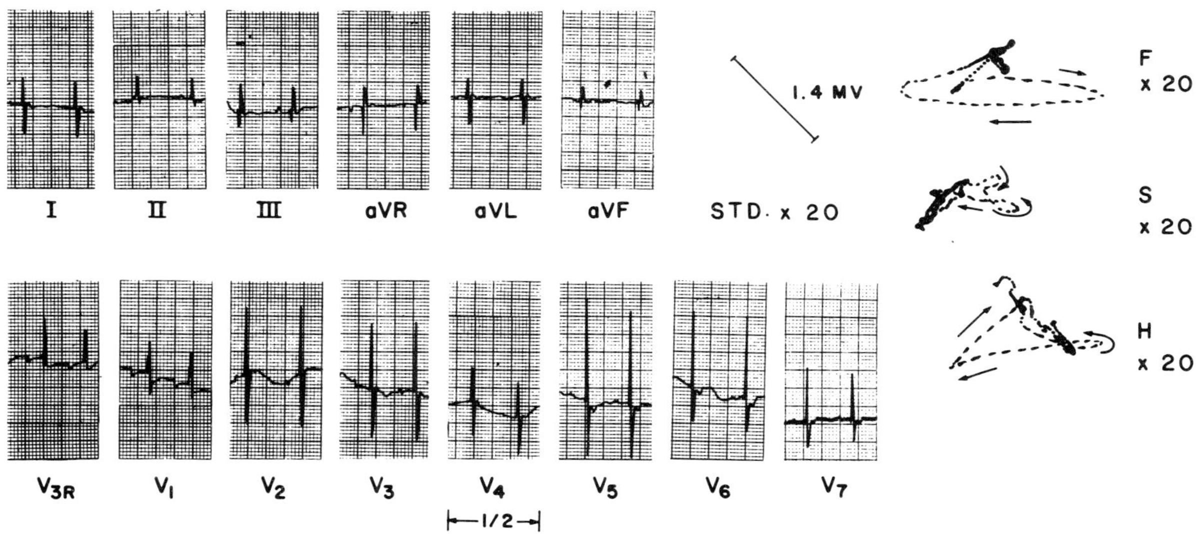

Figure 137. Electrocardiogram of a patient with complete transposition of the great vessels and a large ventricular septal defect. This electrocardiogram indicates biventricular hypertrophy.

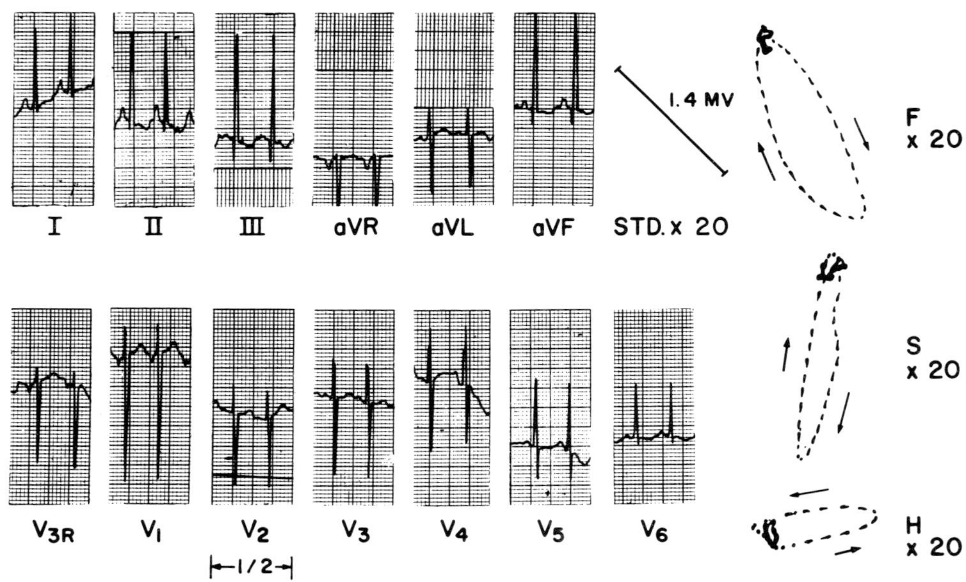

Figure 138. The presence of isolated left ventricular hypertrophy, as shown in this electrocardiogram, suggests that the transposition is part of a complex lesion. In this case, the patient had both a single ventricle and coarctation of the aorta. (From Morgan, A. D., Krovetz, L. J., Schiebler, G. L., Shanklin, D. R., Wheat, M. W., Jr., and Bartley, T. D. 1965. Diagnosis and palliative surgery in complete transposition of the great vessels. Ann. Thorac. Surg. 1:711.)

Table 26. Average life expectancy of children with complete transposition of the great vessels[a]

Type of TGA	Average life expectancy
Simple (patent foramen ovale only)	6 weeks
Atrial septal defect	9 months
Ventricular septal defect	
with increased pulmonary flow	3 months
with pulmonary vascular obstruction	2.0 years
with pulmonic stenosis	4.8 years
Single ventricle	6.8 years

[a] Adapted from Liebman, J., Cullum, L., and Belloc, N. B. 1969. Natural history of transposition of the great arteries. Circulation 60:137–262. By permission of the American Heart Association, Inc.

shortly after birth. It is most common in one of a pair of twins or with placental dysfunction.

Truncus arteriosus has a high incidence of right aortic arch and a wider superior mediastinal shadow than seen in TGA.

Total anomalous pulmonary venous connection has a widely split second sound; these infants are not as cyanotic as patients with TGA.

Any *massive left-to-right shunt in congestive heart failure* may mimic complete transposition of the great arteries, but the cyanosis clears rapidly with oxygen and digitalis.

PROGNOSIS

Infants with *inadequate mixing* have a malignant form of heart disease characterized by marked cyanosis, early tachypnea, poor weight gain, and an enlarging heart. These infants develop congestive heart failure early and are usually dead by 6 months of age (Table 26).

Children with *adequate mixing* have a more benign form and only moderate cyanosis at birth. Their better course and prognosis are usually due to a higher pulmonary resistance or pulmonic stenosis.

MANAGEMENT

Infants in congestive heart failure should be given the usual anticongestive measures (see Chapter 12). In neonates in Group 1, cardiac catheterization should be carried out promptly. After the diagnosis is confirmed, balloon atrial septostomy should be done. A catheter with an inflatable balloon is passed into the left atrium through the foramen ovale. The balloon is inflated with dilute contrast media, and the catheter is rapidly pulled back to the right atrium, tearing the septum. When successful, this technique can alleviate the symptoms, sometimes until the patient reaches an age when corrective surgery is feasible.

In the operation developed by Mustard in 1964, blood from the pulmonary veins is directed through a pericardial tunnel into the right atrium, the right ventricle, and out the aorta. Systemic venous blood enters the right atrium and flows around the pericardial tunnel into the left ventricle and then out the pulmonary artery. This corrects the blood flow pathways except for the coronary sinus return. Although initially this operation was done at 3 to 6 years of age, many centers now have equally good results in infants over 5 kg in weight. The youngest survivor in Stark's series was only 3 days old at the time of surgery.

Long-term results of this operation have been disappointing. Obstruction to caval drainage, residual shunts, and arrhythmias (see Figure 219), as well as late deaths, indicate that better methods for correcting TGA are needed.

High surgical mortality in transposition with VSD and subpulmonic stenosis led Rastelli, in 1969, to develop an alternate to the Mustard repair. In the Rastelli procedure a tunnel is constructed to connect the left ventricle to the aorta. The pulmonary artery is divided and the cardiac end oversewn. A new pulmonary artery is constructed with the use of a graft of ascending aorta, including the aortic or a prosthetic valve, sutured between the distal pulmonary artery and a window opening into the right ventricle.

BIBLIOGRAPHY

Elliott, L. P., Neufeld, H. N., Anderson, R. C., Adams, P., Jr., and Edwards, J. E. 1963. Complete transposition of the great vessels. I. An anatomic study of sixty cases. Circulation 27:1105–1117.

Hagler, D. J., Ritter, D. G., Mair, D. V., Davis, G. D., and McGoon, D. C. 1978. Clinical, angiographic, and hemodynamic assessment of late results after Mustard operation. Circulation 57:1214–1223.

Liebman, J., Cullum, L., and Belloc, N. B. 1969. Natural history of transposition of the great arteries. Circulation 60:237–262.

Mair, D. D., and Ritter, D. G. 1973. Factors influencing systemic arterial oxygen saturation in complete transposition of the great arteries. Am. J. Cardiol. 31:742–747.

Mair, D. D., Ritter, D. G., Ongley, P. A., and Helmholz, H. F., Jr. 1971. Hemodynamics and evaluation for surgery of patients with complete transposition of the great arteries and ventricular septal defect. Am. J. Cardiol. 18:632–640.

Rashkind, W. J., and Miller, W. W. 1966. Creation of atrial septal defect without thoracotomy. A palliative approach to complete transposition of the great arteries. J.A.M.A. 196:991–992.

Rastelli, G. C. 1969. A new approach to "anatomic" repair of transposition of the great arteries. Mayo Clinic Proc. 44:1–12.

Stark, J. 1977. Surgical treatment of patients with transposition of the great arteries. Johns Hopkins Med. J. 140:181–184.

Van Mierop, L. H. S., Alley, R. D., Kausel, H. W., and Stranahan, S. 1963.

Pathogenesis of transposition complexes. I. Embryology of the ventricles and great arteries. Am. J. Cardiol. 12:216–225.
Van Mierop, L. H. S., and Wiglesworth, F. W. 1963. II. Anomalies due to faulty transfer of the posterior great artery. III. True transposition of the great vessels. Am. J. Cardiol. 12:226–239.

chapter 19

VENTRICULAR INVERSION (Congenitally Corrected Transposition of the Great Arteries)

In this anomaly, the ventricles have their left and right relationships inverted. Since the great arteries are anatomically transposed, the aorta arises anteriorly from the left-sided ventricle (anatomically a right ventricle) while the pulmonary artery arises posteriorly from the right-sided ventricle (anatomically a left ventricle). This "corrects" the blood flow pathways so that the systemic venous drainage flows into the pulmonary artery, and pulmonary venous drainage flows into the aorta (Figure 139). Since the inversion of the ventricles is probably the primary embryological error, it seems best to use this term rather than the earlier one of "congenitally corrected transposition of the great arteries."

To understand this malformation, one first has to define two other terms. *Transposition* is an alteration of arterial trunks at their site of origin from the heart. The aorta arises approximately where the pulmonary artery normally sits, and the pulmonary artery where the aorta normally arises. (We reserve the term transposition for those cases where the aorta is anterior to the pulmonary artery. Van Praagh's classification seems to us to be overly complex and not very helpful clinically.) *Inversion* means that an organ (or part of an organ)

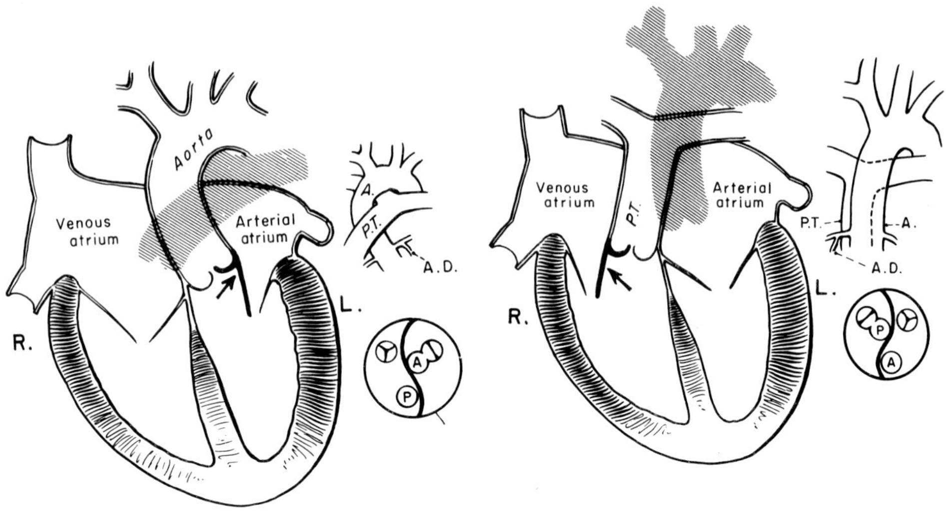

Figure 139. In the normal heart (left) the aortic valve is lower than the pulmonic valve. The anterior mitral valve leaflet (arrow) is intimately related to the aortic valve. The cross-section shows that the pulmonic valve is anterior to the aortic valve and not closely related to the other valves. In ventricular inversion (right), many of the relationships are mirror image. The pulmonic valve has many anatomical resemblances to the normal aortic valve; it is central in the heart and is intimately related to an atrioventricular valve (arrow). The aortic valve is approximately in the position normally occupied by the pulmonic valve, while the pulmonic valve is medial, posterior, and caudad to the aortic valve. The coronary arteries are also inverted and the anterior descending artery is a tributary of the right coronary. (From Schiebler, G. L., Edwards, J. E., Burchell, H. B., DuShane, J. W., Ongley, P. A., and Wood, E. H. 1961. Congenitally corrected transposition of the great vessels. A study of thirty-three cases. Pediatrics 27: (Suppl.):851. Copyright American Academy of Pediatrics, 1961.)

is the mirror image of the normal. Thus, this is an alteration of the side-to-side relationships, but not of the anterior-posterior relationships.

In *ventricular inversion,* the systemic veins, the pulmonary veins, the sinoatrial node, and the atria are normal. The atrioventricular node, the conduction system, both atrioventricular valves, the ventricular musculature, and the coronary arteries are inverted or mirror imaged. The great arteries are transposed, with the aorta anterior to the pulmonary artery.

HISTORICAL NOTES

In 1875, Karl von Rokitansky described the hearts of two infants, a 4-month-old girl and an 11-month-old boy. In discussing these two cases under the topic of transposition of the great vessels, von Rokitansky noted that ''The transposition of the great vessels was corrected by the position of the ventricular septum.'' This change in the position of the septum allowed systemic venous blood to enter the pulmonary artery and arterialized blood to enter the aorta, even though the great vessels were anatomically transposed.

For many years this entity was considered hardly more than a museum curiosity. However, the advent of cardiac catheterization and angiocardiography has resulted in more frequent antemortem diagnosis, as well as elucidation of its clinical, hemodynamic, and surgical peculiarities.

INCIDENCE

Males comprise about two-thirds of the reported cases. In our series, l-loop transposition was found in 2% of our patients with congenital heart lesions, and was frequently associated with a single ventricle. There are no reports of familial occurrence of this entity.

PATHOLOGY

Although ventricular inversion in rare instances occurs as an isolated entity, usually there are associated malformations, especially left-sided atrioventricular valve anomalies or septal defects. Other common lesions are patent ductus arteriosus, coarctation of the aorta, and subpulmonic stenosis.

Left atrioventricular valve anomalies range from atresia to stenosis to insufficiency, and encompass the entire spectrum of atrioventricular valve anomalies. This valve is often displaced, much as in Ebstein's anomaly of the tricuspid valve (see Chapter 24). Edwards states that some degree of displacement of the valve from the annulus is always present, even when not clinically appreciable.

Lev found the sinoatrial node to be in normal position and to have normal histology. The atrioventricular node, although normal histologically, is inverted and is located above and to the left of its normal position. The atrioventricular node and bundle of His are in roughly mirror-image position from their normal locations, and the right and left bundle branches are inverted. The observed propensity to develop heart block may be a result of the longer course of the main AV bundle or of the more superficial location of the left bundle branch on the right side of the ventricular septum.

HEMODYNAMICS

If ventricular inversion is the sole anomaly, there are no alterations in hemodynamics. Alterations in cardiovascular physiology are secondary to associated malformations or atrioventricular conduction anomalies.

CLINICAL FEATURES

The vast majority of patients have symptoms during early life, secondary to the associated defects. A rather common clinical finding is bradycardia caused by atrioventricular block. Even without other associated anomalies, these patients are subject to arrhythmias, Stokes-Adams attacks, and even sudden death.

Auscultation and phonocardiography reflect the associated malformations and are rarely useful in suggesting the diagnosis. The most common murmur is that of "mitral insufficiency." Such a murmur in the presence of atrioventricular block should suggest ventricular inversion as an associated malformation.

On occasion, the second sound in the second left intercostal space is loud and single, suggesting pulmonary hypertension. This is really due to the aortic component of the second sound, which is more prominent than usual because of the anterior position of the aorta. When both components of the second sound are equally loud in the second right intercostal space, one may suspect abnormal locations of the pulmonic and aortic valves.

Associated noncardiac anomalies are uncommon, except for partial or total situs inversus. These latter are to be expected, since ventricular inversion is really "partial situs inversus" of the heart.

ROENTGENOGRAPHIC FEATURES

Absence of the pulmonary artery "knob" in the left upper border of the cardiac silhouette, because of the more medial position of the main and left

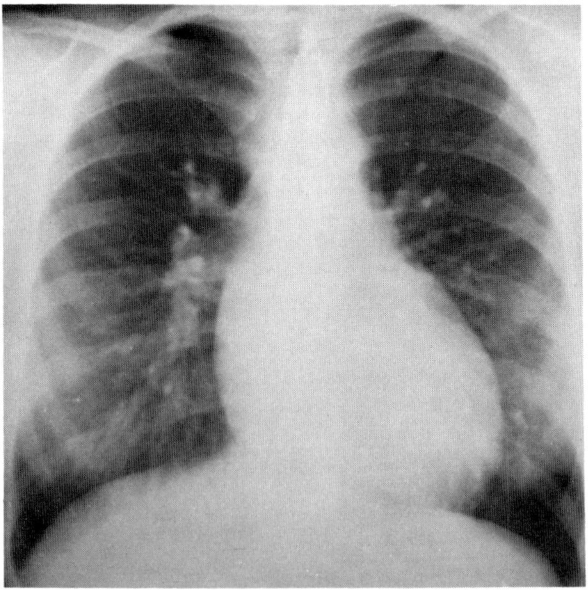

Figure 140. In this x-ray, the right pulmonary artery is prominent, but the main pulmonary artery cannot be distinguished on the left border of the heart. These features by themselves may suggest the correct diagnosis.

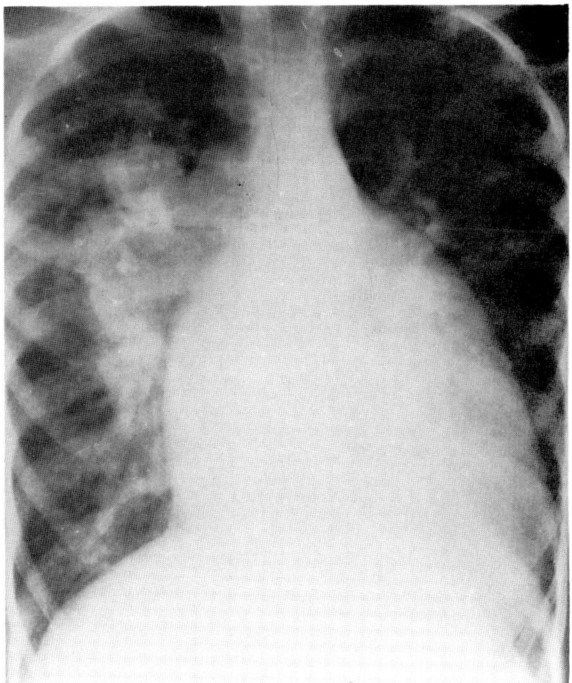

Figure 141. X-ray of a 12-year-old patient with an l-loop transposition of the great arteries and a single ventricle with large pulmonary flow. The right pulmonary artery is enormous in size and has been likened to a waterfall. The prominence of the right pulmonary artery is at least partially due to the fact that the main pulmonary artery is to the right of its normal location. Other features to note are the narrow base and the apparent absence of a main pulmonary artery segment. (From Elliott, L.P., and Gedgaudas, E. 1964. The roentgenologic findings in common ventricle with transposition of the great vessels. Radiology 82:850.)

main pulmonary arteries, suggests the diagnosis (Figures 140 and 141). There may be an indentation of the barium column medially by a large main pulmonary artery. When associated with a single ventricle, the right pulmonary artery may be very prominent (Figure 140).

The smooth upper left border of the heart is formed by the ascending aorta and the usual aortic indentation of the barium column is absent. The base of the heart is often narrow, and left atrial enlargement is common.

ELECTROCARDIOGRAPHY

Delayed atrioventricular conduction, especially complete heart block, should suggest the diagnosis of ventricular inversion. Delayed atrioventricular conduction becomes increasingly common and more severe with age. The Wolff-Parkinson-White electrocardiographic anomaly is occasionally seen, particularly with Ebstein's anomaly of the left atrioventricular valve.

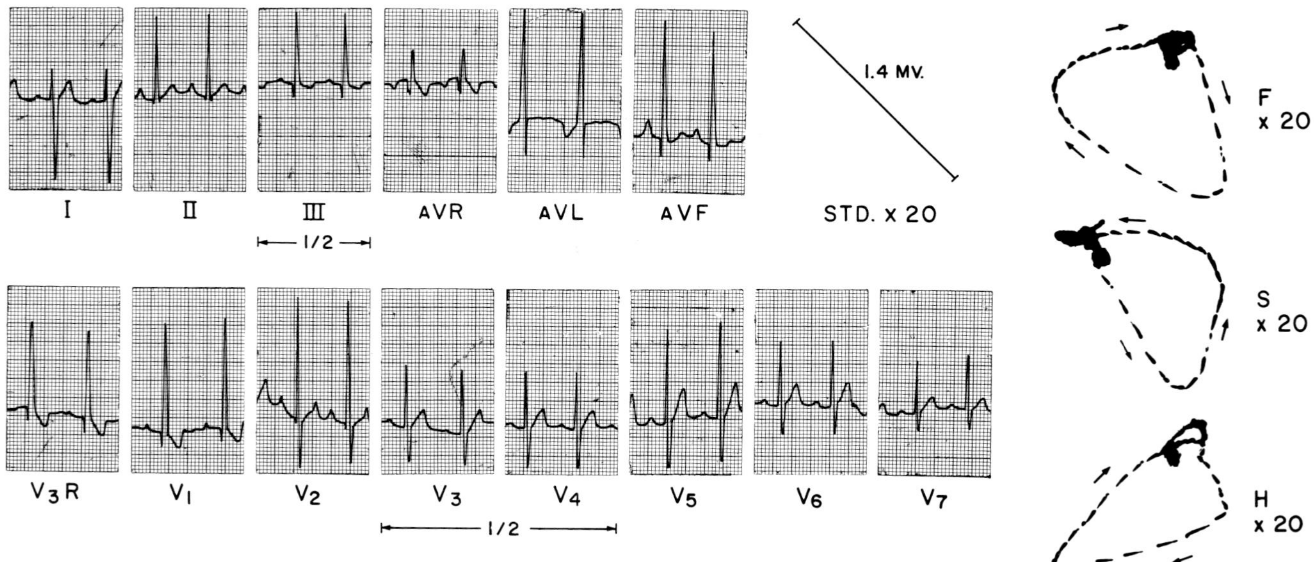

Figure 142. Electrocardiogram of a 30-month-old patient with ventricular inversion. Note the deep q waves in the right precordial leads and leads II, III, and aVF, and the absence of a q wave in the left precordial leads. This pattern should raise the possibility of ventricular inversion, although it is also seen with severe right ventricular hypertrophy and normal arrangement of the great vessels. (From Morgan A. D., Krovetz, L. J., Bartley, T. D., Green, J. R., Jr., Shanklin, D. R., Wheat, M. W., Jr., and Schiebler, G. L. 1966. Clinical features of single ventricle with congenitally corrected transposition. Am. J. Cardiol. 17:379.)

Septal depolarization is directed leftward, superiorly and posteriorly, producing q waves in leads II, III, and aVF and initial negativity in lead V_1. The remainder of the QRS complex reflects the type of ventricular hypertrophy pattern present, if any. For example, if the right-sided ventricle is significantly enlarged, or if the left-sided ventricle is hypoplastic, then the initial q in lead V_1 will be followed by a dominant R giving the well-known qR pattern (Figure 142). Upright T waves in right precordial leads are also commonly present, regardless of the ventricular hypertrophy pattern.

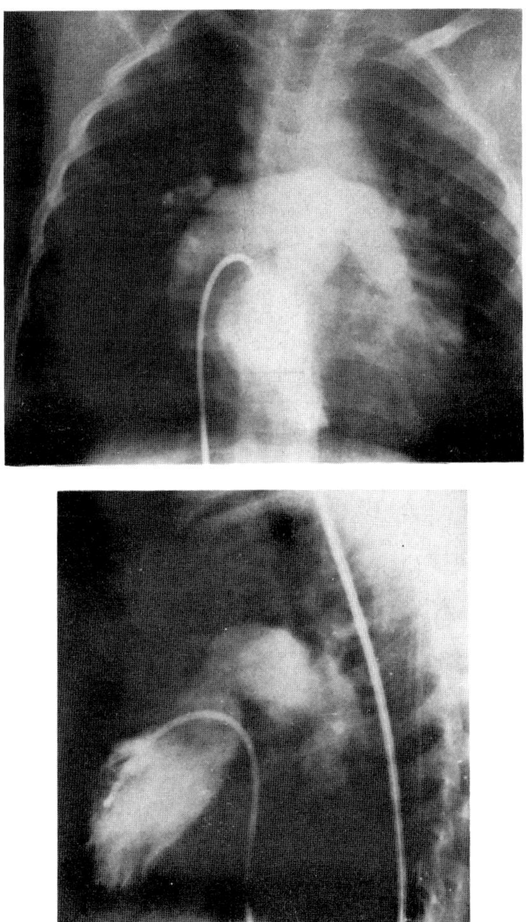

Figure 143. Angiocardiogram of a patient with ventricular inversion and ventricular septal defect with pulmonic stenosis. The catheter is in the venous ventricle (which is morphologically a left ventricle). The pulmonic valve is in the location usually occupied by the aortic valve.

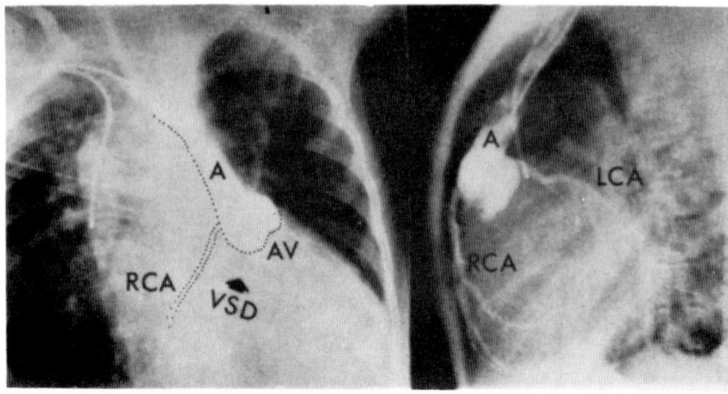

Figure 144. Illustrates the leftward and anterior displacement of the aortic valve. (From Morgan, A. D., Krovetz, L. J., Bartley, T. D., Green, J. R., Jr., Shanklin, D. R., Wheat, M. W., Jr., and Schiebler, G. L. 1966. Clinical features of single ventricle with congenitally corrected transposition. Am. J. Cardiol. 17:379.)

DIFFERENTIAL DIAGNOSIS

Diagnostic problems usually occur when an associated cardiac anomaly has been diagnosed first. The presence of ventricular inversion must be ruled out, since surgical risks are greatly increased by its presence. Furthermore, when a large ventricular septal defect is diagnosed with associated l-loop transposition, a single ventricle must be excluded.

Angiocardiography is the simplest and the most certain way of making the diagnosis. The location of the aortic and pulmonic valves and the contours of the ventricular chambers establish the diagnosis (Figures 143 and 144).

PROGNOSIS

Deaths are usually due to intractable heart failure, recurrent pulmonary infections, or unsuccessful surgical intervention. Sudden deaths, presumably due to arrhythmias, are not uncommon. The median age at death is about 4 years, but individual prognosis depends primarily on the associated defects. Theoretically, one would expect a normal life span in the absence of associated defects. The incidence of atrioventricular conduction anomalies is so great, however, that even without an associated defect a normal life span is rare.

MANAGEMENT

Repair of associated atrial septal defects, pulmonic or aortic valvar stenosis, and extracardiac lesions poses no particular problems, even if the anatomy is not completely defined prior to operation. However, the surgeon should be aware of the high incidence of malformed left-sided atrioventricular valves in this defect.

The risk of inducing heart block during surgery is very high, particularly when closing a ventricular septal defect. Complete heart block has occurred during thoractomy, even prior to manipulation of the heart.

BIBLIOGRAPHY

de la Cruz, M. V., Anselmi, G., Cisneros, F., Reinhold, M., Portillo, B., and Espino-Vela, J. 1959. An embryologic explanation for corrected transposition of the great vessels: Additional description of the main anatomic features of this malformation and its varieties. Am. Heart J. 57:104–117.

Morgan, A. D., Krovetz, L. J., Bartley, T. D., Green, J. R., Jr., Shanklin, D. R., Wheat, M. W., Jr., and Schiebler, G. L. 1966. Clinical features of single ventricle with congenitally corrected transposition. Am. J. Cardiol. 17:379–388.

Schiebler, G. L., Edwards, J. E., Burchell, H. B., DuShane, J. W., Ongley, P. A., and Wood, E. H. 1961. Congenitally corrected transposition of the great vessels. A study of thirty-three cases. Pediatrics 27:(Suppl.):851–888.

Shem-Tov, A., Deutsch, V., Yahini, J. H., Draus, Y., and Neufeld, H. N. 1971. Corrected transposition of the great arteries. Am. J. Cardiol. 27:99–113.

Victoria, B. E., Miller, B. L., and Gessner, I. H. 1973. Electrocardiogram and vectorcardiogram in ventricular inversion (corrected transposition). Am. Heart J. 86:733–744.

chapter 20

TRUNCUS ARTERIOSUS

HISTORICAL NOTES

Isolated cases of persistent truncus arteriosus were reported during the nineteenth century, with the earliest citation apparently ascribable to Buchanan in 1864. A number of reviews [Taruffi (1875), Vierodt (1898), Herxheimer (1910), Abbott (1931), Humphreys (1932), and Lev and Saphir (1942)] have appeared over the years. However, this anomaly was commonly confused with pseudotruncus arteriosus (pulmonic atresia) or aortic atresia until the article by Collett and Edwards in 1949 that did so much to clarify the pathology of this defect.

INCIDENCE

The overall incidence of persistent truncus arteriosus varies from 0.5% to 1% of all congenital heart defects, depending on the nature of the series. A higher incidence will be found in series reporting primarily infants and autopsy statistics, because of the early age of presentation and high mortality rate of this defect.

The sex ratio is equal. Persistent truncus arteriosus has been reported infrequently in siblings.

PATHOLOGY

Collett and Edwards stated that, in order to classify a defect as a persistent truncus arteriosus, the following criteria must be met:

1. There must be only one main arterial trunk leaving the base of the heart (Figure 145).
2. There must be no remnant of an atretic pulmonary trunk or aorta.
3. The single arterial trunk must supply branches of the coronary, pulmonary, and systemic circulations.

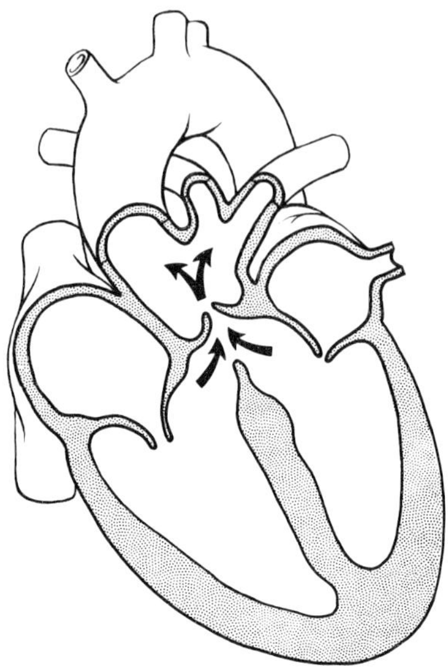

Figure 145. Schema of the intracardiac circulation in persistent truncus arteriosus.

Four anatomic varieties were described by Collett and Edwards. In type I there is a single arterial trunk that gives rise to a main pulmonary trunk, which bifurcates into right and left pulmonary arteries, and an ascending aorta. In type II, the right and left pulmonary arteries arise close together from the posterior wall of the trunk, while in type III either one or both arise from the side of the trunk (Figure 146). In type IV, the main pulmonary arteries are absent, and the circulation to the lungs is furnished by bronchial arteries.

While the classification of Collett and Edwards did much to advance understanding of this defect, their type IV cases have led to both confusion and controversy. Developmentally, persistent truncus arteriosus results from absence of the truncus septum. This prevents closure of the ventricular septum as well, since normally the lower edge of the truncus septum fuses with the conus septum to complete the truncoconal portion of the ventricular septum. Type IV truncus, on the other hand, probably represents the most severe form of tetralogy of Fallot. That is, there is complete obliteration of the right ventricular outflow tract with atresia of the pulmonary trunk. This anomaly has also been called pseudo-truncus arteriosus, a term that we feel should be abandoned because of its potential confusion with persistent truncus arteriosus, since these defects differ considerably.

Type I represents the classical form of persistent truncus arteriosus that accounts for over 90% of cases. Since types II and III are both quite rare, Collett and Edwards' original classification can, in our view, be meaningfully

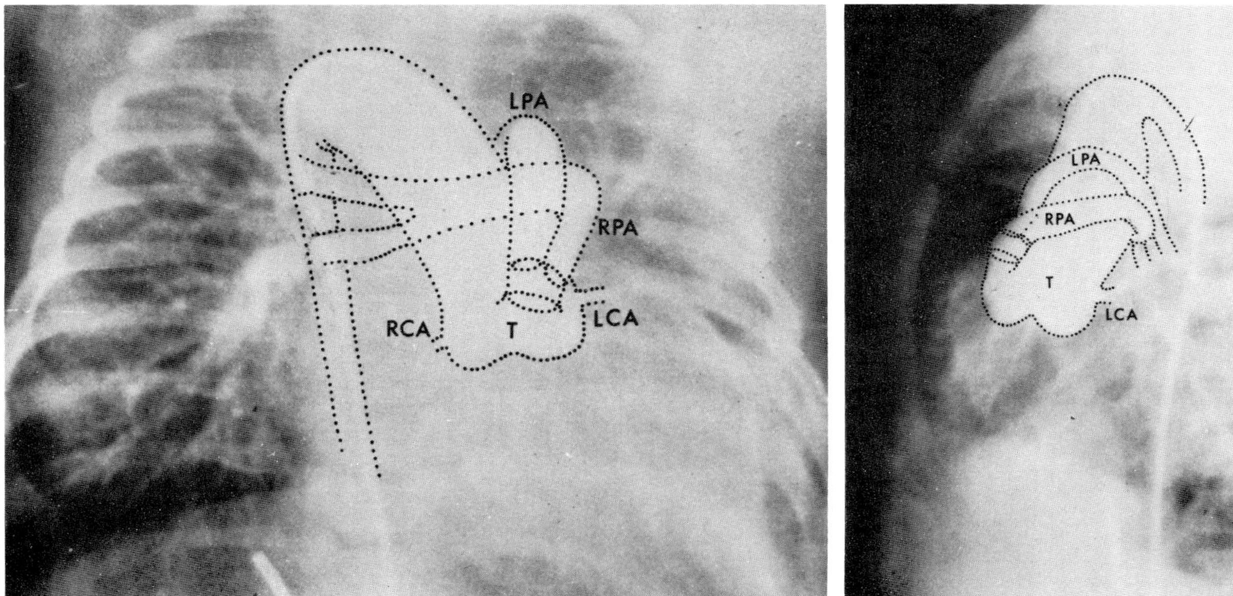

Figure 146. Thoracic aortogram of a 3-month-old female illustrating the massive trunk that gives rise to both the pulmonary arteries and the aorta.

simplified. Types II and III are both characterized by independent origin of the right and left pulmonary arteries from the persistent truncus and for practical purposes can be combined.

A ventricular septal defect is invariably present. The ventricular septal defect is not truly membranous, since it results from the absence of the truncal septum and there is no definable right ventricular outflow tract. (The Van Praaghs discussed two examples without a ventricular septal defect, but we believe that these cases are better classified as aorticopulmonary windows.)

The truncus usually arises approximately equally from both ventricles, although it may originate primarily from either the right or left ventricle (see Figure 145). The truncal valve usually consists of three or four cusps, although this can vary from two to six cusps. In about one-half of patients, the valve is dysplastic and functionally insufficient. Continuity with the mitral valve is expected and is present.

The most common associated cardiovascular anomaly is a right aortic arch, which occurs in approximately 25% of cases. No other defect occurs with any significant frequency, although many have been described, including atrial septal defect, common atrioventricular valve, complete interruption of the aortic arch, and coarctation of the aorta. Collett and Edwards reported that one-fourth of their cases of persistent truncus arteriosus were associated with single ventricle, but this has not been found in any other series.

HEMODYNAMICS

Persistent truncus arteriosus is characterized initially by increased pulmonary blood flow. Ventricular pressures are equal, as are mean aortic and pulmonary trunk pressures. Since both the left and right ventricles empty into the truncus, there usually is a high degree of mixing of the blood streams. Systemic arterial saturation is directly related to the ratio of pulmonary blood flow to systemic blood flow, which at times is so great that systemic arterial oxygen saturation reaches 90% or higher. This high pulmonary flow places a large volume load on the heart as well as on the pulmonary vascular bed.

This combination of high pulmonary arterial flow and pressure leads to early pulmonary vascular bed damage. As pulmonary vascular resistance increases, pulmonary blood flow decreases and arterial saturation falls. When pulmonary resistance is only moderately increased, a reasonable balance may be reached that results in adequate systemic arterial oxygen levels and more tolerable pulmonary blood flows. This situation is temporary, however, since without surgical intervention pulmonary vascular resistance will continue to rise.

In a few patients the right and left pulmonary arteries are small. This situation can be beneficial to the patient since pulmonary blood flow is controlled, thus averting the marked left heart volume load, and pulmonary artery pressure is significantly less than it otherwise would be. These patients may therefore avoid obstructive pulmonary vascular disease, but at the cost of increased cyanosis.

CLINICAL FEATURES

Symptoms usually begin early in infancy and are related to the onset of congestive heart failure. Infants feed poorly, grow slowly, and generally have the characteristic appearance of babies with a large left-to-right shunt. Tachypnea and tachycardia are evident. Extracardiac anomalies are common. Cyanosis is not a major manifestation and the clinician's skill is often challenged to recognize mild systemic desaturation.

Arterial pulses are increased in amplitude, and often bounding, because of the abnormally wide pulse pressure.

The precordium is active, with both left and right ventricular lifts, a systolic thrill, and a harsh systolic murmur similar to that of a ventricular septal defect (Figure 147). A suprasternal notch thrill is uncommon. The first sound is normal and is usually followed by a prominent, constant ejection click. The second sound is of particular importance. One would assume that it will be both loud and single and usually it is. However, in some instances the second sound will have two identifiable components, detectable both by auscultation and by phonocardiography. We have interpreted these as sounds arising from the walls of the aorta and pulmonary trunk. In a few catheterized cases, there has been a pressure drop across the pulmonary trunk orifice, and therefore the pressure wave hitting the pulmonary trunk wall may be delayed.

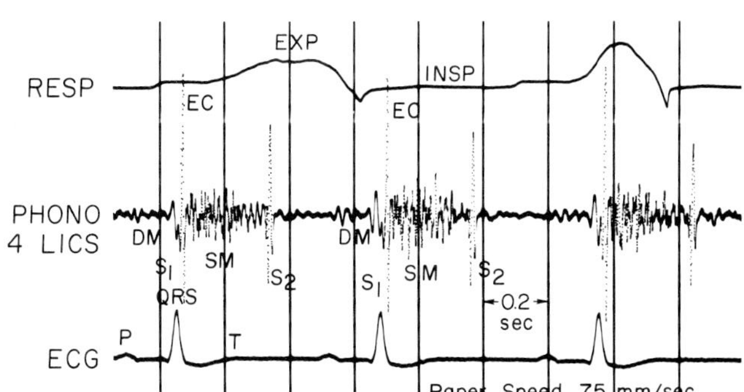

Figure 147. Phonocardiogram of a 1-day-old male with persistent truncus arteriosus. Note that the first sound (S_1) is followed by a very prominent ejection click (EC) that does not vary in intensity with the phases of respiration. This is thought to be the result of the stream of blood suddenly striking the large dilated truncus. The systolic murmur (SM) is secondary to the ventricular septal defect. The second sound (S_2) is usually single, although on occasion there may be two distinct components. The low frequency late diastolic murmur (DM) is common with large pulmonary flow.

This timing, however, will not be changed by respiration and therefore there is no variation in the width of the second sound. Thus while most patients have a single second sound, the presence of narrow, fixed splitting does not rule out the diagnosis of persistent truncus arteriosus.

Diastole is characterized by an early to mid-diastolic rumble of increased mitral valve flow analogous to that heard in association with a ventricular septal defect. The intensity of this murmur is directly related to pulmonary blood flow and left atrial pressure, and, of course, would be diminished by an associated atrial septal defect. A high-frequency decrescendo early diastolic murmur of truncal valve insufficiency (identical with the murmur of aortic insufficiency) may be heard, especially when the valve is dysplastic.

Development of increasing pulmonary vascular resistance alters the clinical findings in proportion to the decrease in pulmonary blood flow. The systolic murmur becomes less intense and shorter in duration, the mitral flow murmur softens or disappears, arterial pulses decrease in amplitude, and cyanosis increases.

ROENTGENOGRAPHIC FEATURES

In a cyanotic infant, a right aortic arch, cardiomegaly, and increased pulmonary arterial markings on chest x-ray strongly suggest a diagnosis of persistent truncus arteriosus (Figure 148). Also commonly seen are left atrial enlargement and straightening of the left heart border resulting from absence of the right ventricular outflow tract and the abnormal position of the pulmonary trunk. At times the right and left pulmonary arteries can be seen to originate at a higher than normal location.

ELECTROCARDIOGRAPHY

The ECG often demonstrates left atrial enlargement and left ventricular hypertrophy early in the course of the disease (Figure 149). Biventricular hypertrophy may be present as a result of volume overload of the left ventricle and pressure overload of the right ventricle (Figure 150). As pulmonary vascular resistance increases and pulmonary blood flow decreases, the pattern changes to one of right atrial enlargement and right ventricular hypertrophy.

DIFFERENTIAL DIAGNOSIS

Patent ductus arteriosus also may present with bounding pulses in an infant with significant congestive heart failure. A continuous murmur is rare in persistent truncus arteriosus, except in the presence of stenosis of the right and left pulmonary arteries comparable (if not identical) with that heard in pulmonary artery coarctation.

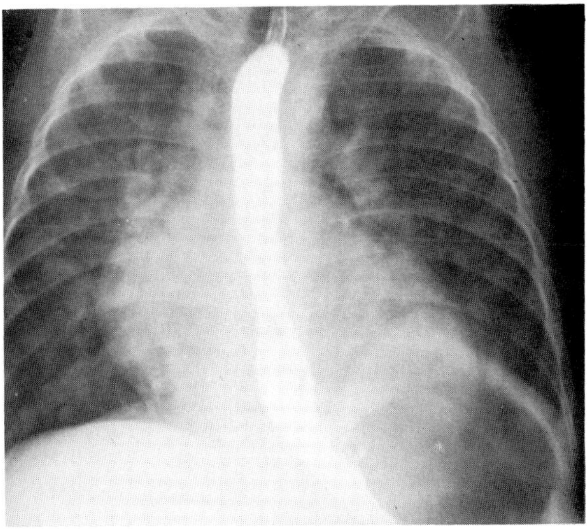

Figure 148. AP roentgenogram of a 19-month-old female with persistent truncus arteriosus. Note the markedly dilated upper mediastinal shadow. The pulmonary arteries have a higher than normal take-off, and there is a marked increase in pulmonary vascularity.

Ventricular septal defect with aortic insufficiency is rare in infancy and is never associated with cyanosis.

PROGNOSIS

Untreated, the majority of patients die in the first 6 months of life. Death is usually due to congestive heart failure and superimposed pneumonia.

Children most likely to survive are those with small pulmonary arteries or those with increased pulmonary vascular resistance. The oldest patient in our series is 12 years, but survival to 43 years has been reported.

Although high mortality rates have been reported for pulmonary artery banding, this procedure remains valuable, particularly since a corrective procedure is now available for children who survive the first year of life.

MANAGEMENT

Initial management is based on reducing the effects of congestive heart failure by standard means (see Chapter 12), followed by early cardiac catheterization. With angiographic demonstration of the defect and assessment of its hemodynamic effects, a decision regarding appropriate surgical therapy is made. Pulmonary artery banding remains a commonly employed approach, although the occasional necessity for banding the right and left pulmonary arteries independently complicates the surgery.

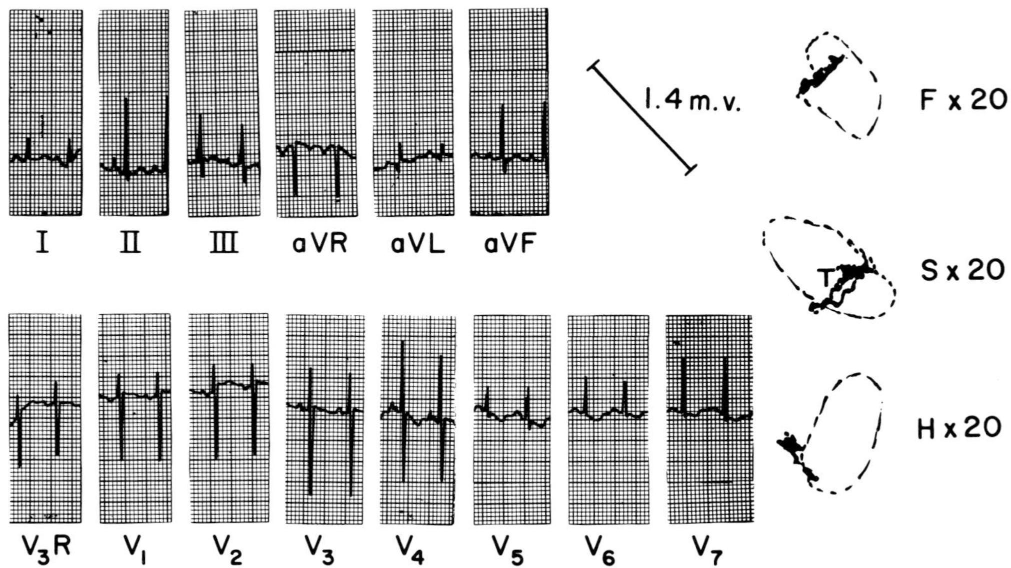

Figure 149. Electrocardiogram of a 1-month-old child with persistent truncus arteriosus, showing left ventricular hypertrophy and left atrial enlargement.

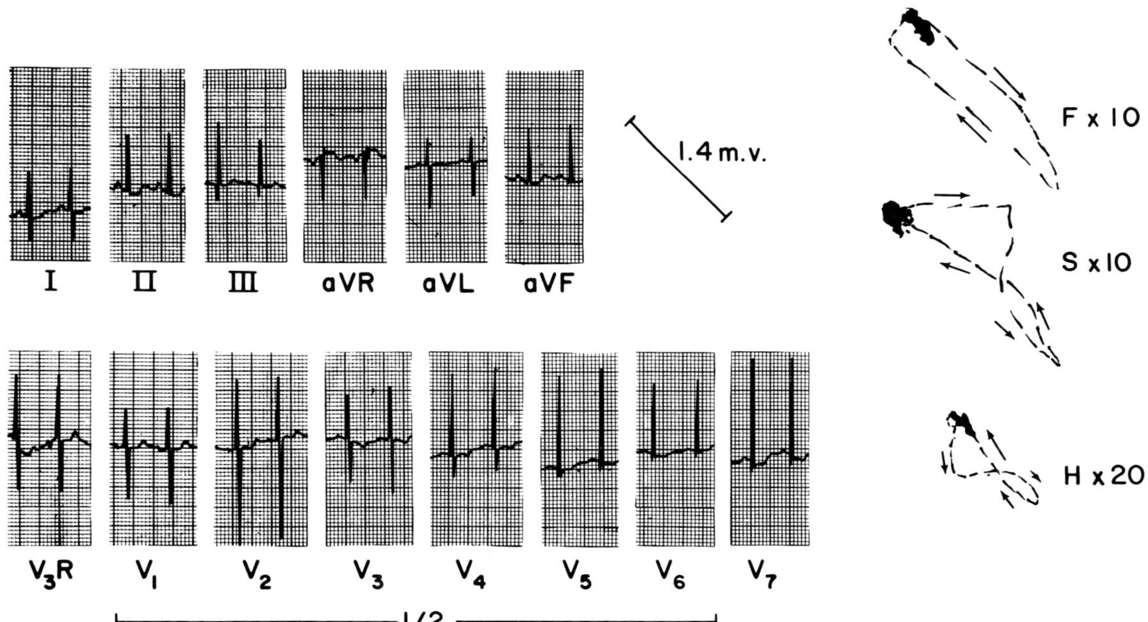

Figure 150. Electrocardiogram of a 3-year-old female with persistent truncus arteriosus. This electrocardiogram exhibits combined ventricular hypertrophy, indistinguishable from that of a ventricular septal defect or a patent ductus.

In recent years a corrective procedure has become available. The ventricular septal defect is closed in such a way as to leave the truncal valve originating from the left ventricle. The pulmonary trunk is detached from the truncus and a valved conduit is placed from the right ventricle to the pulmonary trunk. Significant insufficiency of the truncal valve requires intraoperative attention, but does not appear to add to the early mortality. Pulmonary hyper-resistance unfortunately may develop early in infancy and preclude successful surgery.

BIBLIOGRAPHY

Bailey, W. W., Kirklin, J. W., Bargeon, L. M., Pacifico, A. D., and Kouchoukos, N. T. 1976. Late results with synthetic valved external conduits from venous ventricle to pulmonary arteries. Circulation 56:(Suppl. II):73–79.

Collett, R. W., and Edwards, J. E. 1949. Persistent truncus arteriosus: A classification according to anatomic types. Surg. Clin. North Am. 29:1245–1270.

Mair, D. D., Ritter, D. G., Davis, G. D., Wallace, R. B., Danielson, G. K., and McGoon, D. C. 1974. Selection of patients with truncus arteriosus for surgical correction. Circulation 49:144–151.

Marcolletti, C., McGoon, D. C., Danielson, G. K., Wallace, R. B., and Mair, D. D. 1977. Early and late results of surgical repair of truncus arteriosus. Circulation 55:636–641.

Marcolletti, C., McGoon, D. C., and Mair, D. D. 1976. The natural history of truncus arteriosus. Circulation 54:108–111.

McCue, C. M., Lester, R. G., Bosher, L. H., Jr., and Mauck, H. P., Jr. 1964. Persistent truncus arteriosus, a clinical correlation with the pathologic anatomy. Dis. Chest 46:507–523.

Van Praagh, R., and Van Praagh, S. 1965. The anatomy of common aorticopulmonary trunk (truncus arteriosus communis) and its embryologic implications. A study of 57 necropsy cases. Am. J. Cardiol. 16:406–425.

Victorica, B. E., Krovetz, L. J., Elliott, L. P., Van Mierop, L. H. S., Bartley, T. D., Gessner, I. H., and Schiebler, G. L. 1969. Persistent truncus arteriosus in infancy. A study of 14 cases. Am. Heart J. 77:1–25.

chapter 21

SINGLE VENTRICLE

This is a particularly complicated group of congenital heart lesions. It may occur with either d-loop or l-loop transposition of the great arteries, or, less commonly, with normally related great arteries. In addition, right ventricular outflow tract obstruction and either subpulmonic or pulmonic valve stenosis may be found with either combination (Table 27).

HISTORICAL NOTES

Pathologic description of this entity dates back many years, to Farre, in 1814, and Holmes, in 1824. There has been a bewildering variety of names for it, including cor triloculare biatriatum (Favorite, 1934), cor biloculare (Wood and Williams, 1928), and common ventricle (Abbott, 1936). In 1964, Van Praagh and colleagues used morphologic principles to determine the embryologic origin of the ventricle and helped to clarify the nature of this anomaly.

Clinical recognition has been achieved only recently with the development of selective angiography. Successful surgical repair has become possible only within the last decade (Edie et al. and Ionescu et al., both in 1973).

PATHOLOGY

Taussig suggested in 1939 that single ventricle was simply a very large ventricular septal defect, with contributions from both right and left ventricle to

Table 27. Relationship of the great arteries in single ventricle (combined reports)

	RV obstruction	No RV obstruction
With d-transposition	13	6
With l-transposition	19	10
With normally related great arteries	4	3
Common AV valve	4	1

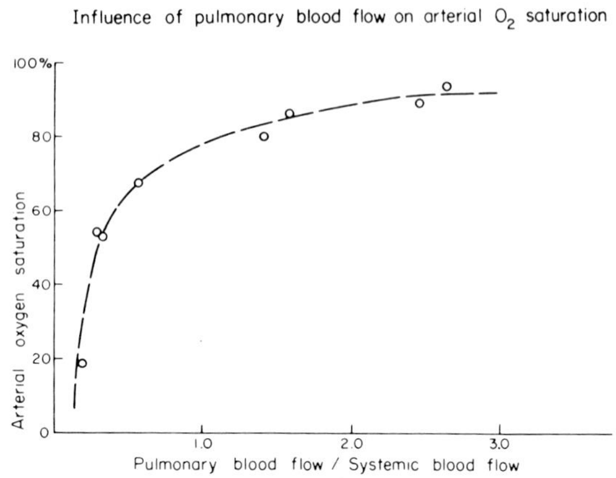

Figure 151. When systemic arterial oxygen saturations are plotted against the ratio of pulmonary blood flow to systemic blood flow, there is an exponential increase with increasing pulmonary flow. (From Krovetz et al. 1970. Circulation 42:953–959. By permission of the American Heart Association, Inc.)

the common chamber. This situation actually forms less than 10% of this grouping. Far more common is one small hypoplastic right ventricle with the effective pumping chamber formed entirely from the left ventricle (Van Praagh's type A). The converse of this, called type B by Van Praagh, is seen in about 5% of cases.

HEMODYNAMICS

Single ventricle without right ventricular obstruction may resemble transposition of the great arteries, with a high pulmonary blood flow and cyanosis; with right ventricular obstruction it may resemble tetralogy of Fallot, with decreased pulmonary vascularity and cyanosis. In individuals with normally related great vessels and no right ventricular obstruction it may mimic large ventricular septal defects.

The degree of arterial saturation is directly related to the ratio of pulmonary blood flow to systemic blood flow. The situation is analogous to a large mixing vessel into which two streams of water are flowing. If one stream is at 100° and the other is at 70°, the final temperature will be determined by the ratio of the waters flowing in these two streams (Figures 151).

CLINICAL FEATURES

As one would expect, the clinical features are extremely variable. In some cases, the patient closely resembles tetralogy of Fallot, and the true nature of the intracardiac shunt is discovered only at cardiac catheterization. The other large group resembles transposition of the great arteries with an extremely variable degree of cyanosis. If the pulmonary blood flow is high enough,

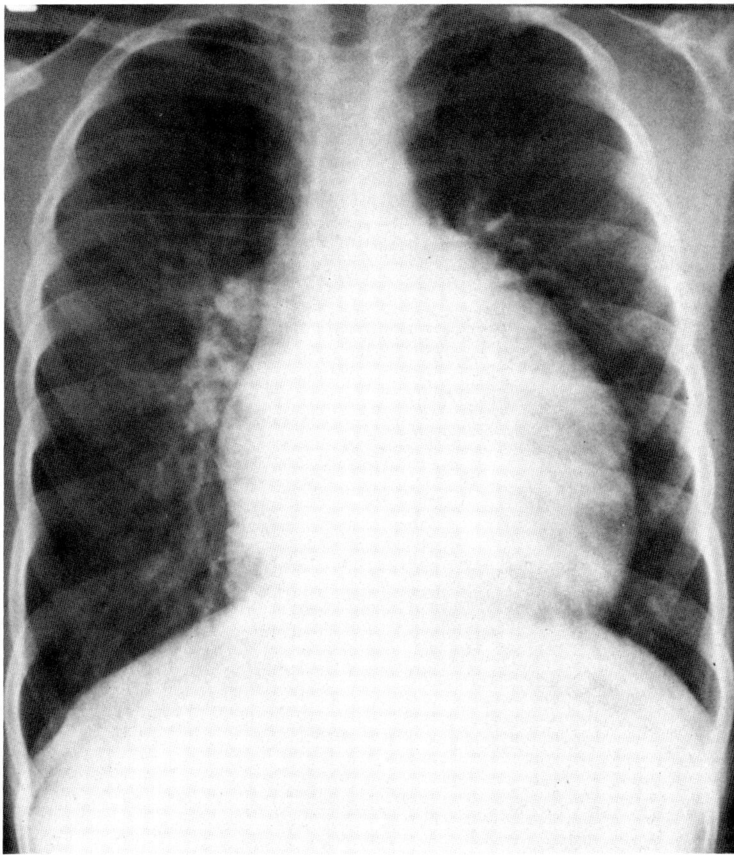

Figure 152. Chest x-ray of a 9-year-old girl with single ventricle and l-loop transposition of the great arteries. Note the large heart, narrow waist, and increased vascularity.

clinically evident cyanosis may be absent and arterial desaturation detected only by laboratory measurements.

The only valuable clue on the physical examination may be the fact that the second sound is single.

ROENTGENOGRAPHIC FEATURES

As would be expected, these are extremely variable. Figures 152 and 153 illustrate this degree of variability.

ELECTROCARDIOGRAM

As would be expected from the variety of lesions seen with single ventricle, either right ventricular hypertrophy or left ventricular hypertrophy may be

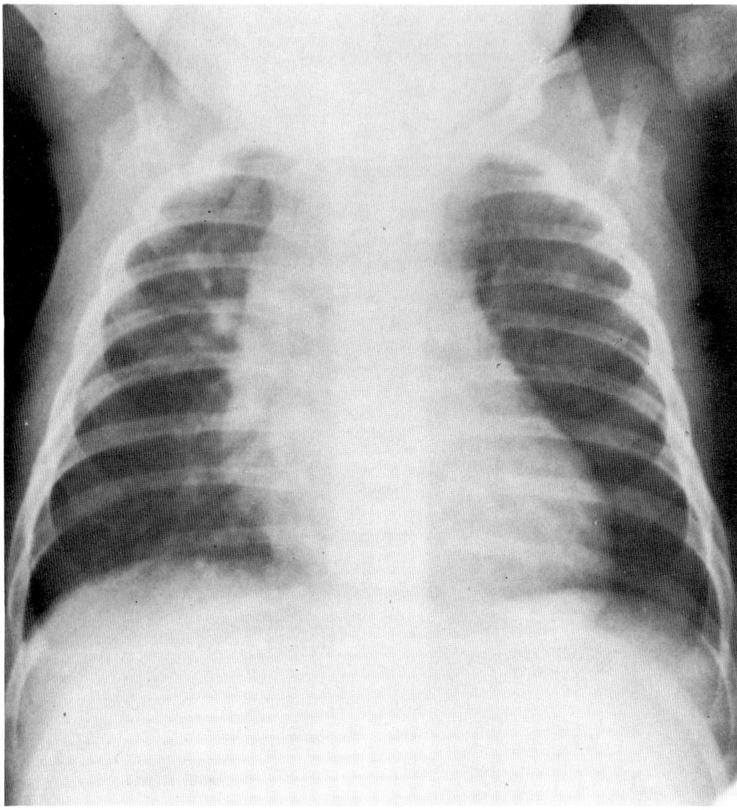

Figure 153. Chest x-ray of a 1-month-old male with single ventricle and pulmonic stenosis. The x-ray is similar to that seen in cyanotic tetralogy of Fallot (See Figure 174).

seen. A qR pattern in the right precordium and no q wave in the left precordial leads (V_5–V_7) is commonly seen with l-loop transposition (ventricular inversion). This normally rightward and anterior force is caused by septal depolarization, and the ventricular septum is either absent or in an abnormal location.

A narrow QRS loop pointing posteriorly is often seen with the asplenia complex (Figure 154). The rS pattern is remarkably similar from leads V_1 through V_6.

DIFFERENTIAL DIAGNOSIS

Since there are so many possible combinations, a high degree of suspicion should be maintained when the second sound is single. The diagnosis is best established by angiocardiography.

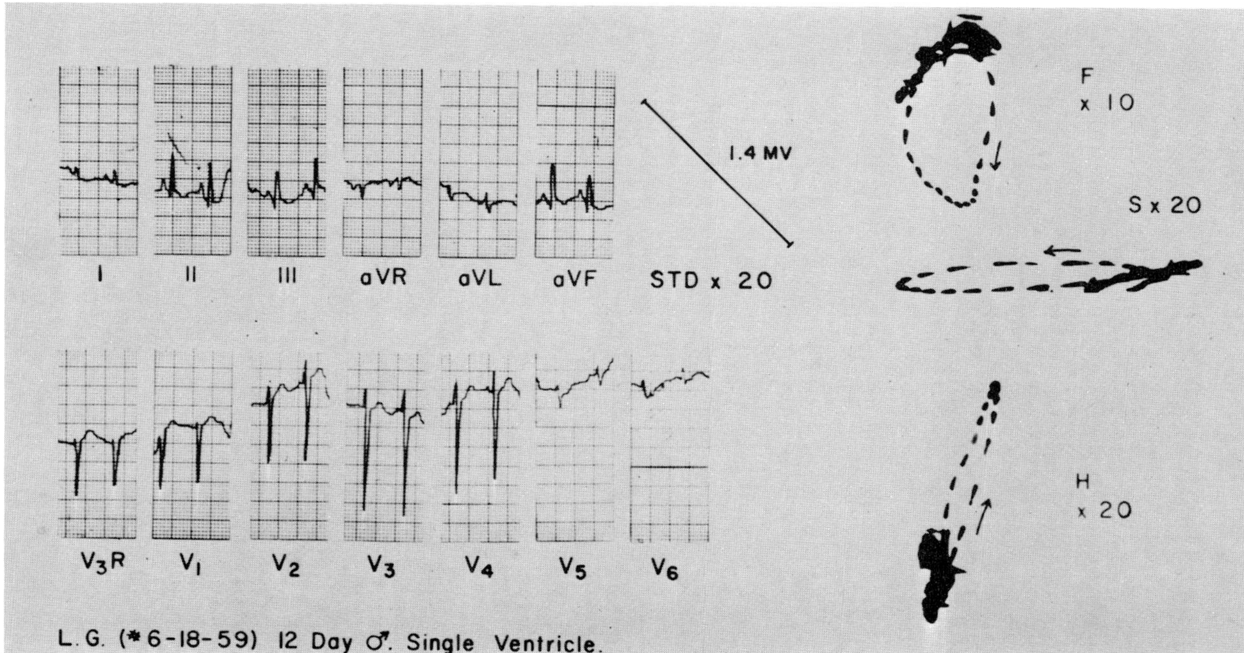

Figure 154. ECG in single ventricle in a 12-day-old male infant. Note the similar QRS complexes from lead V_3R to V_4.

PROGNOSIS

This is extremely variable, with deaths occurring from a few days of age in those resembling transposition to several months in those resembling tetralogy. In rare instances, the degree of right ventricular obstruction is such that pulmonary blood flow is essentially normal and this may be compatible with survival to adulthood.

MANAGEMENT

Appropriate anticongestive measures are needed for patients with high pulmonary blood flow, cardiac overwork, and congestive heart failure. Concurrent chest infections should be treated with appropriate antibiotics. If there is marked cyanosis, cardiac catheterization should be performed promptly. Every effort should be made to establish a complete diagnosis, especially of additional anomalies such as coarctation of the aorta. In the presence of severe unremitting congestive heart failure, pulmonary artery banding is indicated to limit pulmonary blood flow, decrease cardiac work, and protect the lung bed. With severe right ventricular obstruction, a shunt procedure may be appropriate (see Chapter 23).

There have been some recent reports of successful artificial partitioning of the common chamber in children of about 5 to 10 years of age. This clearly justifies the vigor needed in treating these children in infancy to increase their likelihood of survival to an age when appropriate surgery may be carried out.

BIBLIOGRAPHY

Macartney, F. J., Partridge, J. B., Scott, O., and Deverall, P. B. 1976. Common or single ventricle. Circulation 53:543–554.

Seward, J. B., Tajik, A. J., Hagler, D. J., and Ritter, D. G. 1977. Contrast echocardiography in single or common ventricle. Circulation 55:513–519.

Taussig, H. B. 1976. Long-time observations on the Blalock-Taussig operation. IX. Single ventricle (with apex to the left). Johns Hopkins Med. J. 139:69–76.

Van Praagh, R., Ongley, P. A., and Swan, H. J. C. 1964. Anatomic types of single or common ventricle in man. Morphologic and geometric aspects of 60 necropsied cases. Am. J. Cardiol. 13:367–386.

chapter 22

PULMONIC STENOSIS

Pulmonic stenosis may be defined as obstruction to blood flow from the right ventricle. While the most common site of obstruction is at the pulmonic valve, stenosis may also occur proximal or distal to the valve. Obstruction of the right ventricular infundibulum is usually associated with a ventricular septal defect (see Chapter 23), but may occur alone. An anomalous muscle band in the mid–right ventricle is a rare cause of outflow tract obstruction. Narrowings of the peripheral pulmonary arteries may occur at one or two locations or may be multiple and widespread.

Regardless of the site of obstruction, the result is an increase in right ventricular systolic pressure and stroke work. With severe obstruction and an intact ventricular septum, the foramen ovale may be forced open by high right atrial pressure, allowing a right-to-left atrial shunt. This situation is of critical clinical importance and is discussed independently in this chapter. Occasionally, a true ostium secundum atrial septal defect may be present, and, if the obstruction is not severe, shunting may be predominantly left to right.

If a ventricular septal defect accompanies pulmonic stenosis, shunting is determined by the degree of obstruction and may be in either direction. With mild to moderate stenosis, shunting will be from left to right and the clinical features will reflect both anomalies. With severe obstruction, shunting will be from right to left and the findings will mimic those of tetralogy of Fallot (Chapter 23).

HISTORICAL NOTES

Like many of the other cardiac anomalies in this book, narrowing or stenosis of the pulmonic valve was first described by Morgagni in 1761. Diagnosis on clinical grounds was shown to be possible by Taussig in about 1940. The first successful surgery for relief of pulmonic valvar stenosis was performed by Holmes, Sellors, and Brock in 1948.

PULMONIC STENOSIS WITH INTACT SEPTA

Incidence

Isolated pulmonic stenosis constitutes approximately 10% of congenital cardiac anomalies. Fortunately, most patients have only mild or moderate stenosis, and, by our present criteria, fewer than one-third of our patients are recommended for surgical correction. The sex incidence is roughly equal. Dysplastic pulmonic valves are common in the Noonan syndrome.

Etiology

Pulmonic stenosis is occasionally familial. In one series of 125 cases of pulmonic stenosis, a congenital heart defect occurred in six of 282 siblings, but in none of the parents. Of these six siblings, pulmonic stenosis was present in five. Neither maternal age nor birth rank appears to be of etiologic importance. Instances of pulmonic valve stenosis in multiple generations have also been reported.

Pathology

The classical thickened, domed valve with a tight (1 to 3 mm) opening (Figure 155) is seen almost exclusively in infants with severe stenosis. Older indi-

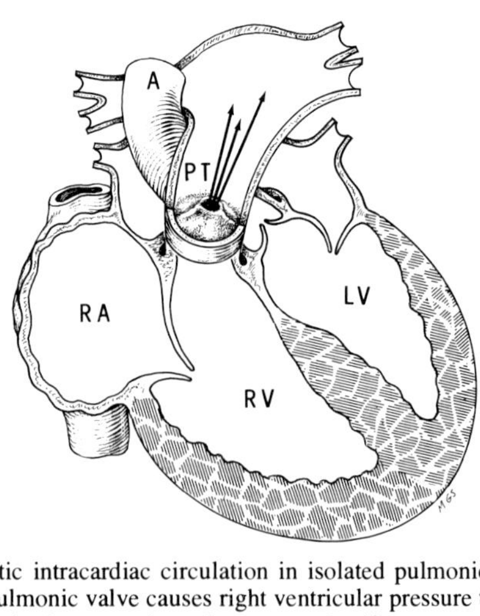

Figure 155. Schematic intracardiac circulation in isolated pulmonic valve stenosis. The narrowed and deformed pulmonic valve causes right ventricular pressure to rise in order to maintain normal cardiac output. At the same time, the narrowed orifice concentrates the energy from the right ventricle into a small cross-sectional area, resulting in a high velocity jet. In time, this jet weakens the wall of the pulmonary artery and causes it to dilate. (From Elliott, L. P., and Schiebler, G. L. 1968. X-Ray Diagnosis of Congenital Cardiac Disease. Courtesy of Charles C Thomas, Publisher, Springfield, Ill.)

viduals usually have less deformity of the valve, with knobby excrescences on the cusp edges and some peripheral cusp fusion. Occasionally, the valve is bicuspid. In isolated infundibular stenosis, there is localized muscular hypertrophy of the outflow tract.

Some degree of right ventricular hypertrophy is always present. Right atrial enlargement is present in severe cases, and may also occur in moderate cases. The aorta almost always arches to the left. Post-stenotic dilatation of the pulmonary artery is not seen with infundibular stenosis or severe obstruction in the young infant. Rarely, the pulmonic valve ring is hypoplastic and the valve is composed of thickened, myxomatous, immobile tissue. Again, little post-stenotic dilatation is seen. This type of dysplastic pulmonic valve is difficult to correct surgically since valvotomy alone is usually not effective.

Hemodynamics

Use of the terms mild, moderate, and severe is based on a combination of clinical differences and catheterization findings. Mild pulmonic stenosis may be defined as right ventricular systolic pressure greater than normal, with a 15-mm pressure drop across the pulmonic valve. Moderate may be defined as a right ventricular systolic pressure that is about 50% of systemic systolic pressure, and severe cases will have a right pressure that is more than 75% of systemic systolic pressure.

With severe obstruction, particularly in the infant, myocardial decompensation may occur, causing cardiac output to fall, and the degree of right ventricular hypertension will no longer correlate as well with the severity of the disease (see Figure 25). Thus, it is important to measure cardiac output when assessing the pressure difference across an obstructed valve.

The diastolic compliance of the right ventricle is reduced and the right atrium must contract more vigorously to empty blood into it. In severe obstruction, right atrial hypertension and enlargement develop. In such cases, the foramen ovale may be forced open, resulting in a right-to-left shunt and systemic arterial desaturation. Left atrial enlargement may be noted under these circumstances.

It is important to keep in mind that when the ventricular septum is intact right ventricular systolic pressure can rise to levels considerably higher than those in the left ventricle. This is not possible in tetralogy of Fallot, since right and left ventricular pressures must be equal in the presence of a large ventricular septal defect. Patients with an intact septum will maintain normal pulmonary blood flows and thus better exercise ability than will patients in whom right-to-left shunting can occur. However, with severe obstruction, these patients may develop very thick right ventricular walls, with resultant myocardial underperfusion and eventually congestive heart failure, a phenomenon that does not occur in tetralogy of Fallot.

Clinical Features

Children with *mild or moderate stenosis* are acyanotic and have normal physical development. Indeed, these children often are chubby or at least stocky in body build. Arterial pulses are normal, as is systemic blood pressure. Palpation reveals a right ventricular lift and a systolic thrill at the second left intercostal space and in the suprasternal notch. An ejection murmur with early systolic accentuation is heard best at the second left intercostal space and radiates to the left shoulder and the left precordium. A systolic ejection click that increases in intensity with expiration, indicating its origin in the pulmonary artery, is usually present. The pulmonic component of S_2 may be normal or slightly reduced in intensity and the duration of splitting of S_2 in expiration varies from 0.04 to 0.06 sec (Figure 156). The intensity of the pulmonic component of the second sound is inversely related, and the width of the second sound splitting directly related, to the severity of the stenosis. Diastolic murmurs are not heard, but a third heart sound may be present.

If an atrial septal defect is present in patients with mild to moderate valvar pulmonic stenosis, clinical diagnosis of this additional defect may be quite difficult. A low-pitched, scratchy tricuspid flow murmur is the only reliable auscultatory feature. Although cyanosis will not be present, a small right-to-left shunt may occur, even though the predominant shunt is left to right. A slight rise in hematocrit or a decrease in arterial pO_2 may indicate such a right-to-left shunt.

Exercise intolerance is sometimes seen in children with *severe stenosis,* but most patients are surprisingly asymptomatic. Prominent jugular "a"

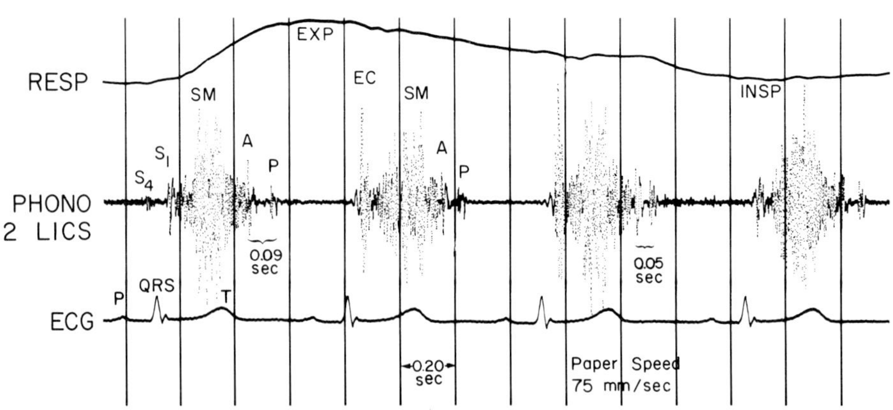

Figure 156. Phonocardiogram of an 11-year-old patient with moderate pulmonic valvar stenosis. Note the crescendo-decrescendo systolic murmur, the wide splitting of S_2, still with respiratory variation, and the only slightly diminished pulmonic component of S_2. A pulmonic systolic ejection click is also present. (Courtesy of Elliott, L. P., and Schiebler, G. L. 1968. X-Ray Diagnosis of Congenital Cardiac Disease. Courtesy of Charles C Thomas, Publisher, Springfield, Ill.)

waves, indicative of increased resistance to right atrial emptying, and a right parasternal heave, indicating right ventricular hypertrophy, are usually found. A systolic thrill is found at the second left intercostal space and in the suprasternal notch, except in infants in congestive heart failure or with very severe stenosis. The duration of the murmur is more prolonged than in moderate cases. The murmur has a late accentuation and usually extends past aortic closure (Figure 157). A systolic ejection click is usually not heard, but if present it is closer to S_1 than in milder degrees of pulmonic stenosis. The pulmonic component of S_2 is soft (occasionally inaudible) and the duration of splitting is widened, to about 0.10 sec. A fourth heart sound at the apex is commonly heard.

Roentgenographic Features

Although radiographs of some cases may be interpreted as normal, right ventricular enlargement and a prominent main and left pulmonary artery are usually detectable (Figures 89 and 158). Overall heart size ranges from normal in mild or moderate cases to marked enlargement in severe cases with failing hearts. Right atrial enlargement is most easily appreciated in severe cases.

Pulmonary arterial vascularity is always normal, although enlargement of the left pulmonary artery may be misinterpreted as indicative of increased vascularity. Since there is no shunt, pulmonary blood flow must be equal to systemic flow; systemic and pulmonary flows are normal unless there is severe congestive heart failure. This is an important differential point for isolated pulmonic stenosis.

X-ray evidence of post-stenotic dilatation of the pulmonary artery occurs, except in those with associated severe infundibular stenosis or in young

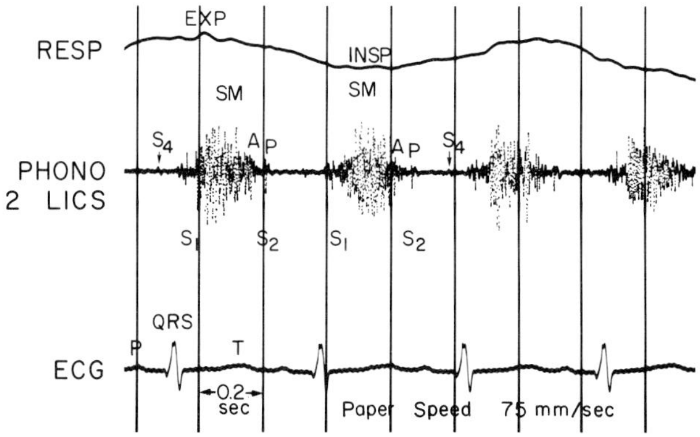

Figure 157. Phonocardiogram of a 2-month-old patient with severe pulmonic stenosis. Note that the systolic murmur tends to peak late in systole and at times overrides aortic component of S_2. Splitting of S_2 is wide and the pulmonic component is reduced in intensity. An ejection click is not seen.

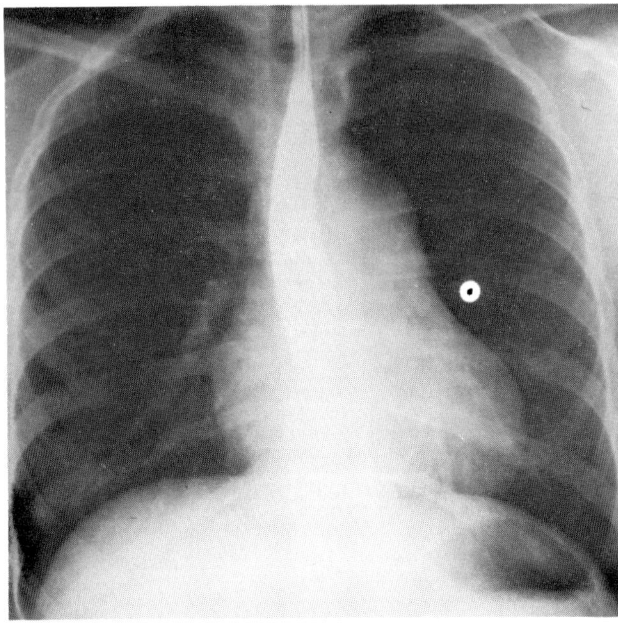

Figure 158. Chest x-ray of a 12-year-old girl with pulmonic valvar stenosis. The pulmonary artery is very prominent. The heart size and pulmonary vascularity are normal.

infants with severe valvar stenosis (see Figure 163). The aortic arch is almost invariably on the left.

Electrocardiography

Patients with *mild to moderate stenosis* usually show some degree of right ventricular hypertrophy (Figure 159). Average frontal plane QRS axis is +110 degrees and P waves are normal in configuration. In some cases, a positive T wave in lead V_1 is the only evidence of right ventricular hypertrophy.

Patients with *severe stenosis* show more severe right ventricular hypertrophy (Figure 160). Marked right axis deviation and right atrial enlargement are common. Tall R waves or even a qR pattern is present in lead V_1. T-wave inversion may be seen from lead V_3R to as far leftward as V_4.

Prognosis

Mild pulmonic stenosis is compatible with a long life, since the right ventricle can tolerate slight increases in pressure work quite well. Serial catheterization data suggest that there is little or no increase of right ventricular pressure with time. In the moderate group, the degree of stenosis may also remain unchanged for many years, although evidence is accumulating that progression

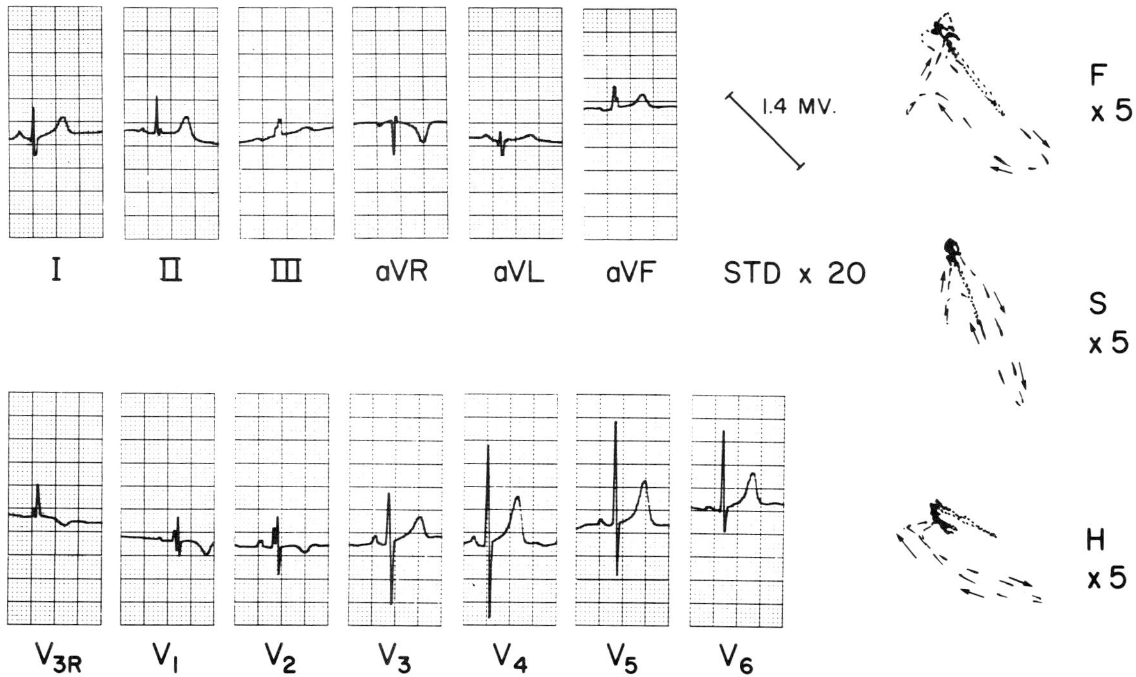

Figure 159. Electrovectorcardiogram of a 10-year-old patient with moderate pulmonic stenosis. Note the 100% R in lead V_3R, the rSR′ in lead V_1, and the clockwise QRS vector in the horizontal plane, all indicating right ventricular hypertrophy.

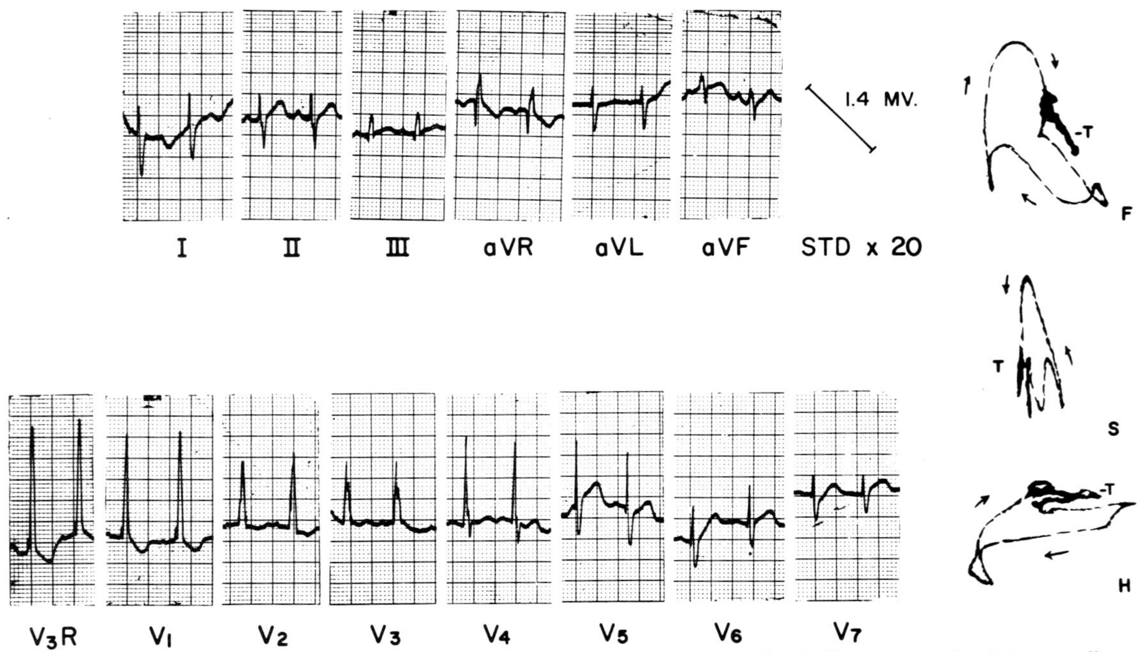

Figure 160. Electrovectorcardiogram of a 5-month-old patient with severe pulmonic stenosis. Note that the R waves over the right precordium are completely upright and that there is a slow progression moving from lead V_3R to V_7 of diminution of the R waves and an increase in the depth of the S waves. This is in contrast to Figure 175. Despite the marked right ventricular hypertrophy, a q wave is still present in lead V_6, indicating the presence of left ventricular activity.

The vectorcardiogram shows rightward and anterior shift of the QRS forces and reversal of inscription of the QRS loop in horizontal and sagittal planes.

of right ventricular pressure, and of symptoms, does occur, especially during the first 2 or 3 years of life.

In the severe group, congestive heart failure is the most important cause of death. Usually occurring during the first year of life, its onset may be abrupt and death may follow rapidly.

Infective endocarditis is a rare but constant hazard, even in the mild forms.

Management

The treatment for severe pulmonic valve stenosis is surgical. Medical management of the patient with congestive heart failure is of little value. While a closed heart approach using a valvulotome is sometimes done in small infants, an open valvotomy using cardiopulmonary bypass allows better visualization of the valve. Currently this procedure can be accomplished with a mortality risk of less than 1%.

Some degree of insufficiency of the valve is usually seen following either procedure. In our experience, based on clinical evaluation and recatheterization of these patients, this has not been a significant problem following open heart repair. Some severe cases, particularly older children and adults, may show persistent right ventricular hypertension postoperatively, as a result of secondary muscular hypertrophy of the infundibulum. Although this will usually regress spontaneously, it has been reported as causing right heart failure and death in the immediate postoperative period. Resection of a portion of this hypertrophic muscle may be necessary in order to avoid this complication. The need for such resection can generally be determined at cardiac catheterization using specific hemodynamic and angiographic criteria. The final decision, however, rests with the surgeon, who must evaluate the right ventricular outflow tract in these severe cases during operation. In addition, the surgeon should inspect the interatrial septum in order not to overlook either an atrial septal defect or a patent foramen ovale. Repair of the atrial septum prevents postoperative right-to-left shunting, a bothersome postoperative complication. Within days after successful valvotomy, striking changes occur in the electrocardiogram, reflecting the changes in right ventricular pressure.

PULMONIC STENOSIS WITH RIGHT-TO-LEFT SHUNT AT THE ATRIAL LEVEL (TRILOGY)

Incidence

Although it is not entirely appropriate to attach the name of Fallot to this defect, this was done in 1950 by Joly, one of his countrymen. Trilogy occurs in between 5% and 10% of patients with pulmonic valve stenosis. This condition thus accounts for less than 1% of all congenital heart disease, being about one-tenth as common as tetralogy of Fallot. Its importance lies in the rapidity with which cardiac failure and death can occur, as well as the fact that it can be readily corrected even in early infancy.

Pathology

When the stenosis is severe, marked right-to-left atrial shunting can occur, and the combination of severe right ventricular pressure overload, decreased pulmonary blood flow, systemic hypoxemia, and congestive failure produces a critical situation that must be treated as a true emergency.

The interatrial communication is usually a patent foramen ovale, but a true atrial defect, most commonly a secundum defect, may occur.

Pulmonic valve atresia with intact ventricular septum is discussed under hypoplastic right heart syndrome (see Chapter 24).

Hemodynamics

We believe that the sequence of adverse events begins with severe right ventricular hypertrophy. By some mechanism, perhaps fibrosis or infarction of the right ventricular myocardium, dilatation of the atrial ring and tricuspid insufficiency develop. With the resultant increase in right atrial pressure, the foramen ovale reopens, a right-to-left shunt occurs, and the left ventricle becomes overloaded. This combination of right ventricular pressure overloading and left ventricular volume overloading is poorly tolerated and the heart fails rapidly.

Clinical Features

These infants often exhibit robust physical development and a healthy appearance that belies the severity of their hemodynamic state. The right-to-left

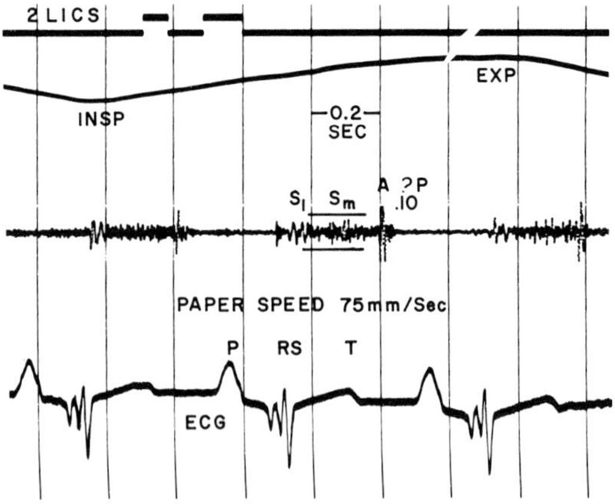

Figure 161. Phonocardiogram of a 25-month-old patient with severe pulmonic stenosis and right-to-left shunt at the atrial level. Note the low intensity systolic murmur and the absent pulmonic component of S_2.

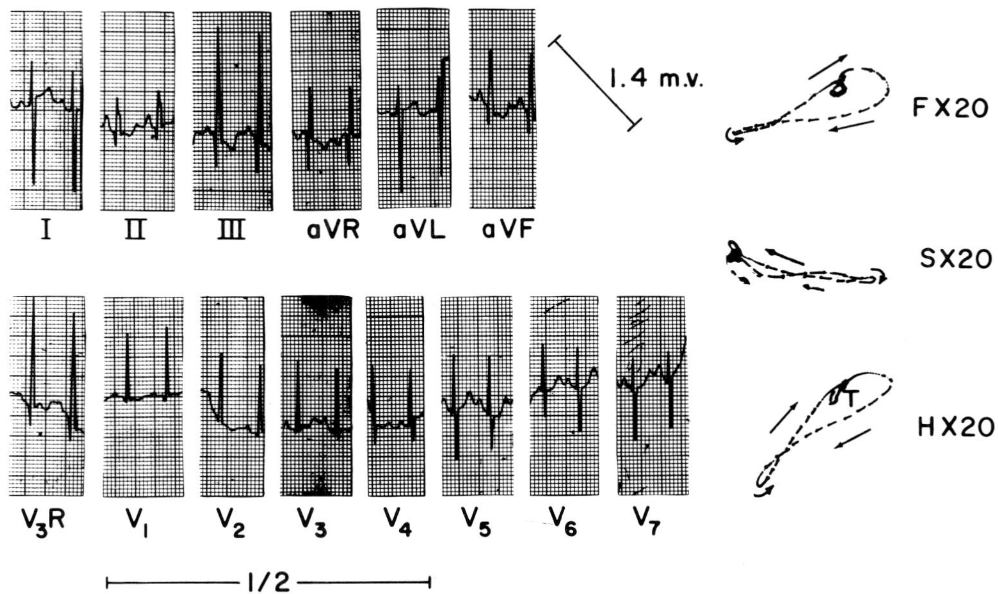

Figure 162. Electrovectorcardiogram of a 7-month-old boy with pulmonic valvar stenosis and a right-to-left shunt at the atrial level. Note the qR pattern and the inversion of the T waves in the right precordium, and the slow progression of totally upright R waves over the right precordium to an RS pattern over the left precordium. Again, contrast this with Figure 175. Right atrial enlargement is present.

The vectorcardiogram shows marked rightward and anterior shift of QRS forces, with a reversal of inscription of the QRS loop in the horizontal plane.

Table 28. Differential diagnosis of trilogy and tetralogy

	Trilogy	Tetralogy
Clinical features		
Congestive heart failure	Common	Rare
Obvious cyanosis and clubbing	Uncommon	Common
Squatting	Never (?)	Common
Physique	Normal	Usually retarded
Giant jugular "a" wave	Common	Rare
Suprasternal notch thrill	Common	Rare
Systolic murmur peaking	Late and overrides aortic closure	Early and ends prior to aortic closure
Pulmonary systolic ejection click	Common	Rare
Paroxysmal hyperpnea	Rare	Common
Roentgenographic features		
Left atrial enlargement	Sometimes	No
Aortic arch	Left	25% right
Main pulmonary artery	Enlarged	Decreased
Pulmonary vascular markings	Decreased	Decreased
Electrocardiogram		
Right atrial enlargement	Common	Rare
Left atrial enlargement	Sometimes	No
Right ventricular hypertrophy	Marked	Less severe; transition to RS in V_2
Right precordial T wave inversion	Common	Rare
Catheterization		
Stenosis	Valvar	Infundibular or valvar
Right ventricle systolic pressure	Greater than systemic (unless in CHF)	Equal to systemic
Tricuspid insufficiency	Common	Rare
Right-to-left shunt	Atrial level	Ventricular level
Echocardiogram		
Right ventricular wall thickening	Marked	Less severe
Large aorta	No	Yes
Discontinuity between septum and aorta	No	Common
Left atrial enlargement	Sometimes	No

shunt may not cause readily apparent cyanosis until rather late, after right heart failure supervenes. The systolic murmur ranges from that typical of pulmonic stenosis to a rather nonspecific, short, grade 1 to 2/6 systolic murmur in extremely severe stenosis (Figure 161). With congestive heart failure, the intensity of the murmur decreases and ventricular filling sounds become louder.

Electrocardiography

Marked right ventricular hypertrophy is a constant finding (Figure 162). In addition, when a right-to-left shunt is present, increased left ventricular forces may be seen. Right atrial enlargement is usually marked, and because of the right-to-left atrial shunt some left atrial enlargement may be present.

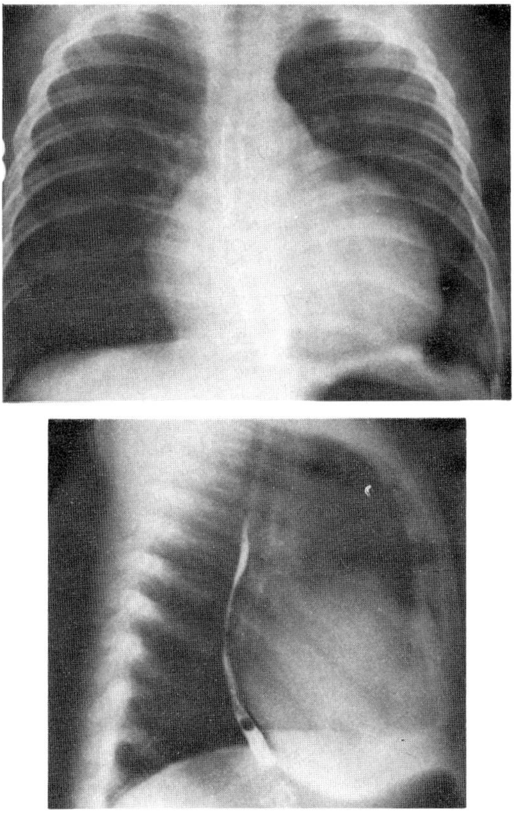

Figure 163. AP and lateral films of an 8-month-old patient with valvar pulmonic stenosis and a right-to-left shunt at the atrial level. Note the marked decrease in pulmonary vascularity that differentiates this entity from isolated pulmonic stenosis. The heart is enlarged and left atrial enlargement is present.

The combination of left atrial enlargement and decreased pulmonary arterial vascularity always suggests a right-to-left shunt at the atrial level.

Differential Diagnosis

Tetralogy of Fallot is the cardiac anomaly most often confused with trilogy prior to the onset of congestive heart failure; the differential diagnosis is detailed in Table 28.

Severe pulmonic stenosis with intact septa is another source of diagnostic confusion. As discussed earlier, if the pulmonary vasculature is clearly diminished on x-ray, pulmonary blood flow must be decreased. This is not compatible with intact septa (Figure 163). The patient must therefore have a right-to-left shunt, even in the absence of clinically obvious cyanosis. An increase in hematocrit also suggests a right-to-left shunt.

Prognosis

Infants with trilogy and congestive heart failure are a medical and surgical emergency. Early recognition of such cases can be literally life saving. Indeed, infants may proceed from apparent well-being to death within a few days.

Management

All too often, parents (and physicians) are misled as to the seriousness of the disease by the generally excellent physical development of these infants and ignore such tell-tale signs as mild, generalized cyanosis. Increasing cardiomegaly on x-ray or increasing signs of right ventricular pressure overloading call for prompt cardiac catheterization. Prompt surgical relief of the obstruction is mandatory. Medical management by itself is of no significant value. Various surgical techniques have been employed, but we prefer open valvotomy through an incision in the pulmonary trunk, using cardiopulmonary bypass.

PULMONARY ARTERY COARCTATION: PERIPHERAL PULMONIC STENOSIS

Incidence and Etiology

This entity, which is being recognized with increasing frequency, may occur as an isolated finding or in conjunction with other cardiovascular anomalies, particularly pulmonic valvar stenosis, tetralogy of Fallot, or patent ductus arteriosus. Recently, association with atrial septal defect has been emphasized. Peripheral pulmonic stenosis is commonly seen in association with the rubella syndrome, where the coarctations are usually multiple. Multiple pulmonary coarctations may also be seen with supravalvar aortic stenosis (see Chapter 25).

Pathology

The coarctations may occur at any point in the pulmonary arterial system. The obstruction may be limited to the origin of the right or left main pulmonary arteries. Sometimes there are several narrowed areas in the major pulmonary artery branches and a diffuse hypoplasia of pulmonary arteries may even occur.

Hemodynamics

If the obstruction is significant, elevation of right ventricular pressure and pulmonary artery pressure proximal to the lesion will occur. Increases in right ventricular pressure range from trivial to systemic, reflecting the severity of the narrowing of the pulmonary arteries.

The finding of a significant pressure difference upon repeated withdrawal of the catheter across the suspected point of coarctation is highly suggestive. Angiocardiographic demonstration provides the most conclusive evidence (Figure 164), although at times the area of narrowing is not easily displayed.

Clinical Features

Symptoms are uncommon. An ejection click is not heard, and the components of the second sound usually split normally. In contrast to valvar stenosis, the

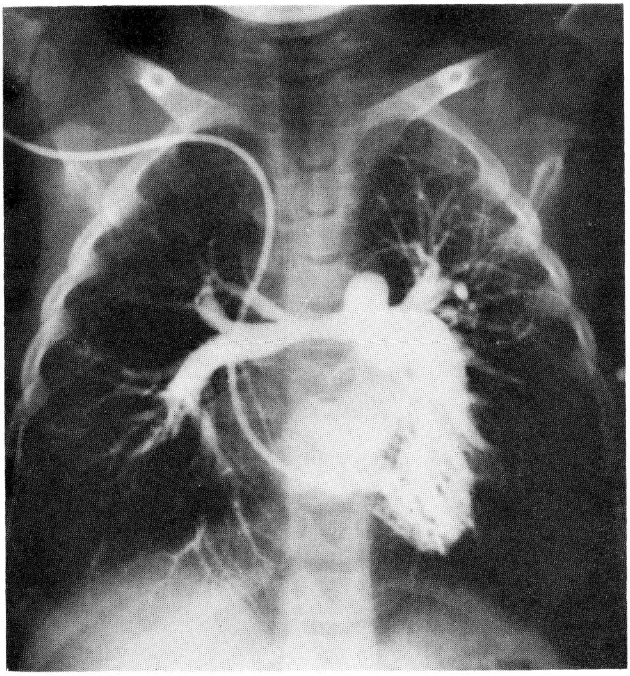

Figure 164. Multiple pulmonary artery coarctations in a 5-year-old patient with post-rubella syndrome. Note the irregularity of the pulmonary arterial system and the hump-shaped pulmonary trunk. There is narrowing of the right pulmonary artery over the vertebral column. Narrowing may also be noted in smaller branches of the entire pulmonary artery bed, causing diffuse irregularity. (Courtesy of Dr. F. A. Hernandez, National Children's Cardiac Hospital, Miami, Florida.)

pulmonic component of the second sound is normal in intensity or slightly accentuated. A grade 2 or 3/6 systolic murmur is present, typically audible over the entire precordium, both axillae, and over the back. This murmur may begin in midsystole and peak in late systole, overriding the second sound. If the obstruction is more severe, a continuous murmur may be heard.

Roentgenographic Features

The pulmonary vascularity is normal. Evidence of mild right ventricular hypertrophy may be present, but not dilatation of the pulmonary trunk or left pulmonary artery.

Electrocardiography

Usually normal, the electrocardiogram will show right ventricular hypertrophy if the obstruction is sufficiently severe. Patients with rubella syndrome may demonstrate a superior frontal QRS axis that is unrelated to the actual anatomy and hemodynamics.

Prognosis

The prognosis has not been fully determined. Progressive right ventricular hypertension may occur in severe cases, but most patients show no significant change in their clinical status.

Management

Since most cases are mild and have multiple sites of coarctation, no treatment is advisable. Surgery is indicated only in severe cases in which there is a discrete coarctation in a proximal vessel (or vessels) accessible to the surgeon. Patients will not be benefited by surgical treatment if they also have multiple peripheral coarctations of equal or greater severity.

BIBLIOGRAPHY

Brodsky, S. J., Krovetz, L. J., and Schiebler, G. L. 1970. Assessment of severity of valvar pulmonic stenosis using isoproterenol. Am. Heart J. 80:660–670.

Danilowicz, D., et al. 1972. Physiologic pressure differences between main and branch pulmonary arteries in infants. Circulation 45:410–419.

Danilowicz, D., Hoffman, J. E., and Rudolph, A. M. 1975. Serial studies of pulmonary stenosis in infancy and childhood. Br. Heart J. 37:808–818.

Dunkle, L. M., and Rowe, R. D. 1972. Transient murmur simulating pulmonary artery stenosis in premature infants. Am. J. Dis. Child. 124:666–670.

Koretzky, E. D., Moller, J. H., Korns, M. E., Schwaltz, C. J., and Edwards, J. E. 1969. Congenital pulmonary stenosis resulting from dysplasia of valve. Circulation 40:43–53.

Mirowski, M., Shah, K. D., Neill, C. A., and Taussig, H. B. 1963. Long-term (10–13 years) follow-up study after transventricular pulmonary valvulotomy for pulmonary stenosis with intact ventricular septum. Circulation 28:906–914.

Rowe, R. D. 1963. Maternal rubella and pulmonary artery stenoses. Report of eleven cases. Pediatrics 32:180–185.

Scherlis, L., Koenker, R. J., and Lee, Y. 1963. Pulmonary stenosis. Electrocardiographic, vectorcardiographic, and catheterization data. Circulation 28:288–305.

Stone, F. M., Bessinger, F. B., Jr., Lucas, R. V., Jr., and Molla, J. H. 1974. Pre- and postoperative rest and exercise hemodynamics in children with pulmonary stenosis. Circulation 49:1102–1106.

Watson, H., and Lowe, K. G. 1962. Ventricular pressure flow relationships in isolated valvular stenosis. Br. Heart J. 24:431–440.

chapter 23

TETRALOGY OF FALLOT

HISTORICAL NOTES

In 1888, Fallot published *The Pathologic Anatomy of the Blue Sickness,* in which he established that one form of cyanosis was due to the cardiac entity now known as the tetralogy of Fallot. Actually, this anomaly was described by Nicholas Stensen in 1671, but Stensen's priority in description was superseded by the scholarship of Fallot's paper, perhaps proving that speed in publishing is not as important as clarity and thoroughness.

The 1940s saw the development of several operations for palliation of tetralogy of Fallot: Blalock-Taussig anastomosis (1945), Potts's operation (1946), and pulmonic valvotomy by Sellors and Brock (1948). The next decade saw the development of open heart surgery, and, in 1955, Lillehei reported the first successful surgical correction of tetralogy of Fallot.

ACYANOTIC TETRALOGY (PULMONIC STENOSIS WITH A LEFT-TO-RIGHT SHUNT)

Pathology

The degree of stenosis is always moderate and the ventricular septal defect large. The obstruction is usually located in the infundibular portion of the right ventricle.

Hemodynamics

The combination of right ventricular outflow obstruction with a ventricular septal defect varies considerably, depending mainly on the severity of the obstruction. At one end of the spectrum is the patient with mild right ventricle obstruction whose shunt is entirely left to right. As the degree of stenosis increases, the left-to-right shunt decreases and right-to-left shunting becomes predominant, characteristic of cyanotic tetralogy of Fallot. As the child and the heart grow, the size of the VSD becomes relatively smaller while the degree of stenosis becomes more severe, and the direction of the shunt may change. Since some patients are acyanotic at rest but become cyanotic with exercise or may become cyanotic as they grow, classification is not always definitive.

Pressures in the right and left ventricles are essentially equal in the presence of the usual large VSD. Patients with acyanotic tetralogy usually have a significant left-to-right shunt, but if the degree of stenosis balances the size of the VSD there may be little or no shunting. Since the stenosis limits pulmonary blood flow, these children generally have fewer clinical problems than patients with only a large ventricular septal defect.

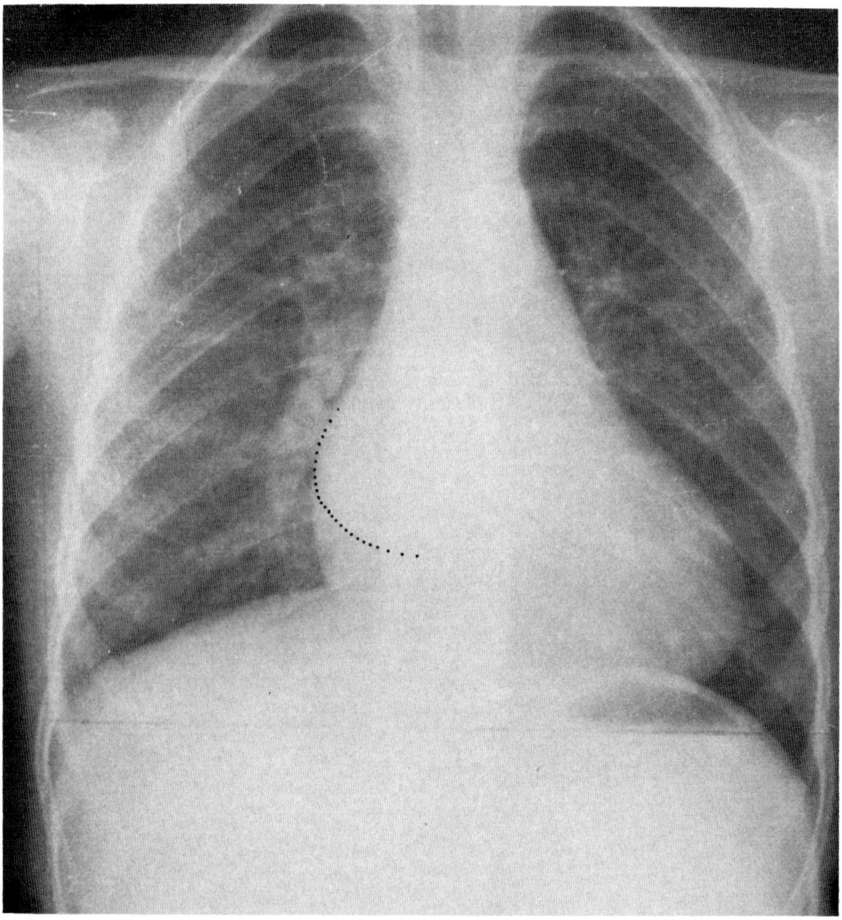

Figure 165. Posteroanterior chest roentgenogram of a 6-year-old girl with a ventricular septal defect and infundibular stenosis with a predominant left-to-right shunt. The concave pulmonary artery segment is seen frequently with infundibular stenosis. There is slight cardiomegaly, with a contour suggesting left or biventricular hypertrophy. Dotted line shows the outline of the slightly enlarged left atrium.

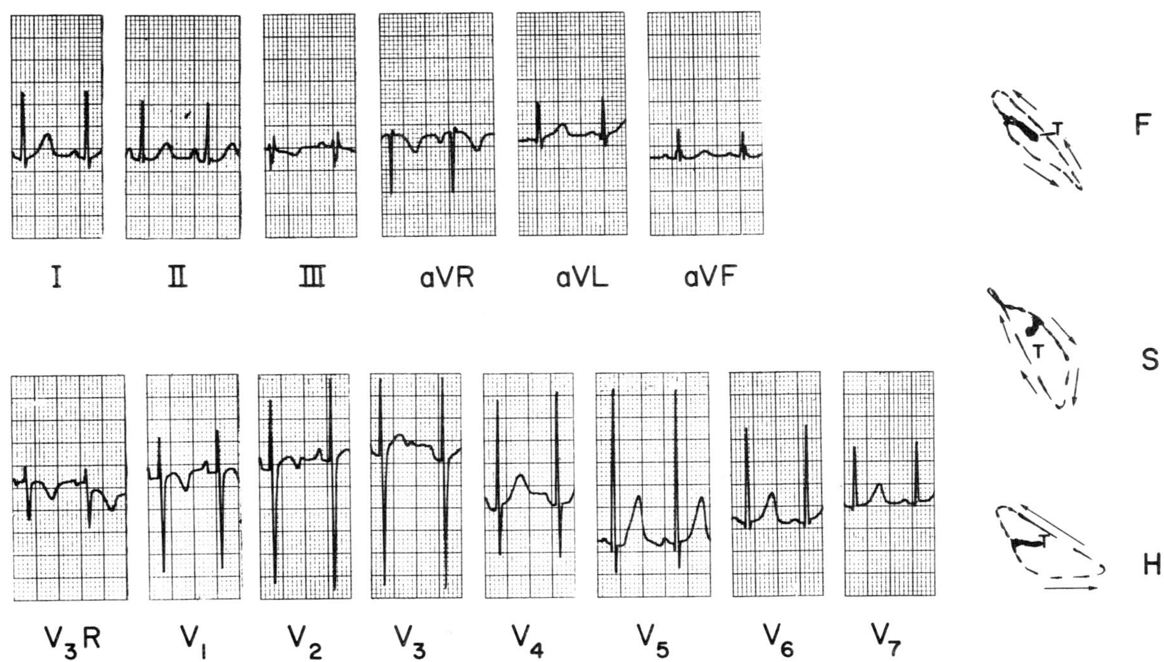

Figure 166. ECG-VCG of a 6-year-old girl with VSD, infundibular stenosis, and predominant left-to-right shunt. The 28-mm S wave in lead V_2 and the 35-mm R wave in lead V_5 with tall, narrow, peaked T waves in leads V_5 and V_6 suggest left ventricular volume overloading. The mid-precordial QRS complexes are not of sufficient magnitude to indicate biventricular hypertrophy.

Clinical Features

By definition, patients are always acyanotic at rest and usually asymptomatic. With mild stenosis they may have symptoms similar to those found with moderate-sized ventricular septal defects. The murmur of right ventricular outflow obstruction is at least a grade 3/6 systolic ejection murmur, slightly higher in pitch than the murmur of isolated valve stenosis. A suprasternal notch thrill or a murmur well transmitted to the neck or left shoulder suggests the presence of pulmonic valve stenosis. It is best heard in the third left intercostal space. Sometimes the murmur from the ventricular septal defect obscures that from the right ventricular outflow obstruction. The second sound is split more widely than normal, with slightly diminished intensity of the pulmonic component. An aortic ejection click is frequently present, suggesting a large aorta.

Roentgenographic Features

Chest x-rays usually show slight enlargement of the left or both ventricles and minor degrees of left atrial enlargement (Figure 165). Pulmonary vascularity may be slightly increased or normal. The contour of the right ventricular outflow tract is sometimes slightly concave.

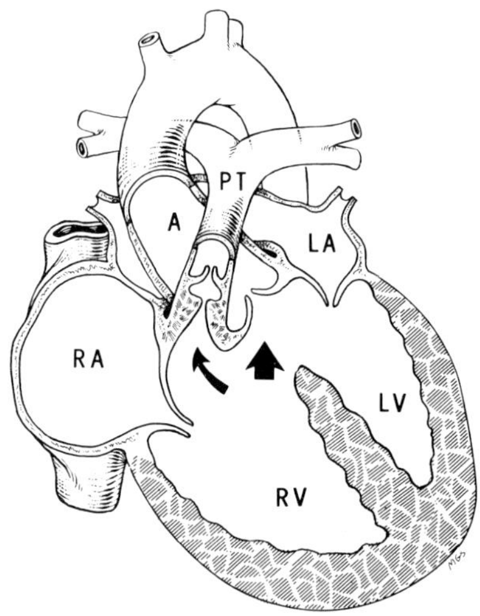

Figure 167. Schematic intracardiac circulation in cyanotic tetralogy of Fallot. Note that systemic venous blood enters the aorta without passing through the body of the left ventricle (heavy arrow). This explains why the burden of pumping blood out the great vessels falls almost entirely on the right ventricle, producing right ventricular hypertrophy and a slightly small left ventricle. (From Elliott, L. P., and Schiebler, G. L. 1968. X-Ray Diagnosis of Congenital Cardiac Disease. Courtesy of Charles C Thomas, Publisher, Springfield, Ill.)

Electrocardiography

Combined ventricular hypertrophy, usually with right ventricular pressure and left ventricular volume overloading, can be found (Figure 166). Less commonly, evidence of only left ventricular hypertrophy is present.

Prognosis

Prognosis during childhood is usually good, since pulmonary blood flow and cardiac stroke work are only slightly increased. Children rarely develop congestive heart failure, but bacterial endocarditis may occasionally occur.

Management

Several reported series of open heart surgery on cases of ventricular septal defect and infundibular pulmonary stenosis with left-to-right shunt have shown operative mortality rates of less than 2%. The results of surgery are generally excellent.

CYANOTIC TETRALOGY OF FALLOT (PULMONIC STENOSIS WITH RIGHT-TO-LEFT SHUNT)

Incidence

In this anomaly, the sex ratio is approximately equal. It comprises about 10% of all congenital heart disease. After age 4, three out of every four children with cyanotic disease have tetralogy of Fallot.

Pathology

The heart with tetralogy of Fallot has certain specific anatomic features (Figure 167). The ventricular septal defect may vary in anatomic location, but is

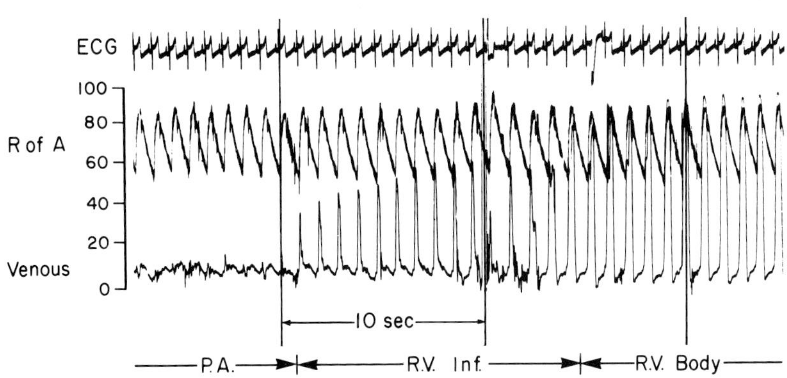

Figure 168. Continuous pressure tracing in a 7-year-old child with tetralogy of Fallot during withdrawal of the catheter from pulmonary artery to right ventricle. Note the initial rise in systolic pressure on withdrawal into the infundibular chamber, followed by further pressure rise in body of right ventricle.

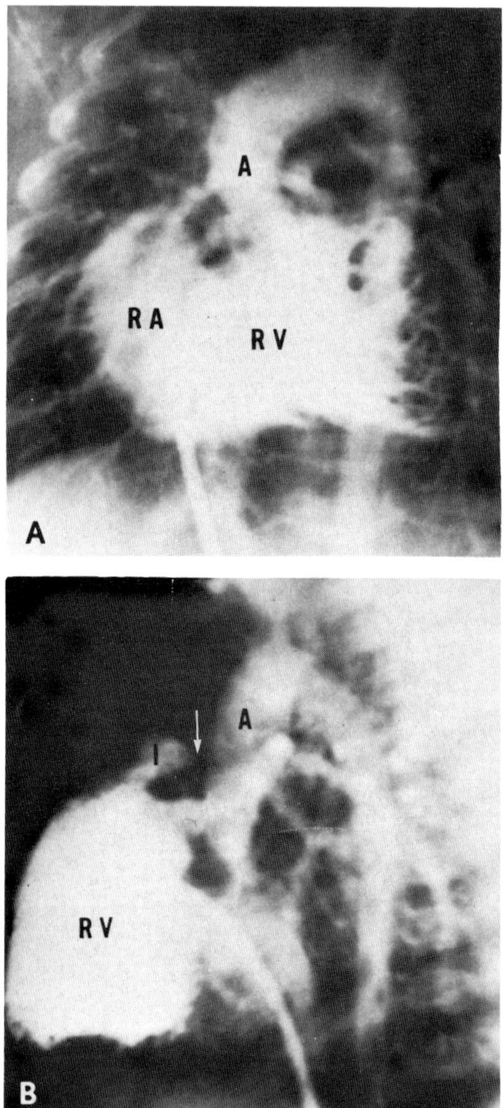

Figure 169. Right ventricular angiocardiograms in Fallot's pulmonary atresia. (A) Frontal and (B) lateral views in a 6-week-old boy. The blind infundibular (I) chamber of the right ventricle (RV) is well demonstrated in the lateral view. The arrow points to location of atretic valve.

Key: A = ascending aorta; RA = right atrium. (From Gleason, D. C., Ferguson, T., Hartmann, A. F., Jr., and Elliott, L. P. 1967. Angiocardiographic differentiation between Fallot's pulmonary atresia and type IV persistent truncus arteriosus. Am. J. Roentgen. 100:312.)

almost invariably large (that is, greater than 1 cm^2/m^2). Typically, the crista supraventricularis (developmentally the conus septum) is hypertrophied and displaced anteriorly. The degree of anterior displacement and hypertrophy initially determines the degree of right ventricular outflow tract obstruction and thus the physiology. Because of the anteriorly displaced crista, the medial papillary muscle of the tricuspid valve is absent, a hallmark of this defect. Anterior conal displacement together with enlargement of the aorta accounts for so-called overriding of the aorta, again a feature that can vary in degree.

Right ventricular outflow obstruction is usually found both in the infundibulum and at the pulmonic valve (Figure 168). Less commonly, there may be obstruction only at the pulmonic valve or only in the right ventricular infundibulum. In any case, the degree of obstruction is severe, resulting in a right-to-left shunt through the ventricular septal defect (Figure 169).

Clinical Features

Patients are rarely overtly cyanotic at birth, unless the right ventricular outflow tract is atretic. Clinically evident cyanosis at rest may not develop for several months. However, once cyanosis appears, it usually becomes progressively more severe. These children are commonly underweight. Extracardiac anomalies, particularly skeletal malformations, are often seen.

Squatting is characteristic of patients with infundibular stenosis. The exact triggering mechanism is unknown, but squatting reduces venous return from the lower extremities and increases systemic resistance, which in turn increases pulmonary blood flow and, therefore, systemic arterial oxygenation.

On physical examination, a right ventricular parasternal lift is observed. A thrill may be palpated along the left sternal border, but rarely in the suprasternal notch.

Auscultatory findings are quite characteristic. A prominent ejection click is heard immediately after the first heart sound (Figure 170). This ejection click is of aortic origin and does not vary with the respiratory cycle. There is a

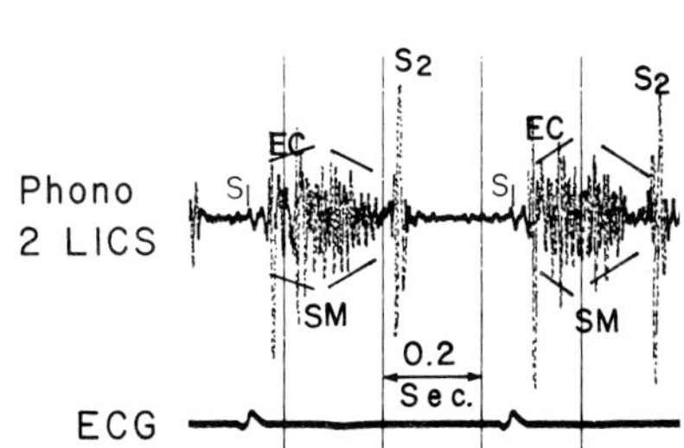

Figure 170. Phonocardiogram of a patient with tetralogy of Fallot and atrial septal defect. Note the prominent, fixed ejection click and early peaking of the systolic murmur. This is in marked contrast to patients with pulmonic stenosis and intact ventricular septa, when the pressure in the right ventricle may remain high and the murmur continues after aortic valve closure.

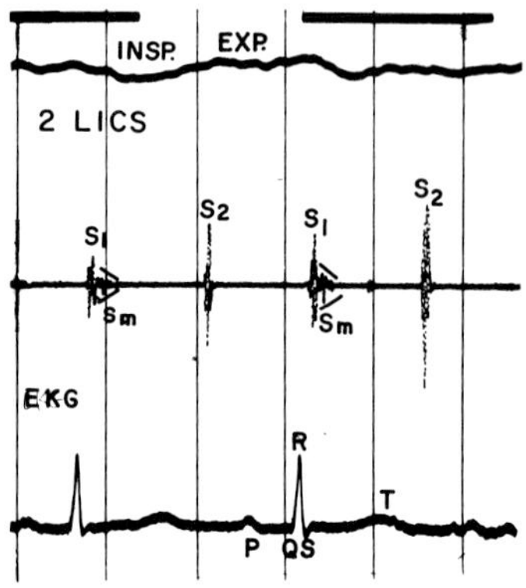

Figure 171. Phonocardiogram of a 2-week-old infant with pulmonic atresia and a ventricular septal defect. In contrast to Figure 170, there is only a short early systolic murmur. The most striking finding is a loud single second sound.

diamond-shaped systolic murmur of medium frequency that reaches its maximum early in systole and ends prior to aortic valve closure. The second sound consists of a single (aortic) component, although the pulmonic component may sometimes be seen on the phonocardiogram. With pulmonic atresia, there is no significant systolic murmur (Figure 171), but sometimes a soft continuous murmur of ductal flow can be detected.

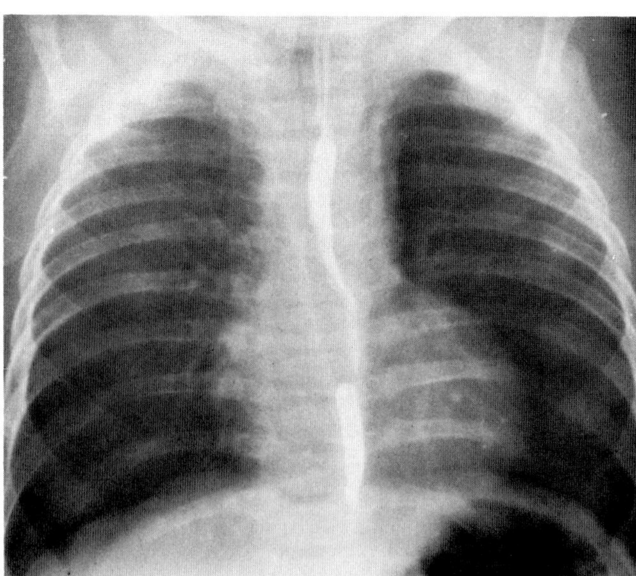

Figure 172. Chest x-ray of a 5-month-old male with classical tetralogy of Fallot. This patient has a left aortic arch.

Roentgenographic Features

Pulmonary arterial markings are decreased on x-ray (Figure 172). On occasion, however, bronchial collateral markings may be so prominent that the vascularity is read as normal or even increased (Figure 94). The characteristic "sheep's nose" appearance is well demonstrated in Figure 172.

Right aortic arch is found in approximately 25% of cases (Figures 89 and 173). The presence of a right aortic arch and decreased vascular markings is virtually diagnostic of tetralogy of Fallot, especially in the older child. In infants, this combination is sometimes seen in tricuspid atresia.

Because the cardiac shadow often is not enlarged, an apparently normal chest x-ray in the presence of clinically obvious cyanosis is strongly suggestive of tetralogy of Fallot (Figure 174).

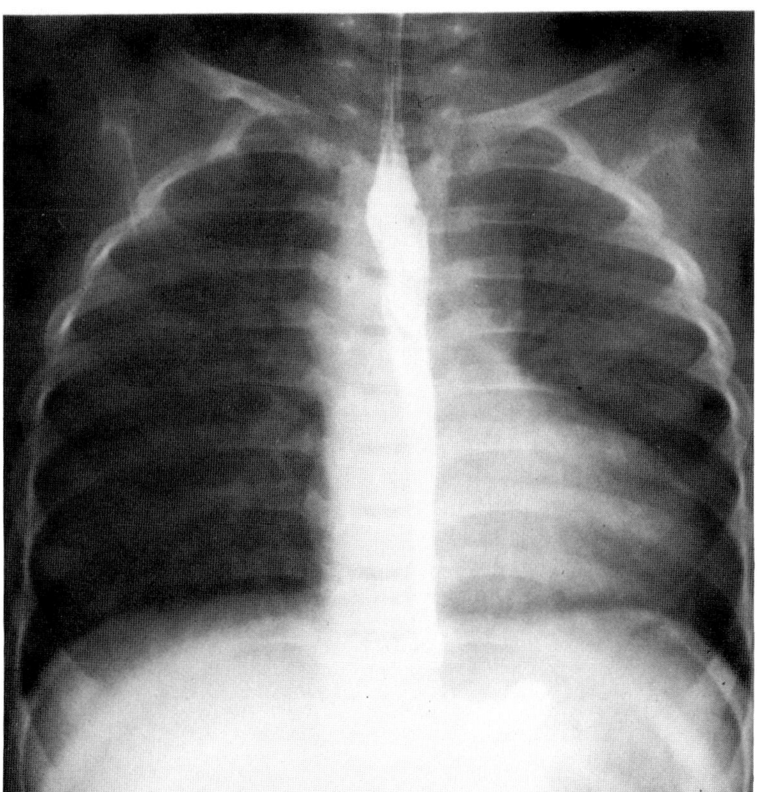

Figure 173. PA view of a 15-month-old boy with cyanotic tetralogy of Fallot and a right aortic arch. Note the superior vena cava pushed to the right by the right arch.

Electrocardiography

There are almost invariably right axis deviation and right ventricular hypertrophy. A characteristic feature of tetralogy is a sudden transition of the QRS complexes between leads V_1 and V_2. In lead V_1, the QRS forces are almost entirely positive, often with a notch on the upstroke, and this changes to an rS pattern in lead V_2 (Figure 175).

Management

Acidosis or anemia should be treated, since these may contribute to the symptoms. Morphine (0.1 mg/kg), propranalol, and oxygen are useful in alleviating hypercyanotic spells.

Although shunt procedures are still recommended by many groups for the infant with severe cyanosis or hyperpneic spells, some larger centers have adopted the approach of total correction of all infants in whom pulmonary arteries are of sufficient size. With unacceptably small pulmonary arteries, these centers would recommend a Blalock-Taussig shunt, but would also recommend patching the right ventricular outflow tract to encourage its growth as well as that of the pulmonic trunk. Side-to-side anastomoses between the descending aorta and the left pulmonary artery (Potts) or between the ascending aorta and the right pulmonary artery (Waterston) are sometimes done when the subclavian artery is inadequate in size. In most centers the operative mortality for shunt procedures in infants is less than 10%.

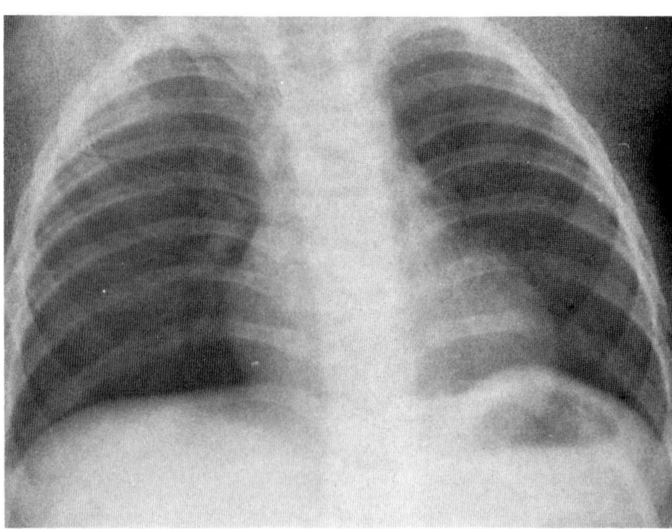

Figure 174. Chest x-ray of an 8-month-old child. In the presence of clinically obvious cyanosis, a nearly normal chest film should suggest tetralogy of Fallot.

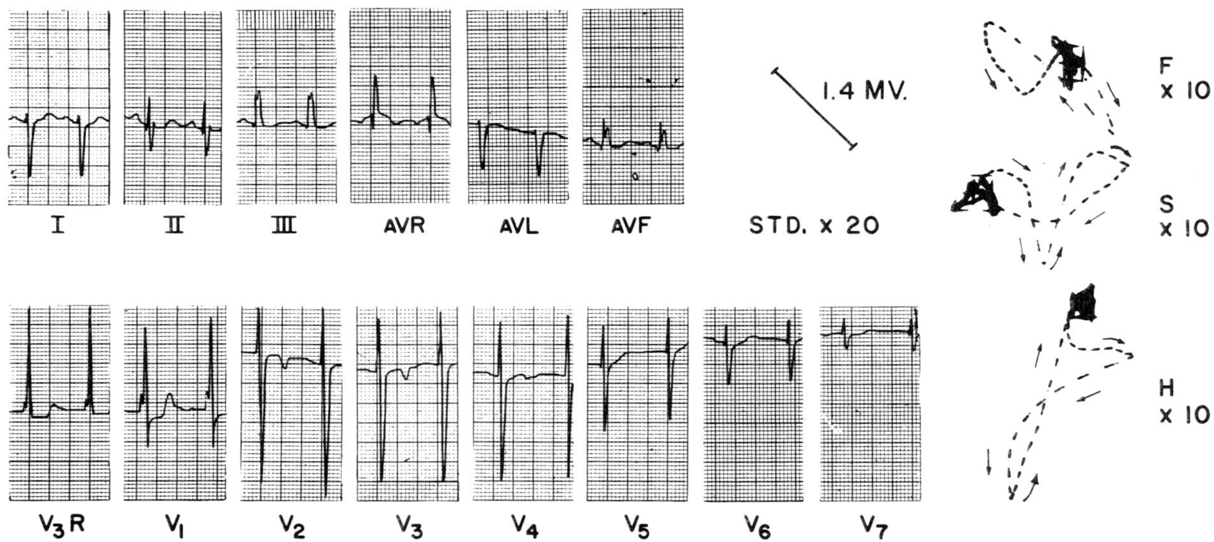

Figure 175. Electrocardiogram of an 11-year-old male with cyanotic tetralogy of Fallot. Note the notching of the R wave upstroke in leads V_3R and V_1. The electrocardiogram changes abruptly between leads V_1 and V_2, indicating a narrow horizontal loop pointed approximately at lead V_1. As the exploring electrode crosses this region, it sees a very marked change. This is so characteristic of cyanotic tetralogy of Fallot that we hesitate to make the diagnosis unless the electrocardiogram is similar to this one.

Open heart repair can be done at any age, although at many centers the preference is to wait until the patient is about 3 to 5 years of age. Recent operative mortality has averaged about 5%, with a slightly higher risk for small infants. Only about 10% of the survivors have a less than satisfactory result.

BIBLIOGRAPHY

Finley, K. H., Buse, S. T., Popper, R. W., Honzik, M. P., Collart, D. S., and Riggs, N. 1974. Intellectual functioning of children with tetralogy of Fallot: Influence of open-heart surgery and earlier palliative operations. J. Pediatr. 85:318–323.

Finnegan, P., Haider, R., Patel, R. G., Abrams, L. D., and Singh, S. P. 1976. Results of total correction of the tetralogy of Fallot. Br. Heart J. 38:934–942.

Guntheroth, W. G., Morgan, B. C., Mullins, G. L., and Baum, D. 1968. Venous return with knee-chest position and squatting in tetralogy of Fallot. Am. Heart J. 75:313–318.

Jarmakani, J. M. M., Graham, T. P., Jr., Canent, R. V., Jr., and Jewett, P. H. 1972. Left heart function in children with tetralogy of Fallot before and after palliative or corrective surgery. Circulation 46:478–490.

Nudel, D. B., Berman, M. A., and Talner, N. S. 1976. Effects of acutely increasing systemic vascular resistance on oxygen tension in tetralogy of Fallot. Pediatrics 58:248–251.

O'Donnell, T. V., and McIlroy, M. B. 1962. The circulatory effects of squatting. Am. Heart J. 64:347–356.

Pacifico, A. D., Bargeron, L. M., and Kirklin, J. W. 1973. Primary total correction of tetralogy of Fallot in children less than four years of age. Circulation 48:1085–1091.

Sunderland, C. O., Matarazzo, R. G., Lees, M. H., Menashe, V. D., Bonchek, L. I., Rosenberg, J. A., and Starr, A. 1973. Total correction of tetralogy of Fallot in infancy. Circulation 48:398–405.

Taussig, H. B., Crocetti, A., Eshaghpour, E., Keinonen, R., Yap, K. N., Bachman, D., Momberger, N., and Kirk, H. 1975. Long-time observations on the Blalock-Taussig operation. VIII. 20 to 28 year follow-up on patients with a tetralogy of Fallot. Johns Hopkins Med. J. 137:13–19.

Truccone, N. J., Bowman, F. O., Jr., Malm, J. R., and Gersony, W. M. 1974. Systemic-pulmonary arterial shunts in the first year of life. Circulation 49:508–511.

chapter 24

HYPOPLASTIC RIGHT HEART

HISTORICAL NOTES

Tricuspid atresia was first described by Holmes in 1824. Peacock described atresia of the pulmonic valve in 1869, and also referred to an earlier description by Hunter, in 1783. Both of these remained little more than curiosities for many years, until the advent of effective surgical therapy stimulated precise description and classification.

INCIDENCE

Tricuspid atresia comprised just over 2% of the diagnoses of all infants with cardiac disease registered in the New England Regional Program from July, 1968, to June, 1974. The sex incidence is approximately equal, and 20% of patients show extracardiac anomalies, particularly of the central nervous system and skeletal system. Tricuspid atresia may be associated with various syndromes, such as asplenia, Down, and cat's-eye.

The incidence of pulmonic atresia is approximately 1% of all congenital heart anomalies.

ETIOLOGY

The etiology of both tricuspid atresia and pulmonic atresia is unknown. Tricuspid atresia can be familial, and we have seen one family in whom two consecutive siblings were born with tricuspid atresia. A third sibling was found at 3 years of age to have an atrial septal defect; at surgery the tricuspid annulus was distinctly small. Tricuspid atresia has been reported after thalidomide ingestion and in association with toxemia of pregnancy and polyhydramnios.

TRICUSPID ATRESIA

Pathology

The tricuspid valve is absent, with its expected position frequently being marked by a dimple in the floor of the right atrium. Absence of a tricuspid orifice necessarily results in absence of the inflow portion of the right ventricle. Therefore, the right ventricle is represented only by its outflow tract. Interatrial communication is usually provided by a stretched foramen ovale, sometimes by a secundum atrial septal defect, and occasionally by an ostium primum defect, particularly in asplenia syndrome.

Although other cardiac defects may be associated with tricuspid atresia, it is simplest to consider tricuspid atresia in relation to the great artery arrangement—i.e., whether or not they are transposed and whether or not there is also pulmonic stenosis (Table 29). Although the size of the ventricular septal defect may influence the clinical situation, we do not discuss this in detail since these nuances are beyond the scope of this book.

Enlargement of the right atrium, the left atrium, and the left ventricle is characteristically present. The ventricular septal defect is usually of small to moderate size and is located in the muscular portion of the septum. In patients with transposition of the great vessels, pulmonic stenosis may be either valvar or subvalvar, and occasionally there is complete atresia of the pulmonic valve.

Hemodynamics

Right atrial pressure is elevated, with marked volume overload of the right atrium. Since all systemic venous blood must cross the atrial septum, the left heart is similarly overloaded. With normally related great vessels, pulmonary blood flow is controlled by the size of the ventricular septal defect and usually is diminished. A patent ductus arteriosus may augment the decreased pulmonic blood flow.

With transposition of the great vessels, pulmonary blood flow is characteristically increased and such patients may develop congestive heart failure. Pulmonic valvar or subvalvar obstruction reduces pulmonary blood flow, with the degree of obstruction determining the particular hemodynamic situation.

Table 29. Simplified classification of tricuspid atresia

Great artery type	Percent of total
Normally related	75
Transposed	
with pulmonic stenosis	8
without pulmonic stenosis	17

Clinical Features

Infants with tricuspid atresia and *normally related great vessels* are usually deeply cyanotic from birth. A systolic murmur caused by flow through the ventricular septal defect is heard at the lower left sternal border. The second sound is usually single. If the ventricular septal defect is quite large, pulmonic blood flow will be increased, in which case cyanosis will be less prominent and congestive heart failure may occur. In this situation a mitral flow murmur may be heard, and the pulmonic component of the second sound is more likely to be audible and perhaps even accentuated.

With time, the ventricular septal defect often becomes smaller, further reducing pulmonary blood flow and increasing cyanosis. The murmur and congestive heart failure, if present, diminish and disappear. Symptoms of increasing hypoxemia become predominant.

In the presence of *transposition of the great vessels,* clinical features are dependent on whether or not pulmonic obstruction is associated. Without obstruction, infants will demonstrate mild cyanosis and congestive heart failure. An ejection click is commonly followed by a systolic murmur caused by flow through the ventricular septal defect. The second sound is single and accentuated because of the anterior aorta and a mitral diastolic flow murmur is present at the apex. If pulmonic obstruction is present, its murmur can be identified, particularly at the apex. Cyanosis is more prominent, but congestive heart failure less likely. In either situation, the ventricular septal defect may gradually become smaller, thus reducing systemic blood flow, sometimes to critical levels.

Roentgenographic Features

In the usual patient, chest radiographs demonstrate decreased pulmonic arterial blood flow in conjunction with right atrial enlargement and a diminished main pulmonary artery segment. A right aortic arch is occasionally present. With transposition of the great arteries, pulmonary arterial vascularity is increased, the heart is generally large, and there may be evidence of left atrial enlargement and left ventricular hypertrophy.

Electrocardiography

The frontal QRS axis is usually leftward and superior, between $-10°$ and $-40°$. Right atrial enlargement is prominent, right ventricular forces are absent, and left ventricular forces are increased. With transposition of the great vessels, left atrial enlargement may be more apparent, and the frontal QRS axis may be leftward and inferior.

Echocardiography

It should be possible to demonstrate the tricuspid valve on a normal echocardiogram. Reduced right ventricular volume and absent tricuspid valve echoes in an infant strongly suggest tricuspid atresia, particularly in the context of other supportive evidence.

Prognosis

With appropriate palliation the majority of patients can survive infancy and early childhood and thus become candidates for corrective procedures. Results with these new procedures have been encouraging, although at the moment the numbers of patients so treated remain relatively small, and follow-up information is necessarily limited.

Management

Surgical management of tricuspid atresia in infancy is palliative. If pulmonary blood flow is critically decreased, a Blalock-Taussig shunt is preferred. Anastomosis of the superior vena cava to the right pulmonary artery (Glenn procedure) is physiologically more appropriate than a Blalock-Taussig shunt, but is technically difficult in the young infant. In patients over 6 months of age, the Glenn procedure is feasible. Patients with transposition of the great vessels may require pulmonary artery banding to control excessive pulmonary blood flow. If a significant pressure difference exists between the atria, atrial septostomy, either by balloon catheter technique or by surgery, is necessary. Some pediatric cardiologists advocate balloon septostomy routinely for all infants less than 3 months old with tricuspid atresia.

A surgical procedure that restores the circulation to more normal physiological state is now possible. Initially devised by Fontan as a valved conduit from the right atrium to the pulmonary artery, the procedure has been modified by others to make use of the hypoplastic right ventricle. If the outlet into the pulmonary artery is adequate, a conduit is placed from the right atrium to the rudimentary right ventricle and the ventricular septal defect is closed. A previously placed Glenn shunt can be left as is. Patients with transposition and tricuspid atresia present a formidable problem for which present surgical techniques are not totally adequate.

PULMONARY ATRESIA WITH INTACT SEPTUM

Pathology

The pathology of this defect is determined to a large extent by what happens at the tricuspid valve. Most commonly, the tricuspid valve is small and competent, and the right ventricular lumen is therefore tiny. Since there is no opportunity for blood to leave the right ventricle either forward or backward, its capacity must remain small.

On the other hand, if the tricuspid valve is insufficient, right ventricular lumen size may be substantial, and at times normal (Figure 176). It should be

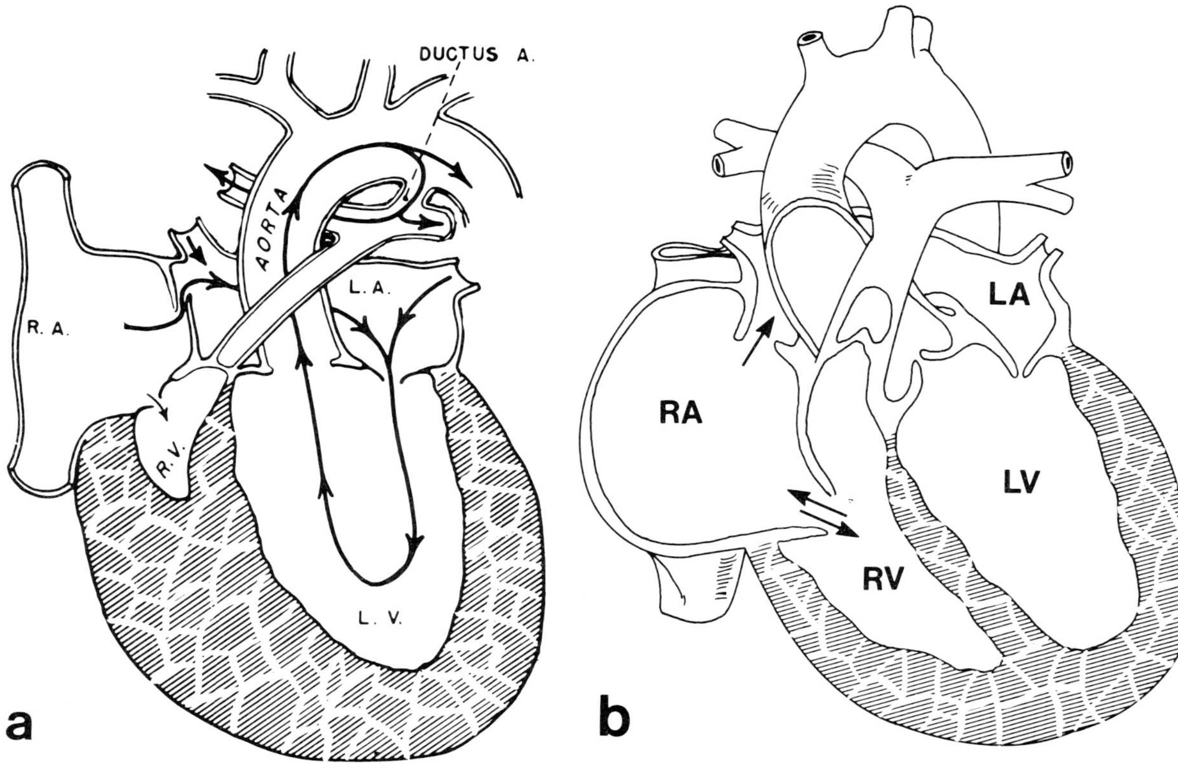

Figure 176. Schema of two types of hypoplastic right ventricle with pulmonic atresia. If the tricuspid valve is competent (a), the right ventricle is tiny and totally nonfunctioning. With tricuspid regurgitation (b), however, the right ventricle is larger, since blood can now flow both into and out of it, although not through the pulmonic valve.

apparent that, if the right ventricular lumen is large, successful definitive surgical therapy is more likely to be achieved. Since the degree of tricuspid insufficiency is variable, a spectrum of right ventricular lumen size exists. Each patient, therefore, must be evaluated individually.

The pulmonic valve cusps are fused, but the valve ring and the pulmonary artery itself are generally of normal size, unlike the small pulmonic trunk usually found in pulmonary atresia with a ventricular septal defect. The right atrium is large, particularly when there is tricuspid insufficiency. A true atrial septal defect may be present, but usually the obligatory interatrial communication is a stretched foramen ovale. Left ventricular volume is increased, as is that of the ascending aorta, and the ductus arteriosus is patent.

In some patients with a small right ventricle and competent tricuspid valve, there is direct communication between the right ventricular lumen and the coronary circulation via dilated sinusoidal channels.

Hemodynamics

As in tricuspid atresia, all systemic venous return must cross the atrial septum and mix with pulmonary venous return. Blood entering the right ventricle can exit only by tricuspid regurgitation or by entrance into coronary sinusoids. Pressure in the right atrium exceeds that in the left atrium, and right ventricular systolic pressure can exceed that in the left ventricle if the tricuspid valve is competent or can be considerably lower in the presence of severe tricuspid insufficiency.

Pulmonary blood flow is controlled by the ductus arteriosus. If the ductus is widely patent, pulmonary blood flow may be large enough to allow reasonable systemic oxygen saturation. Usually, however, pulmonary blood flow is diminished, and the patient is substantially hypoxemic.

Clinical Features

Cyanosis occurs within a few hours after birth in these infants, who otherwise generally are normal in appearance. If tricuspid insufficiency is substantial, resultant right atrial volume overload may cause signs of right-sided congestive failure.

Two murmurs are often heard. The continuous murmur of a patent ductus arteriosus is generally no louder than grade 2/6. With significant tricuspid insufficiency, a systolic thrill and holosystolic murmur are present at the lower left sternal border. The second sound is single. A fourth heart sound may be detected.

Roentgenographic Features

Pulmonary arterial vascularity is significantly decreased (Figure 177). Heart size depends on whether or not tricuspid insufficiency is present and if so to what degree. If substantial, the heart shadow may be markedly enlarged, primarily due to the right atrium. The aortic arch is on the left.

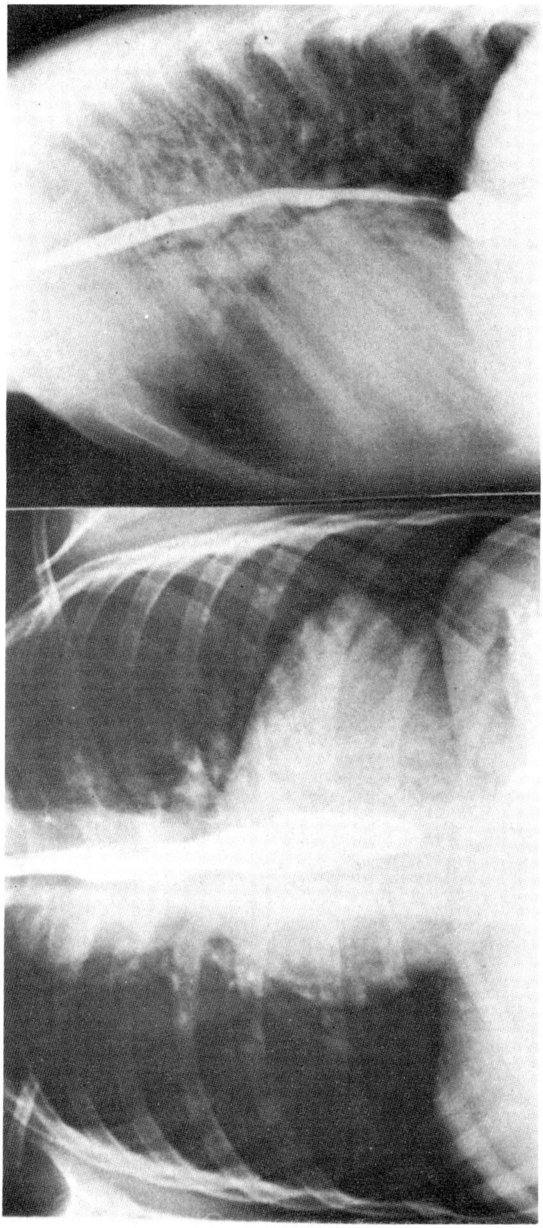

Figure 177. X-ray of a 4½-year-old male with pulmonic atresia. Note the right aortic arch.

Electrocardiography

In those patients without tricuspid insufficiency, the ECG shows right atrial enlargement and left ventricular hypertrophy, with a frontal plane QRS axis directed leftward and inferiorly, between 10° and 60°. The inferior QRS axis may be the major clue that one is dealing with pulmonary atresia rather than tricuspid atresia (Figure 178).

In the presence of significant tricuspid insufficiency, right ventricular QRS forces are more prominent and the ECG will demonstrate biventricular hypertrophy or even isolated right ventricular hypertrophy. *A word of caution is necessary:* patients with right ventricular hypertrophy on ECG do not necessarily have a large volume right ventricle. They may have only a very thick-walled right ventricle with a diminutive lumen. Loudness of the tricuspid insufficiency murmur, heart size on x-ray, and, most importantly, angiography are clearly more definitive measures of right ventricular volume.

Echocardiography

Pulmonary atresia with a small right ventricle will be difficult to distinguish from tricuspid atresia. However, if right ventricular volume is large, this can readily be seen.

Prognosis

Those patients in whom a successful pulmonic valvotomy is accomplished may progress quite satisfactorily. Patients with a small right ventricle have a high mortality even if a successful shunt is performed. Eventually these individuals may be candidates for a right atrium–to–pulmonary artery valved conduit (Fontan procedure).

Management

Rapid diagnosis and appropriate surgical treatment are essential if these infants are to survive. Since the ductus is critical to maintaining life prior to surgery, it is essential that the ductus remain open. Intravenous administration of prostaglandin E-1 has been shown to result in dilation of an already constricted ductus arteriosus and may be given as a continuous infusion prior to surgery. It is expected that this experimental therapy will be generally available within the near future.

Surgical approach depends on the anatomy. Patients with a small right ventricle will require a systemic arterial shunt, such as a Blalock-Taussig procedure. However, if the right ventricle is of adequate size pulmonic valvotomy may provide definitive and long-lasting relief. Although tricuspid insufficiency usually persists after successful valvotomy, it will lessen, and the patient may be clinically well.

In those patients in whom right ventricular volume is not adequate, a combined approach is advocated. Pulmonic valvotomy may allow the right

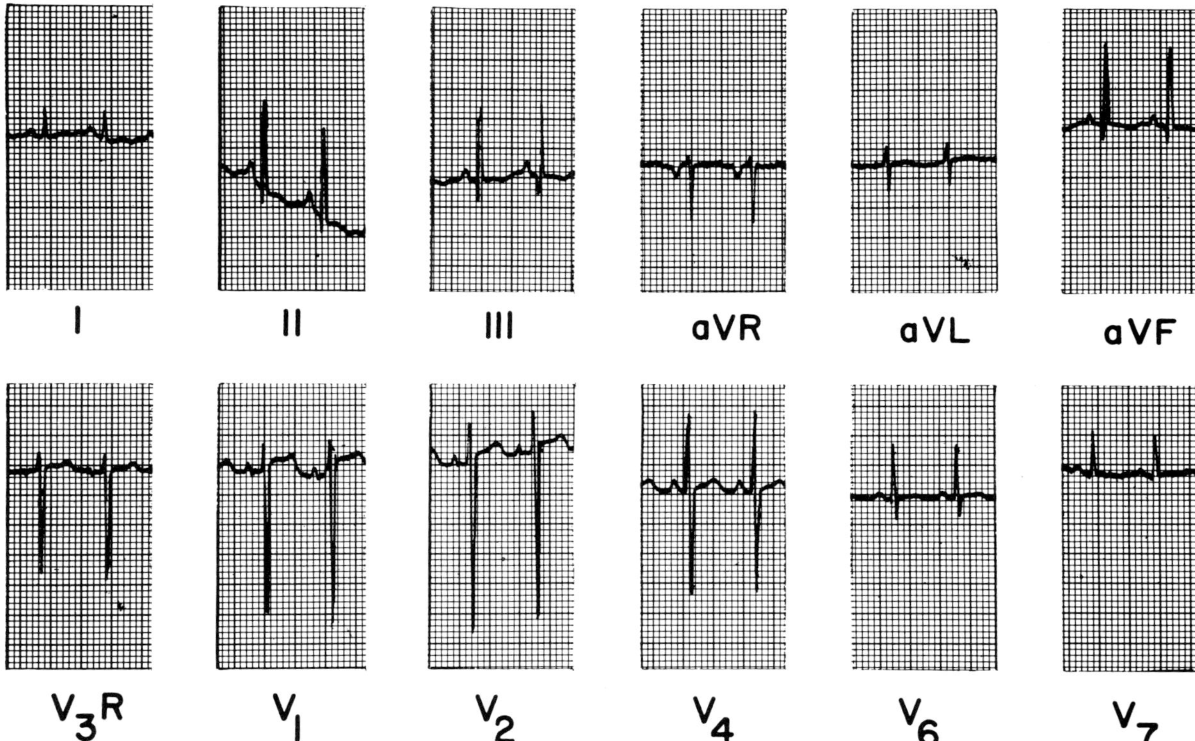

Figure 178. ECG of a newborn infant with pulmonic valve atresia and intact ventricular septum. There is right atrial enlargement, although not severe in degree, and absence of right ventricular forces, suggesting a small right ventricle. The frontal plane QRS axis is inferior, in contrast to infants with tricuspid atresia in whom the frontal plane axis is generally leftward and superior.

ventricle time to increase its volume, while a Blalock-Taussig shunt maintains adequate pulmonary blood flow.

In those patients in whom only a shunt is performed, it has been suggested that balloon atrial septostomy be accomplished at cardiac catheterization, since increasing pulmonary blood flow, and therefore left atrial pressure, by a shunt procedure may impede flow across the foramen ovale.

EBSTEIN'S ANOMALY OF THE TRICUSPID VALVE

In this lesion, the septal and posterior leaflets of the tricuspid valve are displaced downward into the right ventricle for a varying distance (Figure 179). This results in less efficient functioning of the right ventricle, since part of the musculature belonging to the right ventricle is "atrialized" (Figure 180). Although the tricuspid valve is commonly insufficient, it may have relatively normal function or even be stenotic. In extreme examples of this disease, the right ventricle has little or no pumping ability, and the right atrium functions as the pulmonary vascular bed pumper. This is commonly associated with a shunt at the atrial level through an atrial septal defect or a forced-open foramen ovale. Under these circumstances, since the pressure in the right atrium is higher than that in the left atrium, blood will flow from the

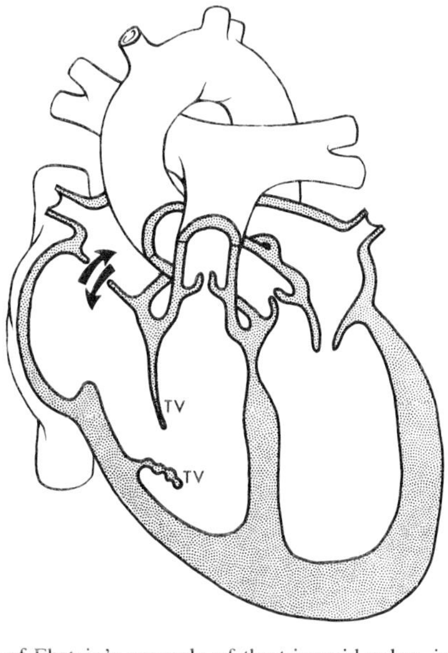

Figure 179. Schema of Ebstein's anomaly of the tricuspid valve, in which one leaflet of the tricuspid valve is displaced downward so that a portion of the right ventricle becomes incorporated into the right atrium. The force of the right ventricle is reduced. In severe cases the cardiac output decreases, pressure in the right atrium rises, and a right-to-left shunt may develop through a patent foramen ovale.

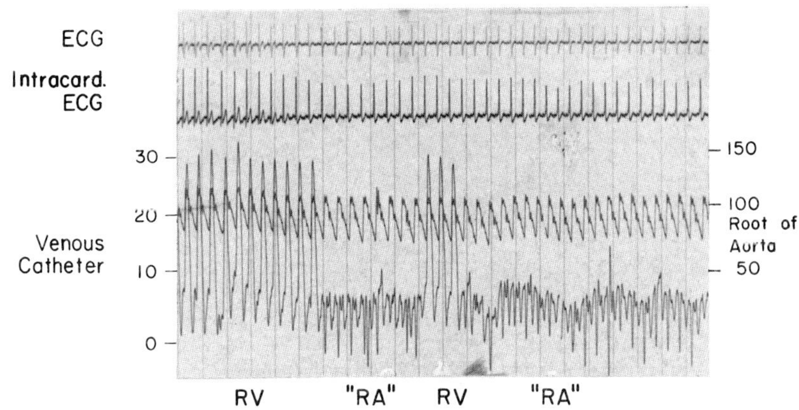

Figure 180. The intracardiac electrocardiogram registers a constant ventricular potential, whereas the pressure tracing varies between a ventricular pressure contour and an atrial pressure contour. The occurrence of an atrial pressure in the presence of a ventricular intracardiac electrocardiographic tracing is diagnostic of Ebstein's anomaly.

right atrium to the left atrium, producing varying degrees of cyanosis. Rarely, the converse may exist and the lesion mimics a left-to-right shunt at the atrial level. Ebstein's anomaly of the tricuspid valve is frequently associated with episodes of supraventricular tachycardia, which further compromises myocardial function.

UHL'S ANOMALY

In this malformation, the right ventricular free wall is extremely thin. It has been described as parchment-like, containing so little musculature that it is translucent. This is an extremely rare anomaly, and we have seen only one example.

As would be expected, this lack of right ventricular musculature means that the entire burden of pumping blood from the great veins out to the pulmonary artery falls upon the right atrium. The clinical roentgenographic and electrocardiographic findings are virtually indistinguishable from those of tricuspid atresia or other forms of hypoplastic right ventricle. Management consists of an appropriate shunt to increase pulmonary blood flow.

BIBLIOGRAPHY

Bialostozsky, D., Horwitz, S., and Espino-Vela, J. 1972. Ebstein's malformation of the tricuspid valve. Am. J. Cardiol. 29:826–836.

Dhanavaravibul, S., Nora, J. J., and McNamara, D. G. 1970. Pulmonary valvular atresia with intact ventricular septum: Problems in diagnosis and results of treatment. J. Pediatr. 77:1010–1016.

Dick, M., Fyler, D. C., and Nadas, A. S. 1975. Tricuspid atresia: the clinical course in 101 patients. Am. J. Cardiol. 36:327–337.

Fontan, F., and Bandet, E. 1971. Surgical repair of tricuspid atresia. Thorax 26:240–248.

Graham, T. P., Jr., Bender, H. W., Atwood, G. F., Page, D. L., and Sell, C. G. R. 1974. Increase in right ventricular volume following valvulotomy for pulmonary atresia or stenosis with intact ventricular septum. Circulation 49:Suppl. II:69–79.

Heymann, M. A., and Rudolph, A. M. 1977. Ductus arteriosus dilatation by prostaglandin E-1 in infants with pulmonary atresia. Pediatrics 59:325–329.

Shams, A., Fowler, R. S., Trusler, G. A., Keith, J. D., and Mustard, W. T. 1971. Pulmonary atresia with intact ventricular septum: report of 50 cases. Pediatrics 47:370–377.

Van Praagh, R., Ando, M., and Dungan, W. T. 1971. Anatomic types of tricuspid atresia: Clinical and developmental implication. Circulation 44:Suppl. II:115.

chapter 25

AORTIC STENOSIS

HISTORICAL NOTES

Riverius, in 1646, was the first to describe a stenotic aortic valve. Bonnet, in 1679, drew attention to the occurrence of sudden death in patients with aortic stenosis. Chevers described discrete subaortic stenosis in 1842.

Monckeberg, in 1907, reported a case of supravalvar aortic stenosis (SVAS). The clinical findings were discussed by Denie and Verheugt in 1958, and the pathological features by Perou in 1961, in a collection of 17 case reports from the world literature. The typical elfin facies of SVAS were first noted by Williams in 1961.

INCIDENCE

Congenital aortic stenosis comprises about 6% of cardiac anomalies. Valvar aortic stenosis usually occurs as an isolated cardiac anomaly. Males predominate by a ratio of between two and four to one. As an incidental finding, bicuspid aortic valves have been reported in about 2% of all males. There are relatively more females with SVAS than in other types of aortic stenosis, but there are too few reported cases to establish a definite male:female ratio.

ETIOLOGY

In children and young adults, valvar aortic stenosis should be presumed to be of congenital origin. Bland and Jones, in their 20-year follow-up of 1000 children with acute rheumatic fever, found only two cases of pure aortic stenosis. (One might question the accuracy of the rheumatic etiology even in these!) The subvalvar form is also a developmental anomaly and commonly has some degree of accompanying insufficiency.

There are two recognized subvarieties of SVAS: *familial* cases transmitted as an autosomal dominant with normal intelligence and normal facies; and a *triad* consisting of supravalvar aortic stenosis, mental retardation, and characteristic elfin-like facies.

Much interest has been generated by the relationship of the nonfamilial supravalvar aortic stenosis syndrome and the infantile hypercalcemia syndrome, particularly since the facies of individuals with these two syndromes are similar. The theory that supravalvar aortic stenosis is related to hypercalcemia has been supported by recent experimental work of Friedman and Roberts. Offspring of rabbits fed large doses of vitamin D during gestation had elevated vitamin D levels, demonstrating transplacental passage, and a significant number had generalized vascular lesions, with some animals showing changes akin to supravalvar aortic stenosis.

AORTIC STENOSIS IN CHILDREN AND YOUNG ADULTS

Pathology

In valvar aortic stenosis, the valve is bicuspid in about 80% of patients, tricuspid in about 15%, and unicuspid in the remaining 5%. Subvalvar stenosis is often the result of a discrete fibrous ring immediately below the valve. In about one-half of patients the subvalvar narrowing consists of a long tubular section. Commonly, the subvalvar ring interferes with valve closure and causes aortic insufficiency.

In SVAS, there is usually a discrete circumferential ridge protruding into the lumen of the aorta above the aortic valve. The narrowing may involve most of the ascending aorta and there may be multiple stenoses in the vascular system, especially in the arteries arising from the aortic arch. The coronary arteries originating below the stenosis are usually normal, but they may be dilated and tortuous. Sometimes one coronary artery is enlarged and the other, obstructed at the ostium, is hypoplastic. The aortic sinuses are usually dilated.

Associated cardiovascular anomalies include aortic valve insufficiency, coarctation of the aorta, hypoplasia of the ascending aortic arch and of the vessels arising from the aortic arch, and mitral insufficiency or stenosis.

Hemodynamics

Aortic stenosis increases left ventricular work and hence the oxygen needs of the myocardium. Coronary blood flow does not increase proportionately and may actually decrease. This decrease may be due to a combination of narrowed coronary ostia, relative decrease in duration of diastole, increased squeezing of coronaries during systole, and possibly a suction effect of the aortic jet stream on coronary ostia. In SVAS, one of the coronary arteries may be hypoplastic, further decreasing the perfusion of the myocardium. All of these produce myocardial ischemia, which may eventually lead to myocardial fibrosis.

Unless there is extremely severe obstruction, the left ventricle is able to maintain a normal cardiac output. Even though the degree of stenosis remains unchanged, the systolic pressure difference across the aortic valve will increase as cardiac output increases as with exercise, fever, or excitement. Thus, the use of resting systolic pressure difference across the valve as the sole criterion of severity may be misleading (see Figure 25).

In children, critical narrowing occurs when the valve orifice is about 0.7 cm^2/m^2 of body surface area. When the valve area is less than this size, left ventricular end diastolic and left atrial pressures increase; isometric contraction time increases and systole is prolonged.

Abnormal aortic valve cusps, particularly in bicuspid valves, through constant traumatization by the blood stream, gradually become fibrotic, less pliable, and even calcified, creating increasingly significant obstruction. The subvalvar form tends to be more rapidly progressive than valvar stenosis.

Clinical Features

Children with aortic stenosis usually have no symptoms, exhibit normal physical development, and often participate in athletics. They are referred generally for evaluation of a loud murmur. This murmur may be heard in the first 48 hr of life and certainly can be heard before 1 year of age. Symptoms, if present, are usually those of mild fatigue, exercise intolerance, and abdominal or precordial pain. Typical anginal pain is rare in pediatric practice. The presence of exertional dyspnea or syncope implies severe obstruction. However, since young children rarely are accurate historians, even vague symptoms deserve careful evaluation. Cyanosis and congestive heart failure are absent, except terminally.

Children with aortic stenosis usually have normal peripheral arterial pulses, both in amplitude and contour. Narrow pulse pressures, anacrotic notches, and an inconspicuous dicrotic notch are more common in adolescents and adults. Prolongation of the left ventricular ejection period is usually associated with significant stenosis.

A sustained left ventricular apical impulse and a systolic precordial thrill are seen in significant obstruction. Conversely, if there is no precordial thrill and no left ventricular lift, the resting systolic pressure difference is almost always less than 30 mm Hg.

A harsh stenotic ejection murmur can be noted maximally in the second right intercostal space, but radiating well to the apex, back, and neck (Figure 181). The murmur is usually maximal in the fourth intercostal space, with subvalvar stenosis. A high frequency diastolic murmur of aortic insufficiency was heard in one-half of our patients with subvalvar aortic stenosis, and in about one-fourth of those with valvar aortic stenosis. One should consider SVAS when the systolic murmur is loudest under the right clavicle and radiates well high into the neck; the murmur may even be louder over the carotid region than in the second right intercostal space. In SVAS, the aortic component of S_2 is often increased in intensity.

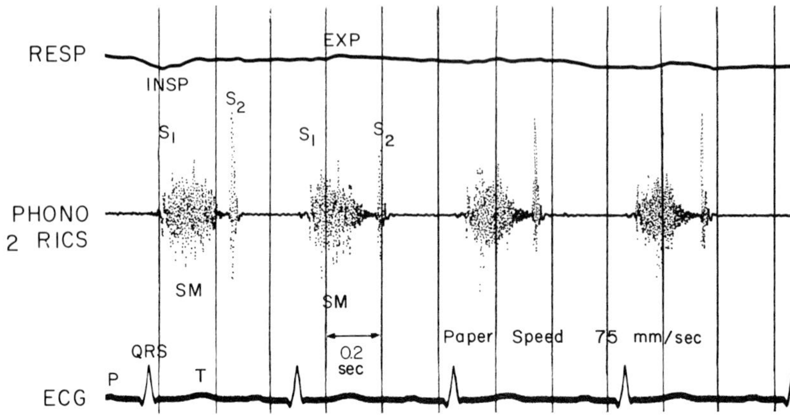

Figure 181. Phonocardiogram of a 2-year-old male with valvar aortic stenosis. The murmur is diamond shaped, i.e., it is soft at the beginning and end of systole and reaches its maximum amplitude about midsystole. (From Elliott, L. P., and Schiebler, G. L. 1968. X-Ray Diagnosis of Congenital Cardiac Disease. Courtesy of Charles C Thomas, Publisher, Springfield, Ill.)

A prominent aortic ejection click that is maximal at the apex is common in mild or moderately severe valvar aortic stenosis. It is not present in the subvalvar or supravalvar varieties. The second sound is narrowly split in inspiration and single in expiration. Paradoxical splitting of the aortic and pulmonic components of S_2 is quite rare even with severe obstruction.

Diastolic sounds, S_3 and S_4, are commonly heard at the apex. Presence or absence of an S_3 has no correlation with peak systolic pressure difference. After age 13, an S_4 usually indicates significant obstruction.

A triad of characteristic facies, mental deficiency, and supravalvar aortic stenosis has been described. The facies have been described as "elfin," with a high, prominent forehead, epicanthal folds, underdeveloped bridge of nose and mandible, and an overhanging upper lip (Figure 182). In addition, these children have dental anomalies, strabismus, and a hoarse voice.

Blood pressure differences between the arms or between the right arm and the legs are relatively common in SVAS. We think this is best explained by the high velocity jet striking the orifice of one of the subclavian arteries and reducing the flow into it (Coanda effect).

Roentgenographic Features

Plain chest films are normal in most cases (see Figure 84). The only clue may be slight enlargement of the ascending aorta or left ventricle (Figure 183); see also Figure 87). Left ventricular hypertrophy produces a globular rounded heart shape but not much increase in overall size. There is little correlation of overall heart size or left ventricular size with systolic pressure difference across the aortic valve. Left atrial enlargement and an apparent slight increase in pulmonary venous vascularity are common.

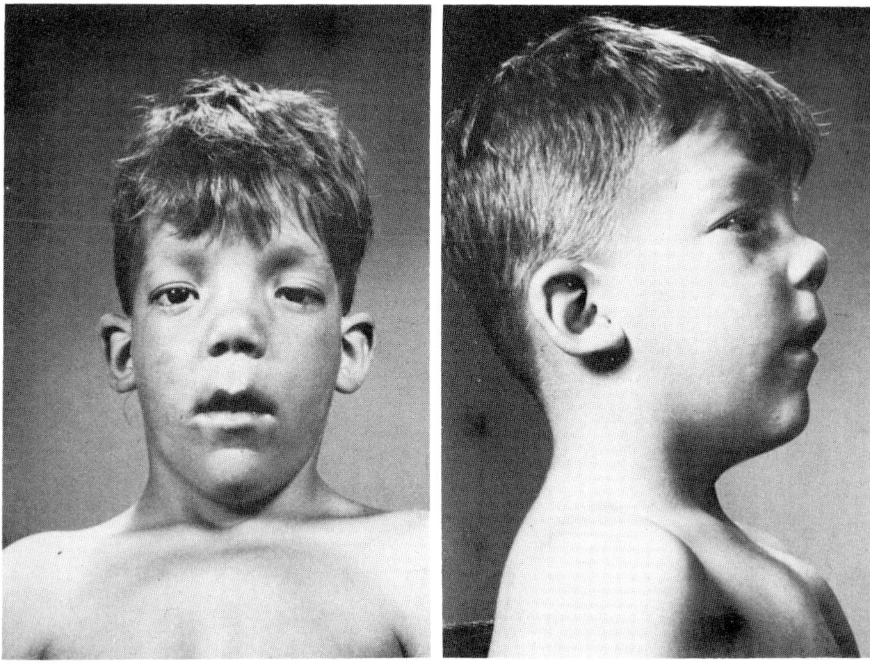

Figure 182. Characteristic facies of a patient with supravalvar aortic stenosis. Note the fullness of the upper lip, the prominence of the cheeks, and the dull facies.

In supravalvar aortic stenosis, post-stenotic dilation of the aorta and enlargement of the aortic knob are not seen. Evidence of residual hypercalcemia, especially dense mineralization of the base of the skull and of the metaphyses of long bones, may be present.

Electrocardiography

Patients with aortic stenosis may have a normal electrocardiogram or may show signs of left ventricular hypertrophy of the pressure-overloading type (Figure 184). The vectorcardiogram usually shows leftward and posterior shift of QRS vector, and an increase in maximal QRS voltage (greater than 0.9 mV).

Left ventricular pressure overloading may be indicated by an anterior and rightward ST vector, causing a positive ST segment in leads aVR and V_1. A T vector less than $-40°$ in the frontal planes or a QRS-T angle greater than $100°$ usually indicates significant obstruction. There may be definite electrocardiographic signs with moderate stenosis or severe stenosis with only equivocal electrocardiographic signs. The electrocardiogram and the vectorcardiogram are at best only crude indicators of the degree of severity of the lesion.

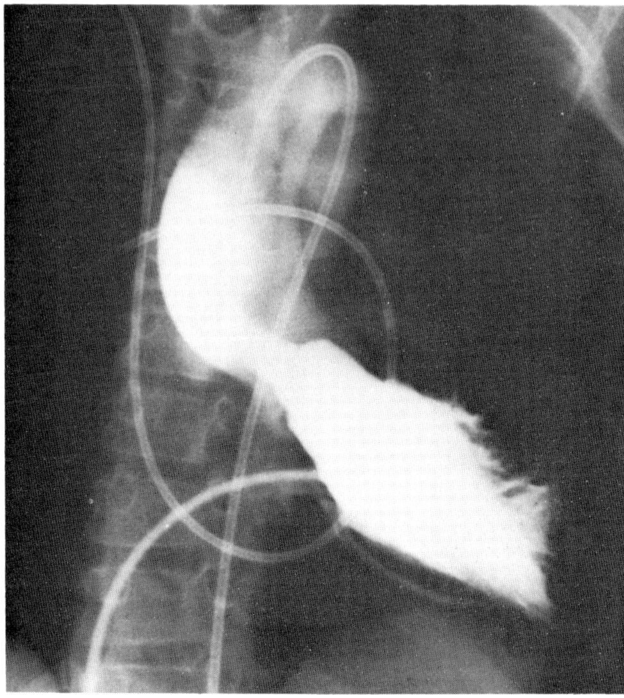

Figure 183. Angiocardiogram of a patient with valvar aortic stenosis. The injection catheter was passed across a small puncture in the atrial septum (trans-septally). Note the jet emerging from the aortic valve and striking the right side of the ascending aorta. The power in such a jet over a period of time can cause weakening and dilatation of this portion of the aorta.

Echocardiography

Since the diameter and wall thickness of the left ventricle increase in proportion to ventricular load, the severity of aortic stenosis can be estimated. These measurements are readily made on echocardiograms. In the absence of myocardial failure, they seem to be a sensitive indicator of severity.

Prognosis

If the patient survives infancy, few difficulties are to be expected during childhood and adolescence. Mild degrees of obstruction are compatible with an active life, but tend to become more severe with time. All patients should be watched carefully for this possibility.

Sudden death, thought to be due to arrhythmias or coronary artery disease, occurs only rarely. It is seen only in patients with severe obstruction, who usually have some warning symptoms and an ECG pattern of significant left ventricular systolic overloading.

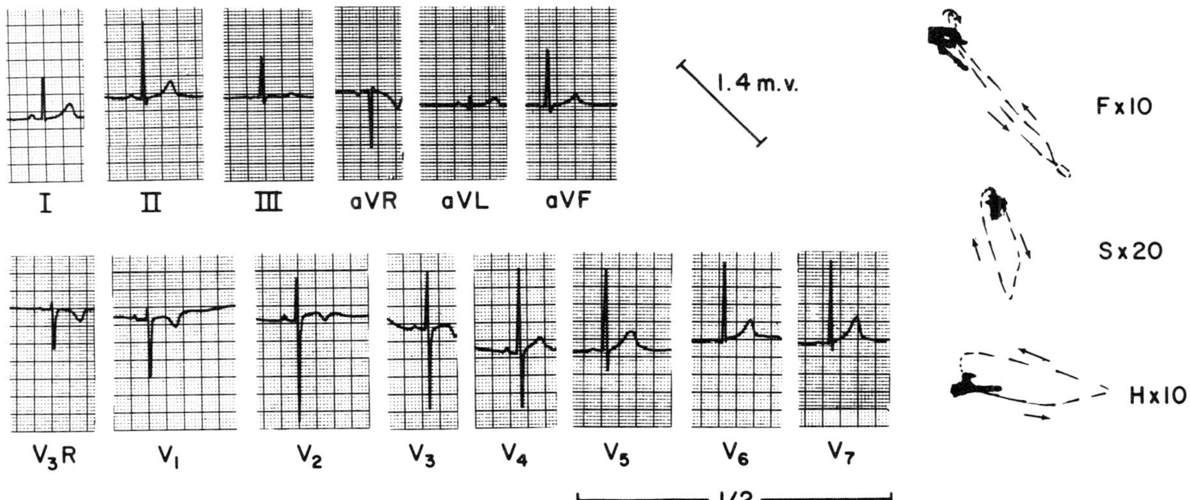

Figure 184. Electrocardiogram of a patient with aortic valvar stenosis. Peak systolic ventricular pressure was 168 mm Hg and the peak aortic systolic pressure was 73 mm Hg. This patient's electrocardiogram has a diminished q wave in leads V_6 and V_7 as the only suggestion of left ventricular systolic overloading.

Bacterial endocarditis is a lifelong threat, especially in the presence of a bicuspid aortic valve. Congestive failure rarely occurs, except as a near-terminal event or after a bout of bacterial endocarditis.

Some degree of left ventricular endocardial thickening is a frequent accompaniment of severe aortic stenosis, but only rarely of such a degree as to embarrass left ventricular function.

The most common causes of death are cardiac failure, myocardial infarction, rupture of the aorta, and bacterial endocarditis.

Management

Indications for cardiac catheterization include the presence of any clinical symptom, such as chest pain, syncope, easy fatigability, or light-headedness. Young children may not be able to describe their symptoms accurately, and a high degree of suspicion should be maintained. ECG evidence of increasing left ventricular pressure overloading, increasing aortic size on x-ray, or increasing left ventricle size on echocardiogram are indications for catheterization. A positive exercise stress test also suggests the need for accurate hemodynamic assessment.

Catheterization reveals a drop in systolic pressure between the body of the left ventricle and the aorta (Figure 185). This change occurs below the valve in subvalvar aortic stenosis, at the valve in the valvar form, and above

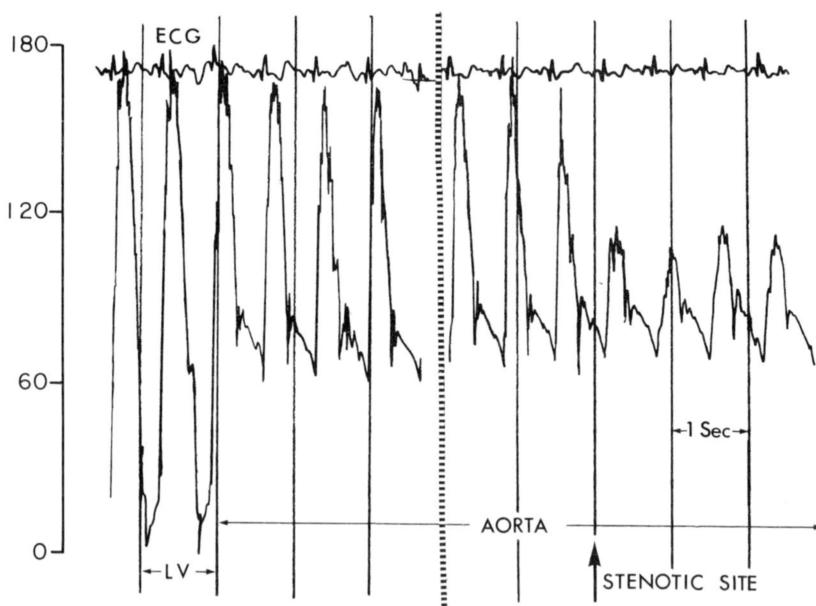

Figure 185. Pullback of catheter from the body of the left ventricle to the aorta in 12-year-old girl with supravalvar aortic stenosis. Note that the change in systolic pressure occurs above the valve.

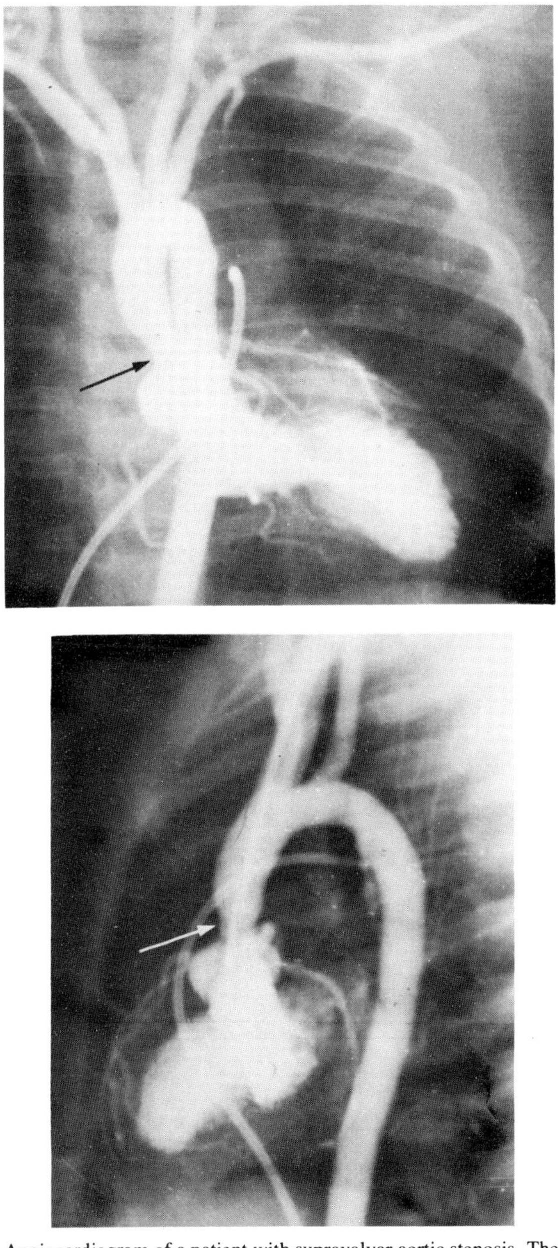

Figure 186. Angiocardiogram of a patient with supravalvar aortic stenosis. The arrows localize the stenotic site.

the valve in SVAS. Angiocardiography will demonstrate the location of the obstruction and the size and route of the coronary arteries (Figure 186).

Our criteria for surgery include: 1) an obviously enlarged heart, unless clearly explained by other pathology; 2) a systolic pressure difference between the left ventricle and the aorta greater than 75 mm Hg, with a normal resting cardiac output; or 3) *the presence of significant symptoms,* such as angina or syncope.

Most centers currently have an operative mortality rate under 5%. In a child, valvotomy should be performed. Rarely, the anatomy of the valve may require its replacement by an artificial valve. The Hancock porcine valve has thus far proven to be an excellent prosthesis.

Postoperative Studies

Successful surgery results in an increase in aortic valve area and a decrease in left ventricular systolic and end diastolic pressures. Hemodynamic and electrocardiographic improvement occurs in about three-fourths of survivors. The operation must be considered palliative, since some degree of aortic incompetence usually is produced and the stenosis is often incompletely relieved. All postoperative patients still are at risk for infective endocarditis and should be managed appropriately.

Postoperative x-rays and electrocardiograms are of little value in determining the success of surgery, nor would we expect them to be, since they are not very helpful in preoperative assessment. We believe that there is a need for postoperative catheterization for proper assessment and management. Thus we recommend hemodynamic evaluation for all patients approximately 1 year after surgery. Although uncommon, restenosis can occur. Subsequent catheterizations may be done as indicated by the specific clinical situation.

SEVERE AORTIC STENOSIS IN INFANCY

Although this is a relatively rare entity, it is a medical and surgical emergency. These critically ill infants usually present prior to 2 months of age with severe congestive heart failure.

Pathology

By definition the aortic valve must be patent since, if it were not, aortic atresia would be present. Since the valve is patent, the ascending aorta is of normal size or may even demonstrate post-stenotic dilatation. Perhaps the most crucial point is the volume of the left ventricle. If the lumen is tiny, the outcome is identical with cases of aortic atresia and it hardly matters that the valve has a pinpoint opening. As the spectrum of cases moves toward a larger lumen size, the point is reached at which the left ventricle can support life and thus valvotomy is not only survivable but indeed life saving.

The aortic valve is often unicuspid, consisting of a mass of thickened endocardial tissue with an eccentric slit orifice. Unfortunately the aortic root is often hypoplastic, and this narrowed annulus may limit lasting surgical relief.

Left ventricular wall thickness is substantially increased, there is some secondary endocardial thickening, and there may be abnormalities of the mitral valve as well. Left atrial wall thickness may also be increased, especially if the atrial septum is intact, and secondary right heart enlargement may be present.

Hemodynamics

Systemic cardiac output is usually reduced, and the pressure difference across the aortic valve does not reflect the magnitude of the obstruction. Thus, a critically ill baby with left heart failure might demonstrate no more than 20- or 30-mm Hg systolic pressure difference. Left ventricular end diastolic pressure and left atrial pressure will be increased, reflecting decreased left ventricular compliance. Secondary right heart hypertension will be noted, and some patients will have a left-to-right shunt at the atrial level.

Clinical Features

Although the infant may appear normal at birth, an ejection murmur maximal at the right base should be audible. Early symptoms are labored respirations, tachypnea, and tachycardia. With varying rapidity, the infant becomes anxious and pale because of falling cardiac output. Intensity of the murmur varies directly with cardiac output. Arterial pulses are present and equal, but weak. The first sound is followed by an aortic ejection click. The second sound is single or narrowly split, and a fourth heart sound is often heard. Rales are usually heard at both lung bases and the liver is enlarged, but not markedly so. Pulmonary edema occurs readily if substantial left heart failure occurs, the infant's condition rapidly deteriorates, and opportunity for successful treatment quickly dissipates.

Roentgenographic Features

The chest x-ray demonstrates significant cardiomegaly and prominent pulmonary venous vascularity. Since a left-to-right atrial shunt may be present, arterial markings may also be increased, but venous markings still predominate. Left atrial enlargement is present.

Electrocardiogram

The neonate may not show significant abnormalities, but by 1 to 2 months of age left ventricular hypertrophy is usually present. Abnormal ST segments and T waves indicate myocardial ischemia.

Echocardiography

Echocardiography is useful in evaluating the size of the left ventricular lumen and its wall thickness, and left ventricular function. Measurement of aortic root diameter in the newborn is critical in distinguishing this condition from aortic atresia.

Differential Diagnosis

Although the murmur resembles that of a *ventricular septal defect,* the murmur of a VSD sufficiently large to cause symptoms in the infant will not be heard during the first few days of life.

Management

In a sick infant in whom the diagnosis of aortic stenosis is considered, cardiac catheterization must be accomplished without delay. Essential information to be obtained includes left ventricular volume and contractility and the size of the aortic root.

Supportive measures, including treatment of congestive heart failure, will be of limited value. Vascular unloading agents, particularly those that can reduce both preload and afterload, may provide more benefit than digitalis and diuretics. Any improvement obtained is temporary. If the left ventricle and aortic root are of reasonable size, aortic valvotomy using cardiopulmonary bypass should be performed immediately. Delay of even a few hours can prove disastrous.

Although many patients will not survive surgery because of poor left ventricular function, those who do may progress quite satisfactorily. Residual aortic stenosis will be present and some aortic insufficiency is generally produced by the operation. Further surgical therapy, including valve replacement, likely will be necessary.

BIBLIOGRAPHY

Bache, R. J., Wang, Y., and Jorgensen, C. R. 1971. Hemodynamic effects of exercise in isolated valvular aortic stenosis. Circulation 44:1003–1013.

Braunwald, E. 1963. Aortic Stenosis: Physiological, Pathological, and Clinical Concepts. Combined Clinical Staff Conference at the National Institutes of Health. Ann. Intern. Med. 58:494–522.

Buckberg, G., Eber, L., Herman, M., and Gorlin, R. 1975. Ischemia in aortic stenosis: Hemodynamic prediction. Am. J. Cardiol. 35:778–784.

Cohen, L. S., Friedman, W. F., and Braunwald, E. 1972. Natural history of mild congenital aortic stenosis elucidated by serial hemodynamic studies. Am. J. Cardiol. 30:1–5.

French, J. W., and Guntheroth, W. G. 1970. An explanation of asymmetric upper extremity blood pressures in supravalvular aortic stenosis. The Coanda effect. Circulation 42:31–36.

Glanz, S., Hellenbrand, W. E., Berman, M. A., and Talner, N. S. 1976. Echocar-

diographic assessment of the severity of aortic stenosis in children and adolescents. Am. J. Cardiol. 38:620-625.
Glew, R. H., Varghese, P. J., Krovetz, L. J., Dorst, J. P., and Rowe, R. D. 1969. Sudden death in congenital aortic stenosis. Am. Heart J. 78:615-625.
Jack, W. D., II, and Kelly, D. T. 1976. Long-term follow-up of valvulotomy for congenital aortic stenosis. Am. J. Cardiol. 38:231-234.
Keane, J. F., Bernhard, W. F., and Nadas, A. S. 1975. Aortic stenosis surgery in infancy. Circulation 52:1138-1143.
Kelly, D. T., Wulfsberg, E., and Rowe, R. D. 1972. Discrete subaortic stenosis. Circulation 42:309-322.
Krovetz, L. J., and Kurlinski, J. P. 1976. Subendocardial blood flow in children with congenital aortic stenosis. Circulation 54:961-965.
Lakier, J. B., Lewis, A. B., Heymann, M. A., Stranger, P., Hoffman, J. I. E., and Rudolph, A. M. 1974. Isolated aortic stenosis in the neonate. Natural history and hemodynamic considerations. Circulation 50:801-808.
Mody, M. R., and Mody, G. T. 1975. Serial hemodynamic observations in congenital valvular and subvalvular aortic stenosis. Am. Heart J. 89:137-143.
Radford, D. J., Bloom, K. R., Izukawa, T., Moes, C. A. F., and Rowe, R. D. 1976. Echocardiographic assessment of bicuspid aortic valves. Angiographic and pathological correlates. Circulation 53:80-85.
Williams, J. C. P., Barratt-Boyes, B. G., and Lowe, J. B. 1961. Supravalvular aortic stenosis. Circulation 24:1311-1318.

chapter 26

IDIOPATHIC HYPERTROPHIC SUBAORTIC STENOSIS: Asymmetric Septal Hypertrophy

HISTORICAL NOTES

Brock, in 1957, described subaortic stenosis as being a result of severe hypertrophy of the left ventricle. This disease entity was named hypertrophic obstructive cardiomyopathy (Hocum) in England, idiopathic hypertrophic subaortic stenosis (IHSS) in the United States, and muscular subaortic stenosis in Canada. During the next decade, Braunwald and associates at the NIH demonstrated the dynamic nature of the obstruction. Recently, patients with similar clinical and angiographic findings but with little or no left ventricular outflow obstruction have come to be recognized. With the development of echocardiography, the characteristic abnormality has been shown to be disproportionate thickening of the ventricular septum as compared with the left ventricular free wall. Thus another designation applied to this group is obstructive asymmetric septal hypertrophy (ASH).

INCIDENCE

This entity constitutes considerably less than 1% of our total clinical experience. A two-to-one predominance of males is found in the obstructive (IHSS) form, but ASH occurs in an equal percentage of both sexes.

ETIOLOGY

Familial occurrence has been documented in slightly less than one-half of the reported cases of IHSS. However, when the specific marker of ASH is considered (Figure 99), the hereditary nature of the disorder becomes clearer. In the study of Henry et al., ASH was demonstrable in at least one first degree relative in each of 28 families when the authors had the opportunity of studying at least three such relatives. A simple Mendelian dominant transmission has been traced in one family for five generations.

Ultrastructural observations suggest that the fundamental defect involves cardiac muscle cell hypertrophy and/or altered cellular morphogenesis. In some patients, the genetic defect will express itself diffusely, eventually causing an incapacitating myopathy. In others, the defect will be restricted largely to the septum, with varying degrees of functional impairment. Variations in severity of left ventricular obstruction, as well as varying involvement of the right ventricular outflow tract, secondary to septal hypertrophy, may be found among members of a single family.

PATHOLOGY

Diffuse hypertrophy of the myocardium, particularly of the ventricular septum, occurs, so that during systole the septum bulges into the left ventricular outflow tract and causes obstruction. Septal displacement of the mitral valve apparatus also commonly causes mitral regurgitation.

HEMODYNAMICS

In interpreting this disease, one must be cognizant of its dynamic nature. Left ventricular–aortic systolic pressure differences are extremely variable and the degree of obstruction may vary from beat to beat. Angiocardiography shows a marked narrowing of subaortic area in systole and a widening of the same area in diastole (Figure 187).

Anything that increases ventricular volume or decreases contractility will decrease the systolic pressure differences; the converse is also true. For example, the systolic pressure difference may be reduced or abolished by general anesthesia. Systolic pressure difference increases after a premature beat and with increased duration of intraventricular conduction time.

Isoproterenol decreases left ventricular end diastolic volume and increases myocardial contractility and, hence, the systolic pressure difference. Mitral insufficiency may also be produced during its infusion.

Methoxamine, an arteriolar constrictor, does not increase myocardial contractile forces. Systolic pressure difference therefore decreases with methoxamine, since it increases left ventricular end diastolic pressure.

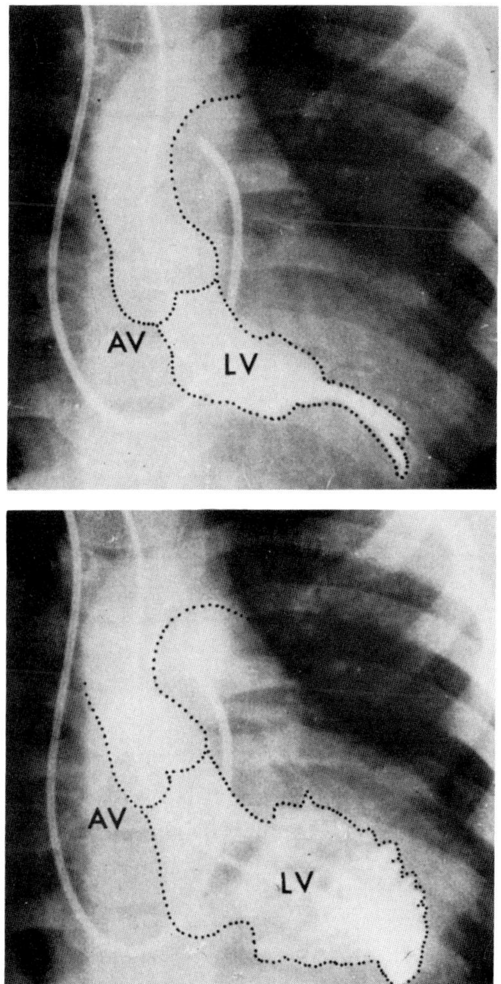

Figure 187. Angiocardiogram of a patient with IHSS that demonstrates the narrowing of the lower portion of the left ventricle in systole (left) and the relatively normal size in diastole (right). This illustrates clearly the dynamic nature of this disease process.

CLINICAL FEATURES

In the usual case, growth and development are normal. A systolic murmur is generally noted in the second decade, followed later by slowly progressive fatigability, dyspnea on exertion, palpitations, angina, and syncope.

Congestive heart failure is rare, but sudden death is common, particularly in the third and fourth decades.

This is the only type of isolated *aortic stenosis with a wide pulse pressure*. Palpitation of the brachial pulse may reveal a double impulse (pulsus bisferiens).

Cardiomegaly, a diffuse cardiac impulse, and prominence of the left chest are found. Systolic ejection murmur and thrill are maximal over mid-precordium and well transmitted to the apex (Figure 188). S_2 may be split paradoxically, with the aortic component being delayed because of prolongation of left ventricle systole. An S_3 and a prominent S_4 are commonly audible. A systolic ejection click is usually not present. A Valsalva maneuver usually increases the severity of the stenosis and the intensity of the murmur.

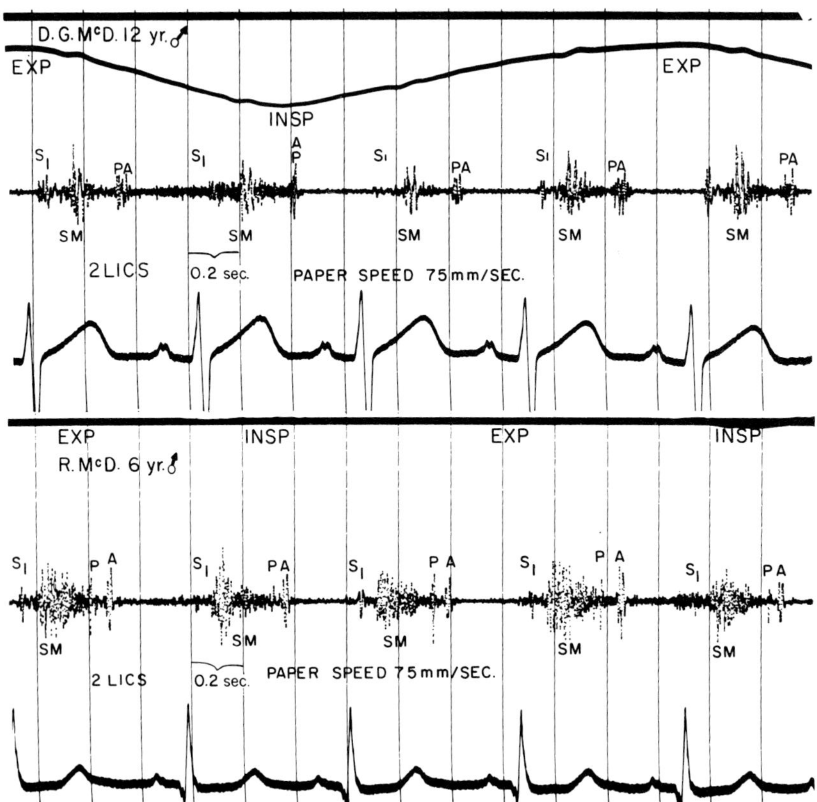

Figure 188. Phonocardiograms of two siblings with idiopathic hypertrophic subaortic stenosis. This murmur is essentially indistinguishable from those due to other types of aortic stenosis, except possibly for a slightly lower location. Paradoxical splitting of S_2 is also seen. (From Wood, R. S., Taylor, W. J., Wheat, M. W., Jr., and Schiebler, G. L. 1962. Muscular subaortic stenosis in childhood. Report of occurrence in three siblings. Pediatrics 30:749. Copyright, American Academy of Pediatrics, 1962.)

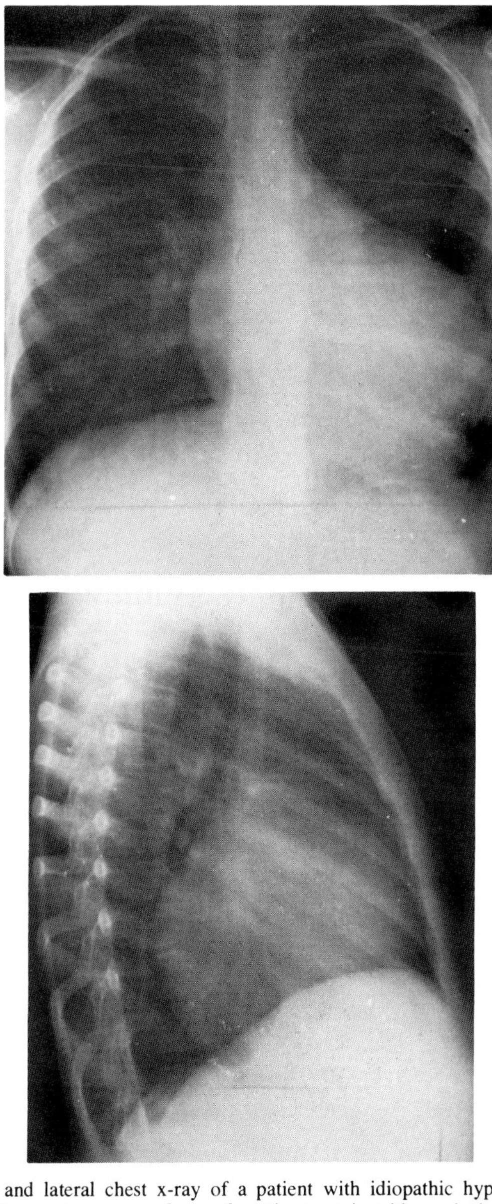

Figure 189. PA and lateral chest x-ray of a patient with idiopathic hypertrophic subaortic stenosis. This is the most common form of aortic stenosis with marked cardiomegaly. The marked degree of left ventricular enlargement without poststenotic dilatation of the aorta is highly suggestive of IHSS.

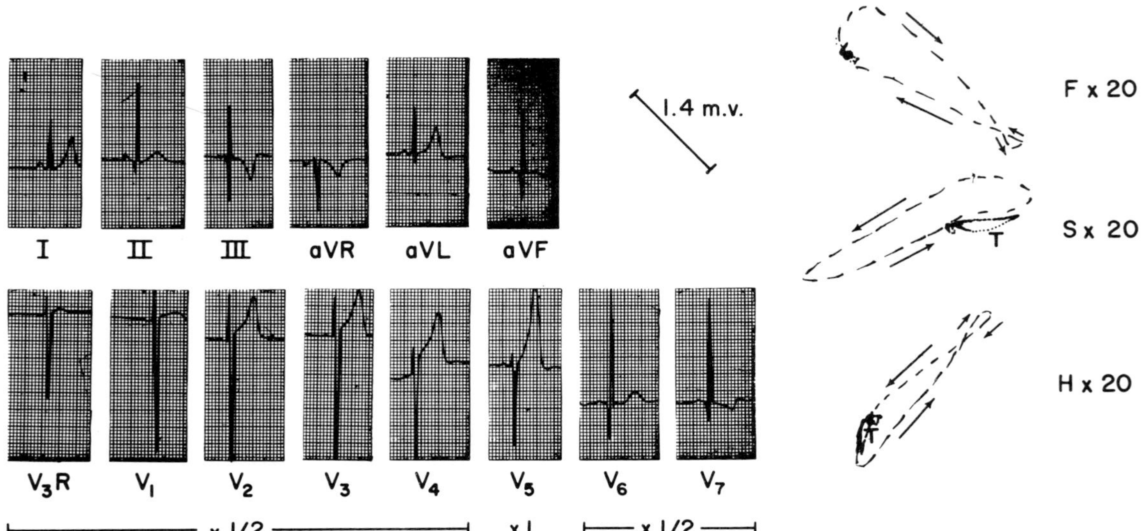

Figure 190. Electrocardiogram of a patient with idiopathic hypertrophic subaortic stenosis that shows marked left ventricular hypertrophy.

ROENTGENOGRAPHIC FEATURES

Cardiac enlargement, mainly concentric hypertrophy of the left ventricle, is present and increases progressively with age. The extent of left ventricular enlargement is greater than in other types of aortic stenosis (Figure 189).

Left atrial enlargement is present, especially if there is concomitant mitral insufficiency. The ascending aorta usually appears normal in size, and there is no valvar calcification.

ELECTROCARDIOGRAPHY

The electrocardiogram usually shows left atrial enlargement, left ventricular hypertrophy, and left ventricular pressure overloading (Figure 190). Partilarly impressive are the deep q waves in left precordial leads. Less frequently, biventricular hypertrophy or the Wolff-Parkinson-White syndrome is present.

ECHOCARDIOGRAPHY

Disproportionate thickening of the interventricular septum in relation to the free wall of the left ventricle is characteristic but not pathognomonic. Normally the septum and free wall of the left ventricle are nearly equal in thickness. In this condition the ratio is greater than 1.3:1 and averages about 1.7:1. An abrupt anterior movement of the mitral valve during midsystole is also commonly seen, and shows a rough correlation with severity. This systolic anterior motion, as well as disproportionate septal thickening, has been reported in a number of other conditions, but both are useful when the clinical picture suggests IHSS.

PROGNOSIS

Maron et al. followed a group of 35 children with ASH for an average of 7.4 years. The clinical course was found to be extremely variable. Two-fifths of the group improved or remained stable, while 29% showed clinical deterioration and 31% died suddenly. A malignant form has been reported in some families, with deaths in the first decade of life.

MANAGEMENT

Propanalol will often reduce the degree of left ventricular outflow obstruction. It appears to be of most value in patients with dyspnea or other symptoms secondary to severe obstruction. The ultimate outcome of the disease does not appear to be affected by drug therapy.

Incision and splitting of the obstructing muscle mass through an aortic valve approach, similar to the operation for pyloric stenosis, has been attempted, with limited success. Of 120 operations reported by Maron, 8% died at surgery, 9% died later of presumed cardiovascular problems, and 12% showed little or no improvement. Furthermore, neither propanalol nor myotomy-myectomy offers complete protection against sudden death in this group of patients.

BIBLIOGRAPHY

Henry, W. L., Clark, C. E., and Epstein, S. E. 1973. Asymmetric septal hypertrophy. Echocardiographic identification of the pathognomonic anatomic abnormality of IHSS. Circulation 47:225–233.

Henry, W. L., Clark, C. E., and Epstein, S. E. 1973. Asymmetric septal hypertrophy (ASH): The unifying link in the IHSS disease spectrum. Observations regarding its pathogenesis, pathophysiology, and course. Circulation 47:827–832.

Henry, W. L., Clark, C. E., Griffith, J. M., and Epstein, S. E. 1975. Mechanism of left ventricular outflow obstruction in patients with obstructive asymmetric septal hypertrophy (idiopathic hypertrophic subaortic stenosis). Am. J. Cardiol. 35:337–345.

Maron, B. J., Henry, W. L., Clark, C. E., Redwood, D. R., Roberts, W. C., and Epstein, S. E. 1976. Asymmetric septal hypertrophy in childhood. Circulation 53:9–19.

Maron, B. J., Merrill, W. H., Freier, P. A., Kent, K. M., Epstein, S. E., and Morrow, A. G. 1978. Long-term clinical course and symptomatic status of patients after operation for hypertrophic subaortic stenosis. Circulation 57:1205–1213.

Morrow, A. G., Reitz, B. A., Epstein, S. E., Henry, W. L., Conkle, D. M., Itscoitz, S. B., and Redwood, D. R. 1975. Operative treatment in hypertrophic subaortic stenosis. Techniques, and the results of pre and postoperative assessments in 83 patients. Circulation 52:88–102.

Ross, J., Jr., Braunwald, E., Gault, J. H., Mason, D. T., and Morrow, A. G. 1966. The mechanism of the intraventricular pressure gradient in idiopathic hypertrophic subaortic stenosis. Circulation 34:558–578.

chapter 27

COARCTATION OF THE AORTA

HISTORICAL NOTES

The earliest description of coarctation of the aorta dates from Morgagni in the year 1760. In that year, Morgagni performed a postmortem examination of a monk and noted a constriction of the aorta a short distance from the heart. Bonnet classified coarctation of the aorta into infantile and adult types in 1903. Surgical correction of coarctation was accomplished simultaneously in 1945 by Gross and Huffnagel in Boston and by Crafoord and Nylin in Stockholm.

INCIDENCE

Coarctation is a moderately common congenital heart defect and accounts for about 6% of all congenital heart anomalies. When coarctation is the sole cardiac anomaly, males predominate by a ratio of roughly two to one; when accompanied by other cardiac anomalies, the sex ratio is more nearly equal. Coarctation of the aorta is apparently rare in Orientals.

ETIOLOGY

Familial occurrence of coarctation is exceedingly rare and we have seen none in our series. Little is known of teratological factors, except for an association with the Turner syndrome. Six of our 277 cases (3%) were associated with Turner syndrome.

PATHOLOGY

In the past (and in the previous edition of this book) aortic coarctation was divided into infantile and adult types, referred to by some as preductal and postductal, respectively. The infantile, or preductal, form characteristically has a diffuse narrowing of the aortic isthmus, whereas the adult type has the more familiar discrete obstruction. It is now apparent that classification into infantile and adult forms is often inappropriate as well as confusing. First, the site of the coarctation cannot be known with certainty until surgery or necropsy. Second, in a significant number of instances, the coarctation is directly opposite to the ductus.

Narrowing of the aortic isthmus in many instances represents a hypoplastic left fourth aortic arch, and is often associated with major intracardiac defects, such as large ventricular septal defect, atrial septal defect, or abnormal mitral valve. Since patients with a hypoplastic aortic arch and intracardiac defect are almost always symptomatic early in life, the origin of the descriptor "infantile" is readily understandable (Table 30). However, the discrete type occasionally also produces symptoms during infancy. For all of these reasons we have elected to discuss the pathology of coarctation of the aorta as either discrete or diffuse narrowing and have divided the clinical presentation into those cases presenting during infancy and those presenting after 1 year of age.

In the *discrete* type of coarctation, the narrowing is usually located at the juncture of the ductus arteriosus and aorta, immediately distal to the origin of the left subclavian artery (Figure 191). However, occasionally it occurs proximal to the left subclavian, between the innominate and the left common carotid arteries, or even in a markedly aberrant location such as the abdominal

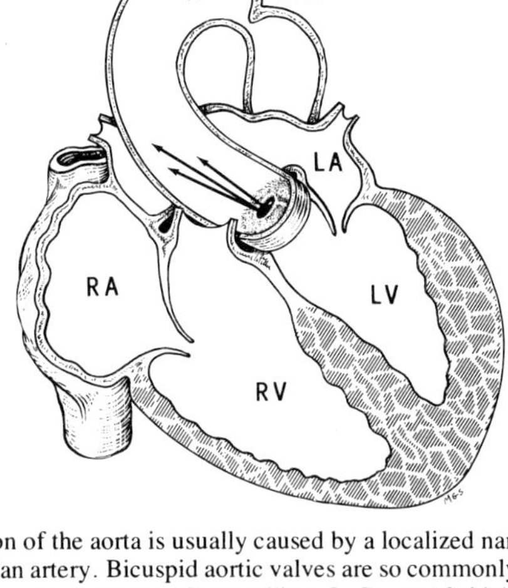

Figure 191. Coarctation of the aorta is usually caused by a localized narrowing just distal to the origin of the left subclavian artery. Bicuspid aortic valves are so commonly associated that one has been added to this schema as a reminder. (From Elliott, L. P., and Schiebler, G. L. 1968. X-Ray Diagnosis of Congenital Cardiac Disease. Courtesy of Charles C Thomas, Publisher, Springfield, Ill.)

Table 30. Major cardiac anomalies associated with coarctation of the aorta (University of Virginia, 1950–1978)

	Infants	1–18 years
Isolated coarctation	22	69
Patent ductus arteriosus (PDA)	17	9
Ventricular septal defect (VSD)	17	8
PDA and VSD	13	5
Atrial septal defect	2	3
Aortic valve disease	9	34
Mitral valve disease	2	7
Transposition of great arteries	4	0
Miscellaneous (one each)	6	0
Totals	92	135

aorta. Coarctations occurring in these locations are obviously more difficult to diagnose. Coarctation of the ascending aorta is best considered as a variety of supravalvar aortic stenosis (see Chapter 25).

Occurrence of intracardiac anomalies in conjunction with discrete coarctations is uncommon, with the exception of a bicuspid aortic valve, which has been reported to occur in as many as 80% of patients with coarctation of the aorta.

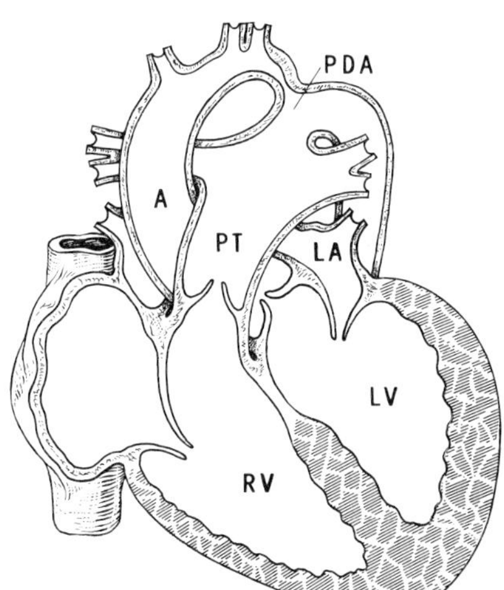

Figure 192. In the so-called infantile type of coarctation of the aorta, the region of narrowing occurs proximal to the location of the ductus arteriosus. Further narrowing and hypoplasia of the aorta commonly occur, and can involve the origin of the left subclavian artery. (From Elliott, L. P., and Schiebler, G. L. 1968. X-Ray Diagnosis of Congenital Cardiac Disease. Courtesy of Charles C Thomas, Publisher, Springfield, Ill.)

In patients with *diffuse narrowing of the aortic isthmus,* the left subclavian artery may arise at the distal end of the narrowed segment and therefore be small or at least demonstrate low pressure (Figure 192). Patency of the ductus arteriosus is common, frequently carrying blood from pulmonary artery to descending aorta. In these instances, of course, the right ventricular pressure is at systemic levels.

In the extreme form of aortic isthmus narrowing, *complete interruption of the aorta* occurs. This interruption is usually just beyond the left common carotid artery (in a left aortic arch). In complete interruption of the aorta, a large ventricular septal defect is almost invariably present, usually supracristal in location. The lower part of the body is perfused by the ductus arteriosus carrying blood from pulmonary artery to aorta (''reversed flow'').

CLINICAL FEATURES

The presence of a discrete coarctation may not be apparent for several years, since such children are generally asymptomatic and the anomaly is quite compatible with athletic supremacy. With growth, the coarctation becomes relatively narrower and the children may then complain of headaches, chest pains, or intermittent claudication (cramp-like pains in the legs following exercise). Major complications, such as cerebrovascular accidents, may occur secondary to severe hypertension and arterial damage, but are fortunately rare in children.

When the anomalies are severe enough to cause symptoms in infancy, affected infants present with poor growth, tachypnea, repeated respiratory infections, congestive heart failure, and, occasionally, peripheral edema.

The blood pressure in the arms, although higher than that in the legs, may be within normal limits. In normal children and adults, the systolic blood pressure in the legs is equal to or slightly higher than that in the arms. A systolic blood pressure higher in the arms than in the legs is the most important diagnostic feature of coarctation. This blood pressure difference may be reduced or absent under certain circumstances:

1. *Another stenotic lesion* upstream from the coarctation, such as aortic stenosis, may reduce the pressure proximal to the coarctation.
2. *Reduced systemic blood flow,* as in congestive heart failure, may cause the coarctation to be missed. The lower the flow past the site of coarctation, the lower will be the pressure drop across the site of narrowing (see Figure 25). It is extremely important to repeat blood pressure measurements after digitalization of infants in congestive heart failure.
3. *Intracardiac left-to-right shunts* will also reduce the flow across the coarctation. For example, coarctation associated with a large ventricular

septal defect will increase the left-to-right shunt and reduce aortic flow, since the resistance to blood flow will be less through the ventricular septal defect than through the coarctation.

4. In *preductal coarctation,* a patent ductus arteriosus enters the aorta below the coarctation and may reduce the blood pressure difference across it. If the pressure in the pulmonary artery is high enough, the ductus may supply blood to the lower extremities at the same pressure that the aorta is supplying blood to the upper half of the body.
5. The orifice of the *left subclavian artery may be stenotic,* involved in the site of coarctation, or arise below the coarctation. In these cases, blood pressure in the left arm will be the same as those in the legs. Rarely, the right subclavian artery arises anomalously below the coarctation. The presence of these possibilities can usually be eliminated by taking blood pressures in all four extremities. Even less commonly, both subclavians may exit below the coarctation, with the right subclavian passing in an aberrant fashion behind the esophagus to the right arm. When this occurs, the presence of the coarctation can be confirmed by palpating the carotid arteries.

The classical murmur for this defect is a harsh ejection murmur extending past the second sound and heard near the angle of the left scapula. However, in many instances the murmur is soft, unimpressive, and easily overlooked unless blood pressures in arms and legs are measured (Figure 193). A suprasternal notch thrill is common, as is a thrill in the second right

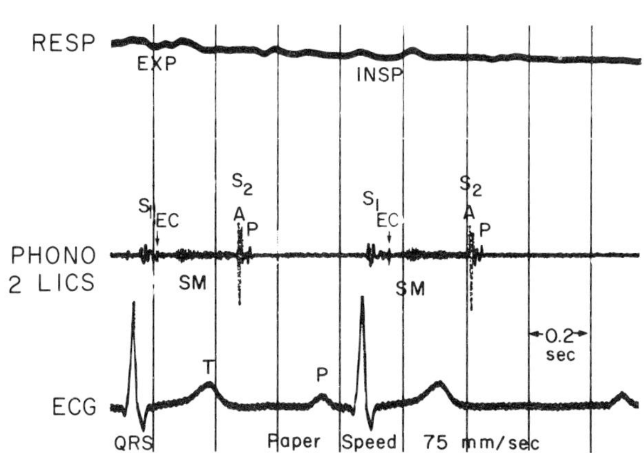

Figure 193. Phonocardiogram of a 6-year-old female with isolated coarctation of the aorta. The murmur of coarctation is often unimpressive, as in this example, and may be overlooked unless the examiner palpates the femoral pulses.

intercostal space near the sternum, and both are usually secondary to an abnormal aortic valve.

ROENTGENOGRAPHIC FEATURES

In older children, there is a concentric type of left ventricular hypertrophy that may be difficult to diagnose as abnormal. The aorta is prominent and one may see a "figure three" sign at the site of narrowing (Figure 194). Notching of the under portion of the third to eighth ribs may be seen in children after the age of 10 (Figure 195).

X-rays of symptomatic infants vary in relation to the associated anomalies, but usually reveal significant cardiomegaly (Figure 196). The left atrium and either one or both ventricles may be enlarged. Pulmonary vascular

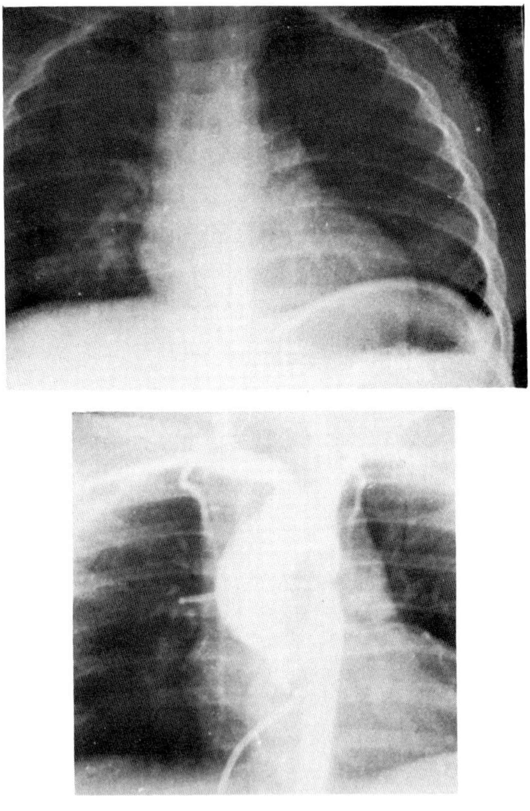

Figure 194. The descending aorta (top) may be seen faintly immediately to the left of the vertebral column. There is an indentation in the aorta that on the thoracic aortogram (bottom) is seen to be the site of the coarctation. Note also the cardiomegaly and the left ventricular hypertrophy.

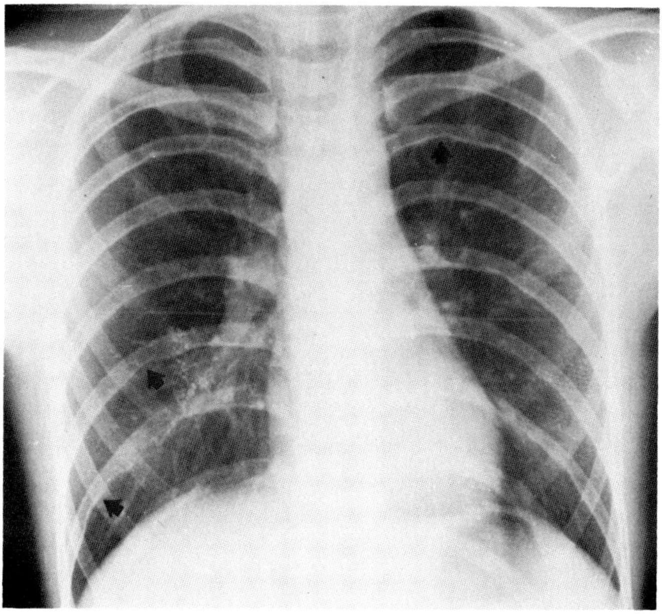

Figure 195. A 12-year-old female with coarctation of the aorta. The arrows point to the prominent rib notches that are always on the lower margin of the ribs. These notches are caused by enlarged, tortuous collateral intercostal arteries, which erode the lower margin of the ribs. The cardiac outline itself is normal.

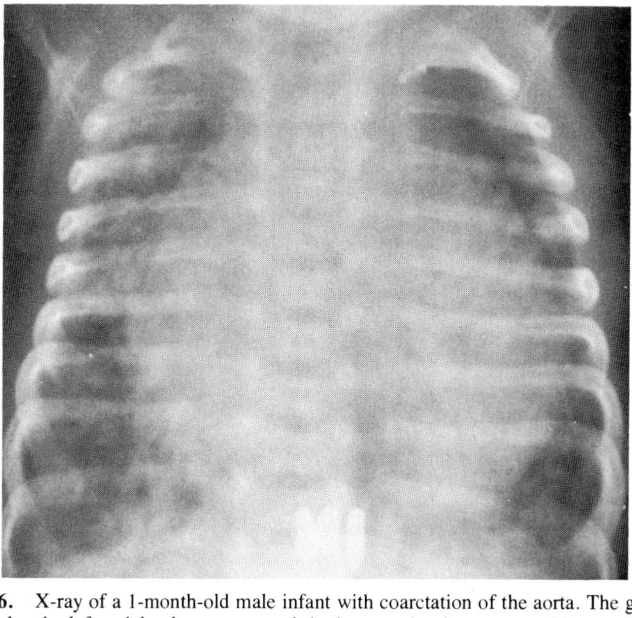

Figure 196. X-ray of a 1-month-old male infant with coarctation of the aorta. The generalized cardiomegaly, the left atrial enlargement, and the increased pulmonary markings are often misdiagnosed as resulting from ventricular septal defect. The proper way to diagnose coarctation in an infant is to feel the femorals. The x-ray is of little help.

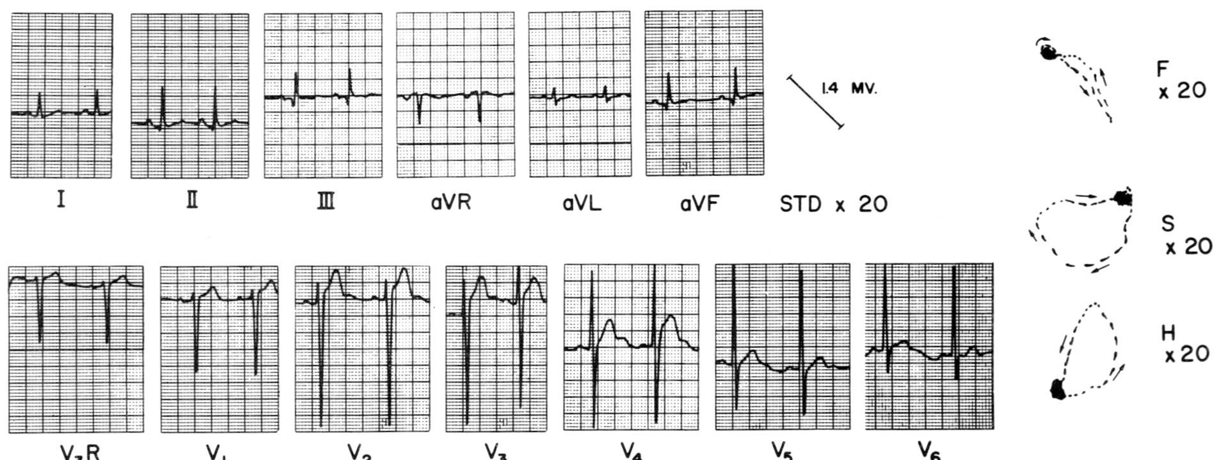

Figure 197. Electrocardiogram of a 15-year-old male with coarctation of the aorta. The absence of a q wave in leads V_5 and V_6, together with tall R waves, suggests left ventricular pressure overloading.

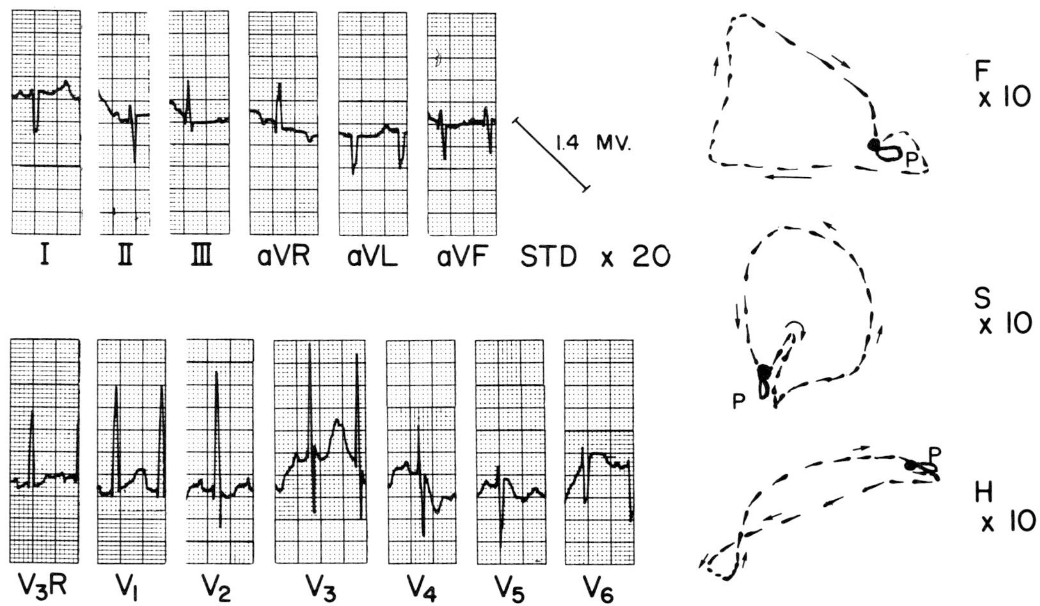

Figure 198. Electrocardiogram of a 3-week-old male with coarctation of the aorta. Right ventricular hypertrophy, seen here, is very common at this age.

markings are usually increased and may be venous in nature because of congestive heart failure, arterial because of an associated left-to-right shunt, or both. The thymic shadow almost invariably obscures the aorta.

ELECTROCARDIOGRAPHY

After 1 year of age, the electrocardiogram may be normal or may show varying degrees of left ventricular hypertrophy (Figure 197). During infancy, the electrocardiogram most commonly shows right ventricular hypertrophy (Figure 198). This is due to the presence of associated defects that in themselves cause right ventricular hypertrophy, a reversing patent ductus arteriosus where the right ventricle becomes the systemic pumper for the lower part of the body, or severe pulmonary hypertension secondary to left heart failure.

PROGNOSIS

The outlook for the child who is asymptomatic during infancy is reasonably good. However, a number of complications may occur and life expectancy even in this group is less than that of normal individuals. They are subject to cerebrovascular accidents, which have occurred even prior to age 2. Bacterial endocarditis is not uncommon, either at the coarctation itself or on a bicuspid aortic valve (see Chapter 37). Associated aortic or mitral valve disease may require additional surgery. There may be advanced degrees of atheromatous changes around the site of the coarctation, and dissecting aneurysms of the aorta are not uncommon. In addition, recent evidence suggests that even following successful surgery the response of the left ventricle to stress remains abnormal.

Coarctation severe enough to be symptomatic during infancy carries a very uncertain prognosis (Table 31). Forty-three percent of the infants treated

Table 31. Results of treatment of infants with coarctation of the aorta

Senior author	Center	Year	Medical treatment only		Surgery	
			Total	Died	Total	Died
Gessner	Gainesville	1966	11	4	18	13
Sinha	Chicago	1969	26	18	28	10
Tawes	Toronto	1969	—	—	179	81
Milner	Transvaal	1972	11	7	18	5
Chen	St. Louis	1977	20	6	16	6
Patel	Birmingham (England)	1977	—	—	61	12
Krovetz	Virginia	1978	19	15	71	21
Totals			87	50 (57%)	391	148 (38%)

Table 32. Effect of associated defects on outcome of treatment in infants (combined reports)

	Medical treatment only		Surgery	
Associated lesion	Total	Died	Total	Died
None	67	10%	34	21%
Patent ductus arteriosus (PDA)	71	72%	91	30%
Ventricular septal defect (VSD)	27	52%	29	48%
VSD and PDA	14	71%	40	55%
Atrial septal defect	9	89%	18	67%
Transposition of great arteries	6	100%	16	69%

by medical means alone survived, whereas sixty-two percent of those operated on survived. It should be pointed out that a number of children in the medical treatment group died before the full effects of therapy could be achieved, and were not always prime candidates for surgery because of the severity of their illness. A second factor working to the detriment of this group was illustrated by Waldhausen et al., who noted that the correct diagnosis was not made in 29% of their cases prior to death or surgery. Finally, no attempt was made in the construction of this table to sort out cases with inoperable defects. On the other hand, patients on medical treatment only were listed as survivors if they were alive at age 1, but still faced additional risks of later medical complications and surgery.

Table 32 considers the effects of associated defects. Infants with an associated patent ductus arteriosus or ventricular septal defect have a guarded prognosis, but those infants who were operated on did slightly better than patients who were treated medically. A combination of these three defects considerably worsens the prognosis—only 28 of 54 infants survived. The presence of an atrial septal defect or transposition of the great arteries is also an ominous sign.

Recent studies suggest that surgical repair of coarctation may not cure preexisting hypertension. Significant elevation of blood pressure may occur at rest and during exercise. Concomitant aortic valve disease may cause further cardiac problems in later life.

MANAGEMENT

For the older child who is essentially asymptomatic, we recommend surgical resection between the ages of 3 and 6 years. At these ages atherosclerosis around the coarctation is still minimal and the chest and great vessels have reached an adequate size. It has been calculated that the aorta will have reached one-half of the adult cross-sectional area by approximately 3 years of age. Surgery after this time carries virtually no risk of restenosis.

For infants in severe congestive heart failure, we recommend a trial of vigorous medical management. Those infants who respond rapidly usually have no associated cardiac defect or one of little hemodynamic significance. Catheterization is done at the first sign of a decline or if the patient is not significantly improved within 24 hr. These infants are emergency cases and should be operated on even though there is a risk of inadequate growth at the suture site. This risk has been considerably reduced by the use of interrupted sutures for the anastomosis.

BIBLIOGRAPHY

James, F. W., and Kaplan, S. 1974. Systolic hypertension during submaximal exercise after correction of coarctation of aorta. Circulation 49: Suppl. II: 27–34.

Malm, J. R., Blumenthal, S., Jameson, A. G., and Humphreys, G. H., II. 1963. Observations on coarctation of the aorta in infants. Arch. Surg. 86:96–103.

Maron, B. J., Humphries, J. O'N., Rowe, R. D., and Mellits, E. D. 1973. Prognosis of surgically corrected coarctation of the aorta. A 20-year postoperative appraisal. Circulation 47:119–126.

Martelle, R. R., and Moss, A. J. 1962. Fifty-three cases of coarctation of the aorta. Am. J. Dis. Child. 103:556–563.

Milner, S., Levin, S. E., Marchand, P. E., and Fuller, D. N. 1974. Coarctation of the aorta in infants under one year of age with particular reference to results of surgery. S. Afr. Med. J. 48:397–400.

Rocchini, A. P., Rosenthal, A., Barger, A. C., Castaneda, A. R., and Nadas, A. S. 1976. Pathogenesis of paradoxical hypertension after coarctation resection. Circulation 54:382–387.

Sinha, S. M., Kardatzke, M. L., Cole, R. B., Muster, A. J., Wessel, H. U., and Paul, M. H. 1969. Coarctation of the aorta in infancy. Circulation 40:385–398.

Tawes, R. L., Jr., Aberdeen, E., Waterston, D. J., and Carter, R. E. B. 1969. Coarctation of the aorta in infants and children: A review of 333 operative cases, including 179 infants. Circulation 39:Suppl. I:173–184.

Waldhausen, J. A., King, H., Nahrwold, D. L., Lurie, P. R., and Shumaker, H. G., Jr. 1964. Management of coarctation in infancy. JAMA 187:270–275.

Wood, W. C., Wood, J. C., Lower, R. R., Bosher, L. H., Jr., and McCue, C. M. 1975. Associated coarctation of the aorta and mitral valve disease: Nine cases with surgical correction of both lesions in three. J. Pediatr. 87:217–220.

chapter 28

HYPOPLASTIC LEFT HEART

HISTORICAL NOTES

The hypoplastic left heart (HLH) syndrome is a term coined by Lev in 1952 to describe a group of diseases having in common underdevelopment of the left side of the heart.

INCIDENCE

The hypoplastic left heart syndrome accounts for slightly more than 1% of all congenital heart disease. However, aortic valve atresia accounts for nearly one-fourth of deaths due to cardiac malformations in the neonatal period. The spectrum of hypoplasia ranges from a vestigial left ventricle in cases with both mitral and aortic valve atresia to only relative underdevelopment of the left ventricle (Table 33).

Table 33. Forms of the hypoplastic left heart syndrome (University of Virginia hospitals, 1970–1978)[a]

	Incidence
Aortic atresia	7
Mitral atresia	8
Aortic and mitral atresia	2
Atresia of transverse aortic arch	5
Hypoplastic aortic arch	28
Cor triatriatum	1
Hypoplastic left heart, not otherwise differentiated	4
Mitral stenosis	4
with transposed great arteries	3

[a] Excluding total anomalous pulmonary venous return.

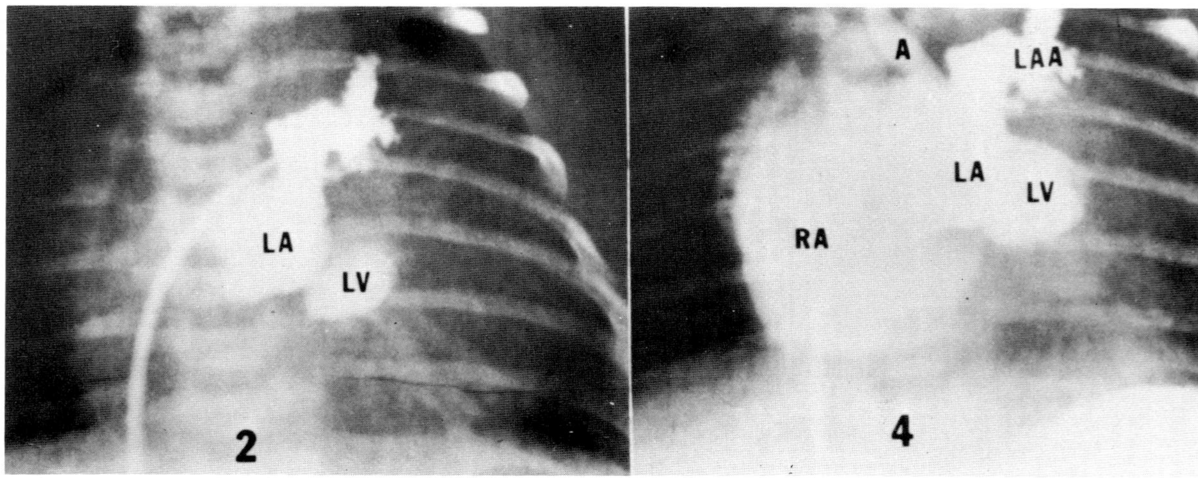

Figure 199. Angiocardiogram of a 2-week-old infant with hypoplastic left heart. Note the small left ventricular (LV) cavity (left) and the small aorta (A) (right). LA = left atrium; LAA = left atrial appendage; RA = right atrium.

PATHOLOGY

Aortic atresia is characterized by complete obstruction of the aortic valve. The left ventricular lumen is small and fibroelastotic. The mitral valve is tiny, with few or no chordae tendineae. In contrast to pulmonic atresia, the mitral valve does not become insufficient. The foramen ovale is open but small in most patients, and the left atrium is thick walled and of small volume. The right ventricle and pulmonary artery are markedly dilated. The ductus arteriosus is widely patent at birth but responds normally by trying to close, which, of course, is catastrophic. A definable coarctation proximal to the entrance of the ductus arteriosus into the aorta is usually present. Proximal to the innominate artery the aorta becomes quite small, since it serves no function other than to supply the coronary arteries (Figure 199).

Isolated mitral atresia is uncommon, but when it occurs the pathology is much like aortic atresia. Usually mitral atresia is associated with a ventricular septal defect, in which case left ventricular size will depend on the size of the VSD. Pulmonic stenosis is common, as is origin of the aorta from the right ventricle. One must be careful in evaluating mitral atresia to be sure of the ventricular interrelationships. For example, if there is ventricular inversion then the atretic left-sided atrioventricular valve is an anatomic tricuspid valve and the lesion is in reality tricuspid atresia. A discussion of these complicated situations is, however, beyond the scope of this book.

HEMODYNAMICS

All of the pulmonary venous return must cross the atrial septum to the right atrium, except in the occasional patient with an intact atrial septum in whom pulmonary blood flow cannot increase after birth, resulting in rapid deterioration and death (Figure 200).

Ductal patency controls the clinical situation, since aortic flow is dependent on right-to-left ductal flow. As the ductus constricts, the patient rapidly manifests inadequate systemic blood flow. If the ductus remains widely patent, the patient may survive for several weeks.

Although this entity has been classified among the cyanotic forms of congenital heart disease, it is more properly classified among the obligatory admixture lesions. In this group of cardiac anomalies, both systemic venous blood and pulmonary venous blood must pass through a common mixing chamber before being distributed to the pulmonary and systemic vascular beds.

The amount of blood flowing through each vascular bed is determined primarily by the resistance of that bed. The other important factor is the size of the communication between the right and left atria. If the interatrial communication is inadequate in size, or absent, this causes severe pulmonary venous

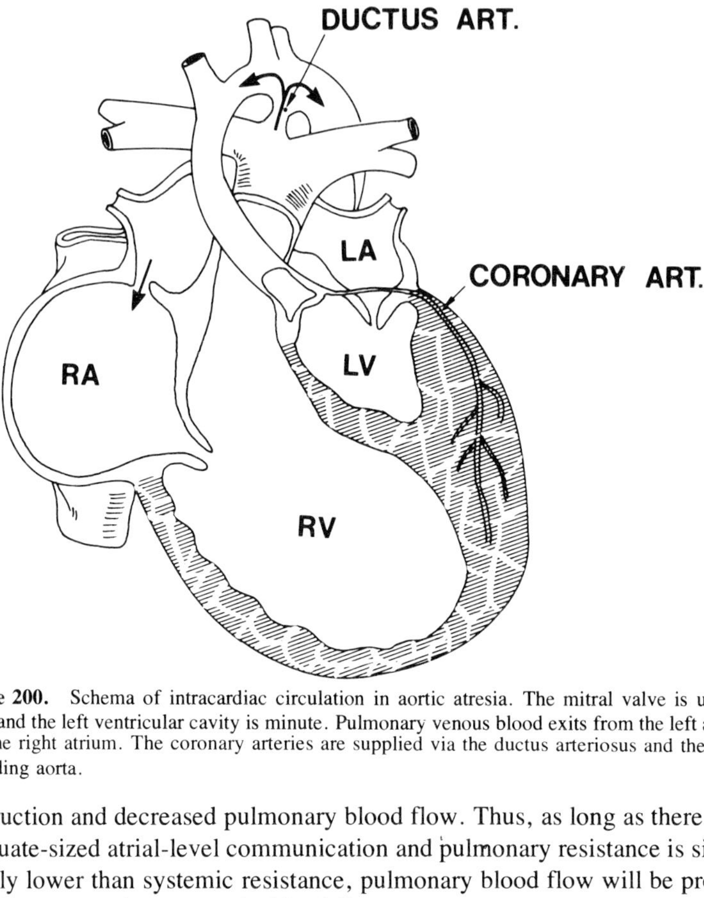

Figure 200. Schema of intracardiac circulation in aortic atresia. The mitral valve is usually small and the left ventricular cavity is minute. Pulmonary venous blood exits from the left atrium into the right atrium. The coronary arteries are supplied via the ductus arteriosus and the small ascending aorta.

obstruction and decreased pulmonary blood flow. Thus, as long as there is an adequate-sized atrial-level communication and pulmonary resistance is significantly lower than systemic resistance, pulmonary blood flow will be proportionally greater than systemic blood flow.

Although pulmonary congestion is commonly seen, there is usually no difficulty in oxygenation of the blood in these infants, and fully saturated blood returns from the pulmonary veins. There is an excellent correlation of systemic arterial saturation with the ratio of pulmonary to systemic blood flow. That is, as in other admixture lesions, the lower the pulmonary vascular resistance the greater the pulmonary blood flow and the higher the arterial oxygen saturation.

CLINICAL FEATURES

The infant appears healthy at birth, but within a few hours to a day or two rapid deterioration occurs. Tachypnea and labored breathing are accompanied by what has been described as "gray cyanosis," the result of both systemic desaturation and low cardiac output. Congestive heart failure is rapidly pro-

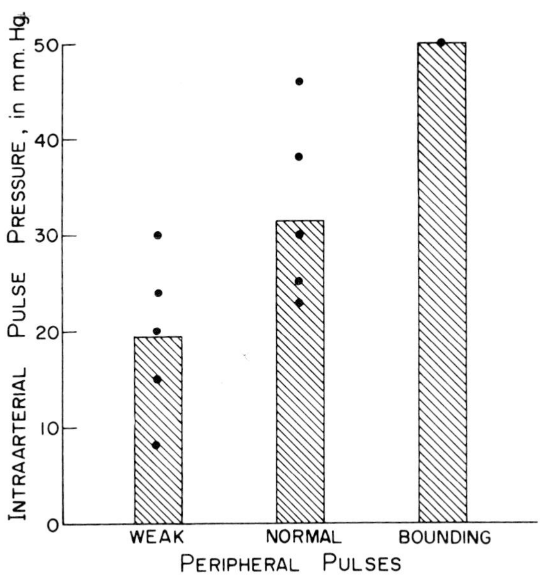

Figure 201. The clinical observation of weak pulses in association with aortic atresia is best explained by decreased pulse pressure. In the five infants with weak or decreased pulses, intra-arterial pulse pressures averaged 19 mm Hg, as compared with an average of 32 mm Hg in five infants with normal pulses and 50 mm Hg in one patient with "bounding" pulses.

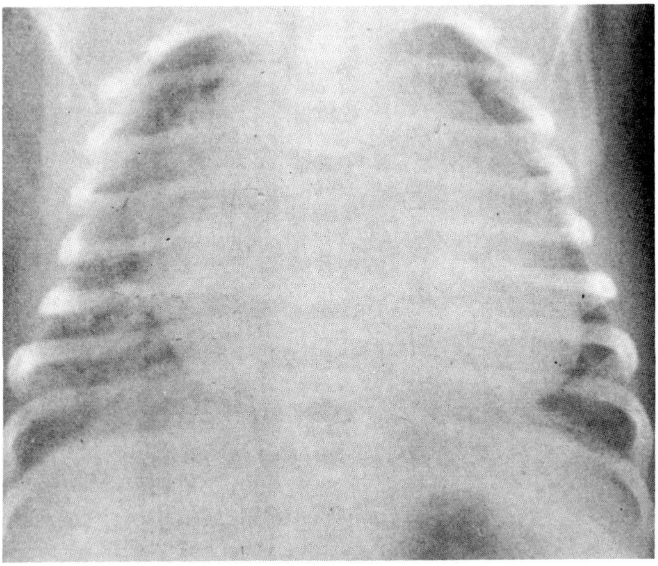

Figure 202. PA view of a 2-week-old female infant with hypoplastic left heart syndrome. There are marked cardiomegaly and pulmonary venous engorgement.

gressive, manifested by tachycardia and massive hepatomegaly. Increased right heart activity may be apparent. Murmurs are insignificant, although at times the continuous murmur of a patent ductus arteriosus is audible. The second sound is loud and single and a prominent fourth heart sound is frequent.

One of the striking physical findings in aortic valve atresia is the poor quality of the peripheral pulses, especially in the presence of severe congestive heart failure. This is presumably due to low cardiac output, with a resulting low pulse pressure (Figure 201).

ROENTGENOGRAPHIC FEATURES

There is usually moderate to severe cardiac enlargement. The hilar shadows are increased and congested, with many patients showing distinct pulmonary venous congestion (Figure 202).

ELECTROCARDIOGRAPHY

All tracings show evidence of right ventricular hypertrophy. In aortic atresia, ductal constriction may produce myocardial ischemia and T wave changes, especially in left precordial leads.

ECHOCARDIOGRAPHY

The echocardiogram has become a valuable diagnostic procedure, and many investigators now advocate it as the definitive means of confirming the diagnosis. A diminutive aortic root, abnormal mitral valve excursion, and a small left ventricle virtually establish the diagnosis.

DIFFERENTIAL DIAGNOSIS

This diagnosis should be entertained in any infant who develops heart failure in the first week of life. Gray cyanosis, weak pulses, cardiomegaly, and ECG evidence of marked right ventricular hypertrophy help to establish the diagnosis.

Critical aortic stenosis usually shows left ventricular hypertrophy with strain, but severe right ventricular hypertrophy is not uncommon.

Neonates with *myocarditis* usually show low ECG voltages and ST-T segments changes.

Obstructed forms of *total anomalous pulmonary venous return* usually show intense cyanosis and no cardiomegaly.

Coarctation of the aorta may present with severe heart failure and similar X-ray and ECG findings. The pulse discrepancy between upper and lower extremities may not become apparent until the heart failure improves.

PROGNOSIS

The average age at death is 4 to 5 days. Furthermore, the majority of these infants die within 48 hr of recognition. Occasional survival to a few weeks of age may occur when ductal patency persists.

MANAGEMENT

Management of these infants is primarily diagnostic, since all such patients die, usually within a few days. Palliative surgical measures have been suggested and accomplished by some groups, but with no substantial success. We do not believe it is justifiable to subject an infant to complex surgery, and the infant's family to the accompanying stress, with little hope for a meaningful result. This is not a repressive approach on our part, but a considered judgment that current methodology is inadequate to deal with this defect. (Perhaps one can make a case for a few large centers, engaged in experimental surgery, to study new methods in these babies provided that the parents are aware that what is being done is experimental.)

Once the diagnosis is confirmed, the findings should be explained to the parents and the hopelessness of the situation presented.

BIBLIOGRAPHY

Cayler, G. G., Smeloff, E. A., and Miller, G. E., Jr. 1970. Surgical palliation of hypoplastic left side of the heart. N. Engl. J. Med. 282:780–783.

Elliott, L. P., Best, E. B., and Schiebler, G. L. 1961. Aortic atresia: A case report and a review. Am. Heart J. 62:821–829.

Friedman, S., Murphy, L., and Ash, R. 1955. Congenital mitral atresia with hypoplastic nonfunctioning left heart. Am. J. Dis. Child. 90:176–188.

Krovetz, L. J., Rowe, R. D., and Schiebler, G. L. 1970. Hemodynamics of aortic valve atresia. Circulation 42:953–959.

Lambert, E. C., Canent, R. V., and Hohn, A. R. 1966. Congenital cardiac anomalies in the newborn: A review of conditions causing death or severe distress in the first month of life. Pediatrics 37:343–351.

Lev, M. 1952. Pathologic anatomy and interrelationship of hypoplasia of the aortic tract complexes. Lab Invest. 1:61–70.

Noonan, J. A., and Nadas, A. S. 1958. The hypoplastic left heart syndrome. Pediatr. Clin. North Am. 5:1029–1056.

Peterson, C. R., Bramwit, D. N., Craig, D. E., and Jones, R. C. 1969. Aortic valvular atresia and premature closure of the foramen ovale. J. Thorac. Cardiovasc. Surg. 58:79–83.

Watson, D. G., and Rowe, R. D. 1962. Aortic-valve atresia: Report of 43 cases. JAMA 179:14–18.

chapter 29

MITRAL VALVE PROLAPSE

HISTORICAL NOTES

Although Osler, in 1880, and Cuffer and Barbillon, in 1887, described the typical clinical findings of mitral valve prolapse, late systolic murmurs were thought to be innocent, and midsystolic or late systolic clicks and systolic whoops were considered to be extracardiac in origin. Not until Barlow, in 1963, demonstrated angiographically the association of mitral regurgitation with the clinical syndrome of systolic click and late systolic murmur was this established as a separate clinical entity.

INCIDENCE

This is a common entity, occurring in about 10% of children referred for cardiac evaluation. It appears to increase in frequency with age, and is most common in early adolescence and young adulthood. It is apparently two to three times as common in females as in males. The prolapsing mitral valve is also seen with various forms of congenital heart disease, particularly secundum atrial septal defect.

PATHOLOGY

The described features are obviously based on those with more severe involvement. In most patients, this is a benign condition and the autopsy material obviously represents those with more severe involvement. In autopsied patients, the mitral valve is thickened and redundant, bulging into the left atrium. The posterior valve leaflet is more severely involved than the anterior.

CLINICAL FEATURES

The vast majority of patients are asymptomatic and are referred for evaluation because of findings detected during a routine physical examination. However,

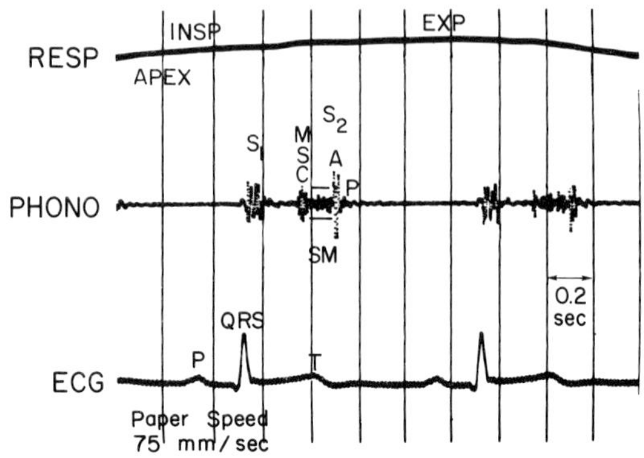

Figure 203. A midsystolic click (MSC) followed by a late systolic murmur (SM).

the click or murmur may be so loud that the parents request the examination after hearing various strange sounds emanating from the child's chest. These sounds may be heard at a distance from the patient, particularly in a quiet room. It is not uncommon for the child himself to be aware of these sounds.

There are striking variations in auscultatory findings with changes in posture. Typically, there is a quiet period following the first heart sound and then a mid- to late systolic click. This is often followed by a late systolic murmur (Figure 203). The murmur may become holosystolic with changes in position. In some patients, the murmur has a quality of a "whoop" (Figure 204). Such murmurs typically diminish or even disappear in the supine position, and may be loudest with the patient standing, squatting, or sitting leaning forward.

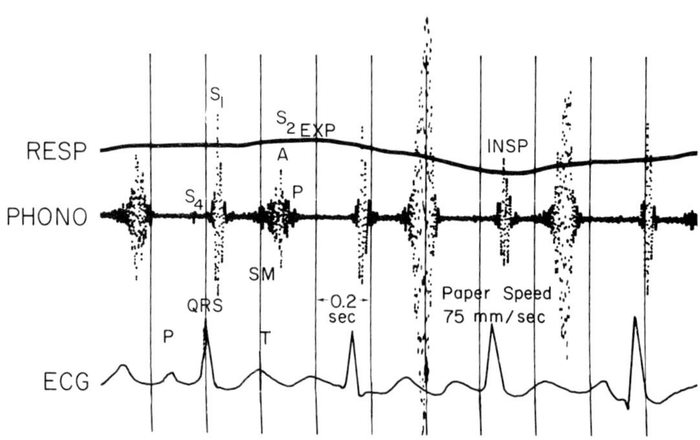

Figure 204. A very rare, but impressive, type of murmur is the "systolic whoop," recorded here in a 20-year-old female. These murmurs usually sound superficial and are of short duration, as in the case above, where the murmur occupies only late systole and encompasses the second sound (S_2). Variation in intensity with respiration is common.

The systolic clicks tend to move toward the first heard sound with sitting and standing, in some cases apparently merging with them.

ROENTGENOGRAPHIC FEATURES

Cardiac size and contour are normal, except in those patients with significant mitral regurgitation.

ELECTROCARDIOGRAPHY

Repolarization abnormalities, disorders of conduction, and arrhythmias have been reported to occur in many patients. The electrophysiologic basis for these observations remains obscure. Since mitral valve prolapse, particularly as an isolated echocardiographic finding, has been reported in 10%–40% of otherwise healthy patients, the association may be fortuitous.

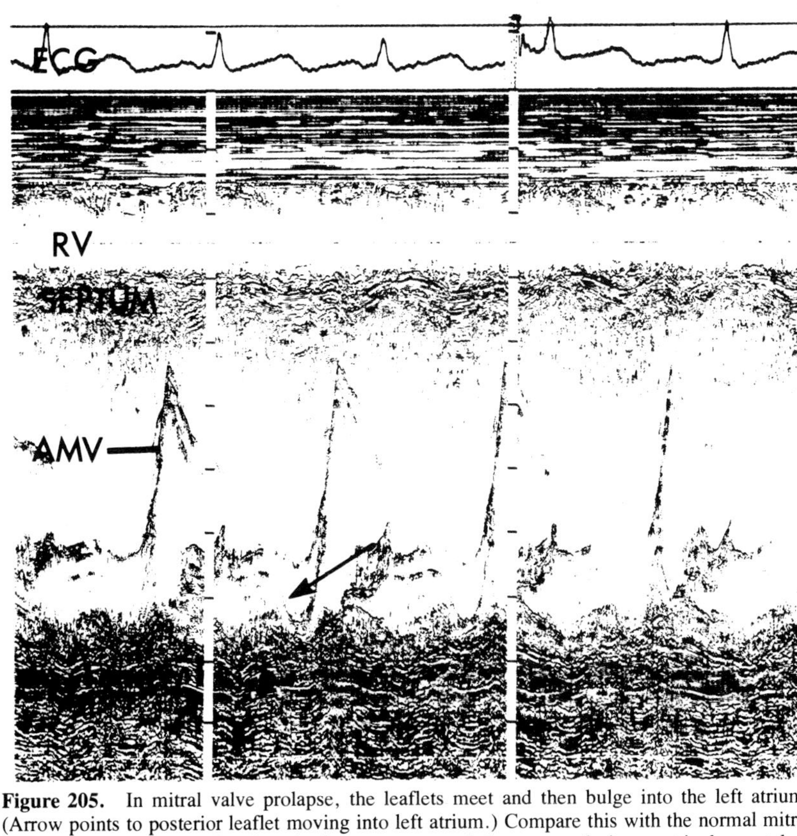

Figure 205. In mitral valve prolapse, the leaflets meet and then bulge into the left atrium. (Arrow points to posterior leaflet moving into left atrium.) Compare this with the normal mitral valve motion in Figure 97, where leaflets move toward the septum during ventricular systole.

ECHOCARDIOGRAPHY

Typically, the posterior mitral valve leaflet may be seen to prolapse in late systole (Figure 205). Less commonly, both leaflets prolapse into the left atrium. Prolapsing of the valve, like the murmurs, may be appreciated best in certain positions. Caution is needed in interpretation, since false positives and false negatives are not uncommon.

PROGNOSIS

Patients with isolated midsystolic clicks appear to have a mild form of prolapse and probably have a normal life expectancy. Patients with midsystolic click and a late systolic murmur should probably have antibiotic prophylaxis against infective endocarditis. Progressive mitral regurgitation has also been reported, and patients with midsystolic click and a late systolic murmur should be followed carefully.

Atypical chest pain, without a constant relationship to effort or emotion and usually of short duration, has been reported in varying degrees of frequency. Many patients who were considered to have neurocirculatory asthenia in earlier years may well have had this syndrome. Sudden death due to arrhythmias has also been reported, but is fortunately rare.

MANAGEMENT

Patients with chest pain need careful explanation of its significance. Our current recommendation is to use antibiotic prophylaxis for patients with midsystolic clicks and late systolic murmurs, although it must be recognized that this may very well change. It seems wisest for patients with ECG changes to refrain from strenuous athletic competition, since the nonspecific T wave changes have been reported to revert to normal after training has stopped.

BIBLIOGRAPHY

Allen, H., Harris, A., and Leatham, A. 1974. Significance and prognosis of an isolated late systolic murmur: A 9- to 22-year follow-up. Br. Heart J. 36:525–532.

Barlow, J. B., and Pocock, W. A. 1975. The problem of nonejection systolic clicks and associated mitral systolic murmurs: Emphasis on the billowing mitral leaflet syndrome. Am. Heart J. 90:636–655.

Fontana, M. E., Pence, H. L., Leighton, R. F., and Wooley, C. F. 1970. The varying clinical spectrum of the systolic click–late systolic murmur syndrome. Circulation 41:807–816.

Mills, P., Rose, J., Hollingsworth, J., Amara, I., and Craige, E. 1977. Long-term prognosis of mitral-valve prolapse. N. Engl. J. Med. 297:13–18.

Procacci, P. M., Savran, S. V., Schreiter, S. L., and Bryson, A. L. 1976. Prevalence of clinical mitral-valve prolapse in 1169 young women. N. Engl. J. Med. 294:1086–1118.

Sahn, D. J., Wood, J., Allen, H. D., Peoples, W., and Goldberg, S. J. 1977. Echocardiographic spectrum of mitral valve motion in children with and without mitral valve prolapse: The nature of false positive diagnosis. Am. J. Cardiol. 39:422–431.

Weiss, A. N., Mimbs, J. W., Ludbrook, P. A., and Sobel, B. E. 1975. Echocardiographic detection of mitral valve prolapse. Circulation 52:1091–1096.

chapter 30

DIFFERENTIAL DIAGNOSIS OF COMMON CARDIAC ANOMALIES: How to Diagnose Congenital Heart Disease in One Easy Lesson

This section summarizes the main features of some of the cardiac anomalies that comprise the vast majority of congenital cardiac malformations (Table 34). Any such condensation is fraught with hazards, the greatest being that the attempt to do so will be misused by the reader as a literal and always accurate guide. A prime requisite in utilizing the information in this section is to realize that it has many exceptions. In no way should it obviate careful utilization of all the standard methods of acquiring information about a child with heart disease. However, a novice must begin somewhere (and the experts will no doubt already have turned elsewhere for their information).

The surprise value of this section is in how often one can arrive at a logical and intelligent differential diagnosis using only the basic tools of history, physical examination, chest radiograph, and electrocardiogram (Figure 206). The reader must realize that this schema has numerous exceptions and exclusive use may lead to erroneous diagnosis.

Table 37. Most common cardiac malformations in infants under one year of age (percentages)

Malformation	Catheterized[a]	Symptomatic[b]	Clinical[c]
Transposition of great arteries	20	7	13
Ventricular septal defect	11	30	20
Patent ductus arteriosus	9	7	6
Coarctation of the aorta	9	13	10
Hypoplastic left heart	9	5	11
Hypoplastic right heart	7	4.5	3
Truncus arteriosus	7	5	11
Tetralogy of Fallot	5	8	4
AV canals	—	8	10
Totals	77	87.5	88

[a] Varghese, P. J., et al. 1969. Cardiac catheterization in the newborn. Pediatrics 44:24–29.
[b] Coleman, E. N. 1969. Progress report on infants with serious cardiac malformations. Br. Heart J. 31:441–446.
[c] Landtman, B. 1971. Clinical and morphological studies in congenital heart disease. Acta Paediatr. Scand. [Suppl.] 213.

VENTRICULAR SEPTAL DEFECT

Infancy	Childhood
Common cause in congestive heart failure in infancy	Most common defect; marked variation in size and associated symptoms
Murmur commonly not heard until 4–6 weeks; then harsh systolic murmur and thrill maximal along lower left sternal border	Harsh systolic murmur, and often thrill maximal along lower left sternal border
X-ray: biventricular hypertrophy, left atrial enlargement, large pulmonary artery, small aorta, and increased pulmonary vascular markings	X-ray: large pulmonary artery, small aorta, increased pulmonary vasculature and left atrial enlargement
ECG: biventricular hypertrophy, left atrial enlargement	ECG: normal or left atrial enlargement with biventricular or left ventricular hypertrophy

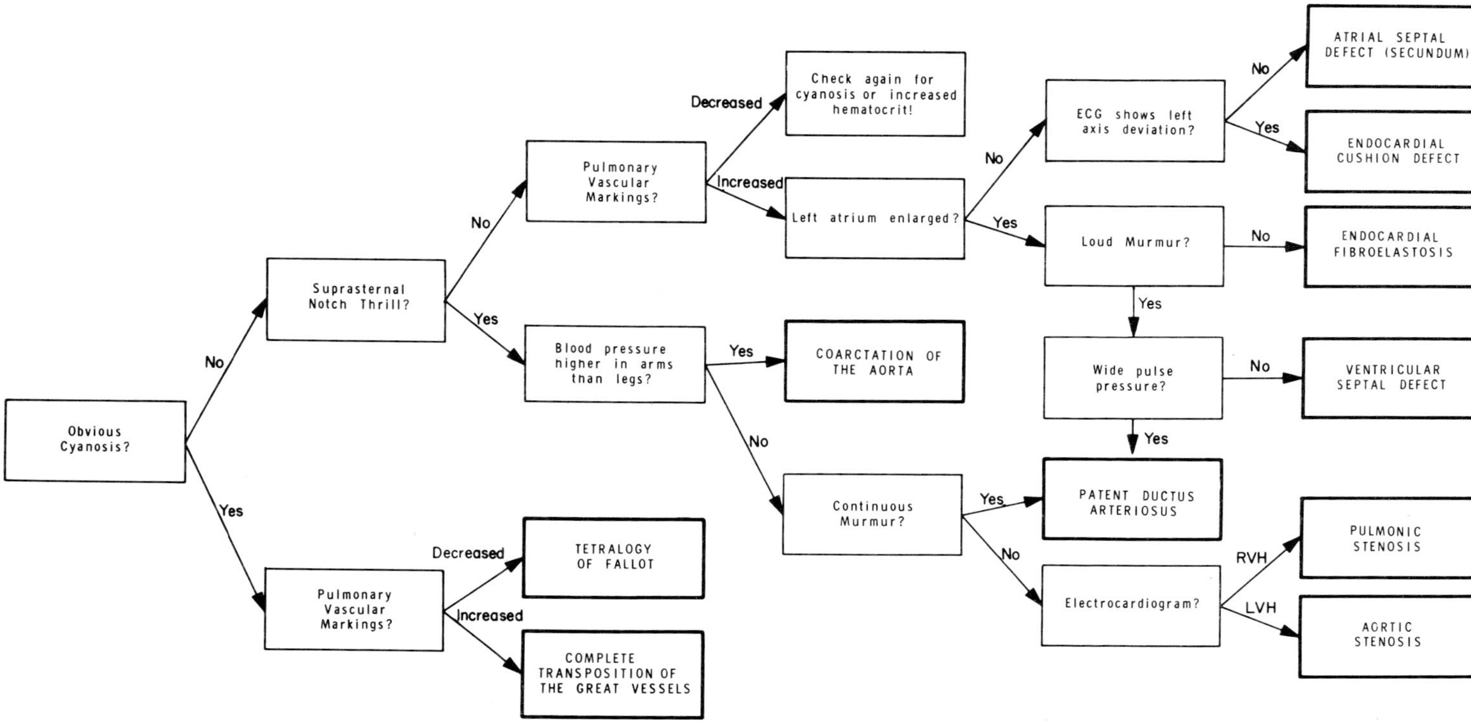

Figure 206. Schema of differential diagnoses after 1 year of age.

PATENT DUCTUS ARTERIOSUS

Infancy	Childhood
High index of suspicion with 1. history of rubella in pregnancy 2. prematurity 3. females	Usually asymptomatic, females predominating
Wide pulse pressure causing bounding pulses, even in the presence of congestive heart failure	
Continuous murmur or pansystolic murmur common, but may have nonspecific murmurs	Systolic thrill and continuous murmur encompassing S_2
X-ray: increased pulmonary vascular markings, cardiomegaly, left atrial enlargement	X-ray: often normal but may show large aorta, left ventricular hypertrophy, and left atrial enlargement
ECG: biventricular hypertrophy, left atrial enlargement	ECG: normal or left ventricular hypertrophy and left atrial enlargement

ATRIAL SEPTAL DEFECT

Infancy	Childhood
Frequent respiratory infections	Asymptomatic slender female
Acyanotic	No thrill, but right ventricular impulse: widely split and fixed S_2
Widely split and fixed S_2	
Right ventricular heave	Systolic murmur of increased pulmonary valve flow that may sound innocent; diastolic tricuspid flow murmur virtually pathognomic when heard
X-ray: increased pulmonary arterial markings, normal aorta and left atrium	X-ray: large pulmonary artery, increased pulmonary arterial markings, normal aorta and left atrium
ECG: right ventricular hypertrophy, right atrial enlargement	ECG: right ventricular hypertrophy with rSR′ and V_1

ENDOCARDIAL CUSHION DEFECT

Infancy	Childhood
Defect causing early symptoms, usually complete AV canal; one-third of cases occur in mongolism	Usually ostium primum ASD with cleft mitral valve
Severe congestive failure, repeated upper respiratory infections, and poor physical development	
Murmurs resemble a ventricular septal defect with mitral insufficiency	Murmurs resemble secundum atrial septal defect, except a mitral insufficiency murmur may be heard
X-ray: large heart, increased pulmonary vasculature, both arterial and venous	X-ray: similar to secundum ASD; may have larger heart and left atrial enlargement (if mitral insufficiency is present)
ECG: left axis deviation, biventricular hypertrophy, and prolonged P-R interval	ECG: left axis deviation, rsR′ pattern in V_1, and prolonged P-R interval

AORTIC STENOSIS

Infancy	Childhood
Critically ill infant in severe congestive heart failure	Robust male with few or no symptoms
Large heart, mainly left ventricle and left atrium	
Variable murmurs that may increase as the infant comes out of failure; poor pulses	Systolic murmur and thrill maximal over midsternum or second right intercostal space transmitted to suprasternal notch and neck
	Narrower splitting of S_2 than normal
X-ray: Cardiomegaly	X-ray: enlargement of aorta and left ventricular contour usually only clue
ECG: left ventricular hypertrophy and ST segment changes	ECG: variable degree of left ventricular hypertrophy

COARCTATION OF THE AORTA

Infancy	**Childhood**
High index of suspicion warranted in any infant with congestive heart failure	Asymptomatic, robust male
Blood pressure higher in arms than in legs, with diminished leg pulses. B.P. in arms may increase with R_x of congestive heart failure	Blood pressure higher in arms than legs, with diminished or absent leg pulses
Murmur is variable—may sound innocent or consist of a systolic murmur and thrill at base of heart heard equally well or better in back	Systolic thrill and murmur at base of heart that may be loudest in back
X-ray: cardiomegaly, increased pulmonary vascularity, left atrial enlargement	X-ray: normal size heart with large aorta indented at site of coarctation; rib notching in older children
ECG: right ventricular hypertrophy, or biventricular hypertrophy, left atrial enlargement	ECG: variable degree of left ventricular hypertrophy

PULMONIC VALVAR STENOSIS

Infancy (Trilogy)	**Childhood**
Chubby infant with round face, mild cyanosis, and congestive heart failure	Moon facies
Rough systolic ejection murmur in second left intercostal space that may be heard at birth	Systolic thrill and rough murmur, maximal at second left intercostal space, transmitted to suprasternal notch and left deltoid
	S_2 widely split but varies with respiration with decreased pulmonic component
X-ray: right heart enlargement	X-ray: large main and left pulmonary artery with normal peripheral pulmonary vascular markings
ECG: severe right ventricular hypertrophy and ST segment changes	ECG: right ventricular hypertrophy, pressure overloading type

TOTAL ANOMALOUS PULMONARY VENOUS CONNECTION

Mild cyanosis and congestive heart failure in first months of life (with severe pulmonary venous obstruction, intense cyanosis)
Murmurs similar to ASD; wide fixed splitting of S_2; "venous hum" in back over site of anomalous insertion of veins
X-ray: "snowman" contour; right heart enlargement, increased pulmonary vascularity, and no left atrial enlargement
ECG: right ventricular hypertrophy and right atrial enlargement

DIFFERENTIATING FEATURES OF THE TWO MOST COMMON CYANOTIC CONGENITAL CARDIAC ABNORMALITIES

Feature	Tetralogy of Fallot	Complete transposition of the great vessels
Congestive heart failure	Rare	Common
Associated extracardiac anomalies	Common	Rare
Right aortic arch	Common	Rare
Pulmonary vascular markings	Decreased	Increased
Birth weight	Lower than average	Average
Sex ratio	Equal	Predominantly males
X-ray	Boot-shaped heart	Narrow waist above an egg-shaped heart
Onset of cyanosis	May not be evident for several months	Obvious (within a few days after birth)
Murmur	Harsh	Usually faint or absent (unless VSD or PS present)
Paroxysmal anoxic episodes	Common	Rare
Familial tendency	Occasional	Rare

DIFFERENTIATING ANOMALIES ACCORDING TO DEGREE AND TIME OF ONSET OF CYANOSIS

Severely cyanotic from birth
- Tricuspid atresia
- Transposition of great arteries (inadequate mixing)
- Pulmonic atresia, especially with small right ventricular chamber

Moderately cyanotic at birth or during first week
- Transposition of great arteries (better mixing)
- Pulmonic atresia with VSD
- Respiratory distress syndrome

Increasingly obvious cyanosis
- Tetralogy of Fallot
- Total anomalous pulmonary venous return
- Truncus arteriosus

Cyanosis developing after infancy
- Eisenmenger's syndrome
- Congestive heart failure
- Methemoglobinemia

DIFFERENTIATING ANOMALIES ACCORDING TO ROENTGENOGRAPHIC PULMONARY VASCULAR MARKINGS

- Normal vascular markings
  - Obstructive lesions (aortic stenosis, pulmonic stenosis)
  - Myocarditis
  - Cardiomyopathy
- Increased pulmonary arterial vascular markings
  - Left-to-right shunts (see Table 12)
  - Obligatory admixture lesions
    - Single ventricle
    - Truncus arteriosus
    - Transposition of great arteries
- Decreased pulmonary arterial vascular markings
  - Right-to-left shunts with pulmonary outflow obstruction
- Increased pulmonary venous markings
  - Pulmonary venous obstruction
    - Mitral stenosis
    - Total anomalous pulmonary venous return, with obstruction
  - Left heart dysfunction
    - Mitral insufficiency (severe)
    - Aortic stenosis (severe)
    - Cardiomyopathy (severe)
    - Myocarditis (severe)

DIFFERENTIATING ANOMALIES ACCORDING TO TIME OF ONSET OF CONGESTIVE FAILURE

- In the first week of life
  - Hypoplastic left heart syndrome
  - Coarctation of the aorta
  - Rhythm disturbances
- Later in the newborn period
  - Ventricular septal defect
  - Patent ductus arteriosus
  - Truncus arteriosus
  - Transposition of the great arteries

PART III
Acquired Heart Disease

In this section, we discuss the cardiac diseases that most commonly develop following birth. In some instances these may occur in the neonatal period (e.g., purulent pericarditis), but most are much more common after 2 years of age.

Although there may be a genetic predisposition for these anomalies, or for complications of cyanotic congenital heart disease, we consider that the disease process itself is acquired. One interesting aspect of this area of pediatric cardiology is that more stress may be placed on prevention.

chapter 31

RHEUMATIC FEVER

HISTORICAL NOTES

Although he did not publish his findings, David Pitcairn first recognized the relationship between organic heart disease and rheumatic fever in 1788. Baillie also reported on this relationship in 1797, but the first clear concepts of rheumatic fever and rheumatic endocarditis are attributed to Wells (1810) and Bouilland (1832).

Trousseau, in 1865, noted that rheumatic fever often followed scarlet fever. Haig-Brown, in 1886, identified the latent period between a sore throat and the onset of rheumatic fever. However, not until Todd devised the antistreptolysin O test in 1932 and Lancefield identified the group A hemolytic streptococcus as the chief cause of streptococcal disease in man in 1944 did evidence begin to accumulate indicating that rheumatic fever was causally related to a prior streptococcal infection.

INCIDENCE

Acute rheumatic fever affects approximately one of every 2000 children of ages 5 to 15 years. Rheumatic fever is uncommon in children less than 5 and rare before 2 years of age. Although recent evidence suggests that both the incidence and severity of rheumatic fever are declining, it is still the most common cause of acquired heart disease in children. Part of the reason for the declining incidence of rheumatic fever probably is greater diagnostic precision.

ETIOLOGY

An infection with a group A β-hemolytic streptococcus, which may be asymptomatic, always occurs prior to the onset of acute rheumatic fever.

Patients with rheumatic fever frequently have some of the following predisposing factors:

1. Positive family history
2. Poor socioeconomic environment
3. A previous attack of rheumatic fever

It has been postulated that rheumatic fever is a hypersensitivity disease. The basis for this theory may be summarized as follows. Rabbit antiserum prepared against the cell wall of a group A streptococcus cross-reacts with human heart tissue. The antigenic components are located in the cardiac myofibers in both normal and rheumatic hearts. Binding of gamma-globulin can be demonstrated in the myofibers, the vessel walls, and the interstitial cardiac muscle tissue of many rheumatic fever patients, consistent with the hypothesis that gamma-globulin binding is specifically associated with myofibril injury.

PATHOLOGY

A recent necropsy study of patients dying of acute rheumatic fever suggested that the Aschoff body is a diseased lymphatic channel, and that damage to the myocardium and impairment of its function are secondary to obstructive lymphangitis. Aschoff bodies are frequently found in biopsies of left atrial appendages taken at the time of surgery from patients with rheumatic heart disease who have no other evidence of clinical activity. In studies involving over 3000 such patients, Aschoff bodies were found in about 40%. Since the Aschoff body becomes apparent about 5 weeks after onset of the disease and its life cycle is generally completed in 6 to 8 months, this has been interpreted as evidence that low-grade rheumatic activity can persist for many years.

Rheumatic endocarditis is manifested by verrucae on valve cusps, thickening of valves, and thickening and shortening of chordae tendineae. In children, mitral insufficiency is the most common valvar disturbance, followed by aortic insufficiency. Mitral stenosis is uncommon, since it usually takes years to develop. Isolated aortic stenosis in childhood is almost always congenital in origin. Angiocardiographic studies have established that the Graham-Steel murmur of "relative pulmonic insufficiency" may be due to organic aortic insufficiency. In children, the pulmonic and tricuspid valves are rarely affected.

CLINICAL FEATURES

The latent period between a streptococcal infection and the onset of rheumatic fever is 1 to 3 weeks, except for chorea, which may not appear for 6 months. Arthritis is by far the most common presenting complaint (approximately

75%), and this is usually a migratory polyarthritis. Carditis is the sole major clinical feature in about 15% and chorea in about 5% of diagnosed rheumatic fever.

Among patients with carditis alone, fever is the most common presenting complaint. Dyspnea, cough, or chest or abdominal pain also occurs, especially with severe carditis.

Carditis occurs in 40% to 50% of all patients with acute rheumatic fever. Its diagnosis should be based on one or more of the following features:

1. An *organic heart murmur*. Mitral insufficiency usually produces a systolic murmur of at least grade 2, loudest at the apex and transmitted to the axilla and back. Its intensity is not markedly affected by inspiration or changes in position. The murmur often has a blowing, high-pitched character that mimics the cry of a seagull. The murmur generally begins immediately after the first heart sound and extends through most of systole (Figure 207). In addition, there may be a low-pitched apical mid-diastolic murmur, resulting from increased diastolic flow across the mitral valve secondary to the regurgitation. This latter murmur begins after the third heart sound and is of short duration.

   The diastolic murmur of aortic insufficiency begins immediately after the aortic component of the second sound. It is usually high-pitched and best heard at end expiration in the third intercostal space at the left sternal border, with the patient leaning forward.

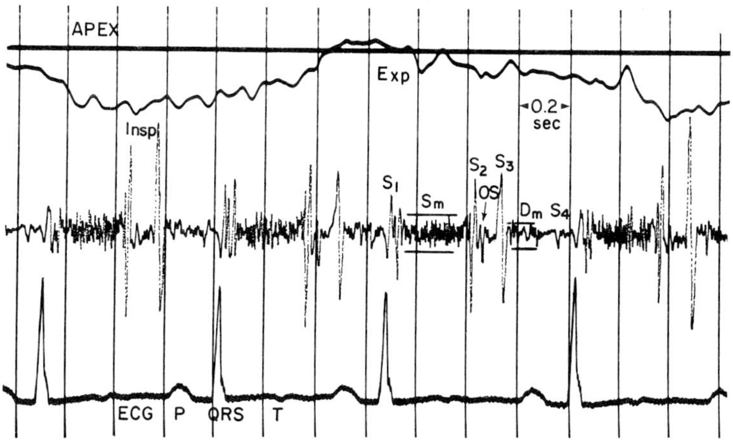

Figure 207. Phonocardiogram of a patient with rheumatic mitral insufficiency. There is a pansystolic murmur as well as a diastolic murmur. Note also the presence of an opening snap that occurs in the presence of severe mitral insufficiency.

Key: Insp = inspiration; Exp = expiration; S_1, S_2, S_3, and S_4 = 1st, 2nd, 3rd, and 4th heart sounds; S_m = systolic murmur; D_m = diastolic murmur; OS = opening snap; AP = aortic and pulmonic components of S_2.

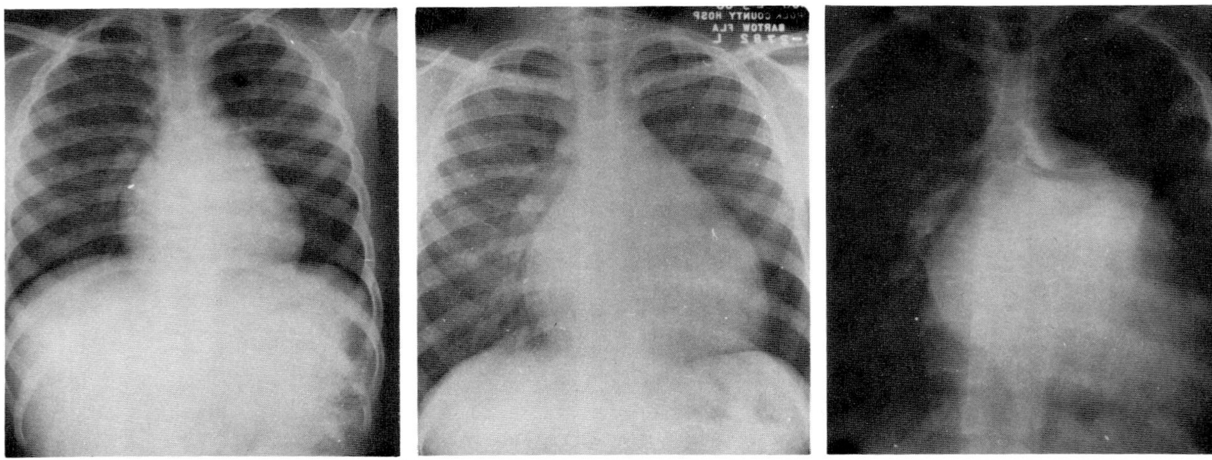

Figure 208. The progress of rheumatic mitral insufficiency in a young Negro male, as documented by serial chest roentgenograms. (Left) Shows the patient at the age of 9, 2 years after his initial attack of acute rheumatic fever. There is slight left atrial, as well as cardiac, enlargement present at this time. (Middle) Shows the patient at the age of 11. During this 2-year period, marked cardiomegaly has appeared. (Right) Shows patient at age 15. This film was deliberately overexposed to show the shadow of the gigantic left atrium within the overall cardiac silhouette. Note also that the left main stem bronchus is markedly elevated, another sign of left atrial enlargement.

2. *Pericarditis* should be documented by detection of a pericardial friction rub or an unequivocal effusion, demonstrated by echocardiography or pericardiocentesis.
3. *Increasing cardiac enlargement,* determined by x-ray examination, is diagnostic of active carditis (Figure 208). Some investigators also accept an obviously enlarged heart that remains enlarged as indicative of carditis. Cardiomegaly occurs in one-third of patients with a mitral murmur, but not in those with only aortic murmurs.
4. *Congestive heart failure* occurs in 5% to 10% of first attacks of rheumatic carditis. It is more common in children under 6 years of age and in recurring attacks of rheumatic carditis. Patients with congestive heart failure almost always have significant murmurs and cardiomegaly.

In one study of 275 initial attacks of rheumatic fever, carditis was present in 115 (Feinstein and Spagnuolo, 1962). A murmur of mitral origin was found in 80 patients, an aortic murmur in 16, and both in 16. Almost all of the acute features of carditis were present at the time of admission, and rarely worsened after admission. The severity of the carditis tended to be inversely related to the severity of the arthritis. Carditis was slightly more frequent in females.

NONCARDIAC MANIFESTATIONS OF RHEUMATIC FEVER

Arthritis is present in three-quarters of all patients. The joints are painful, red, warm, and swollen and remain affected for 1 to 5 days. The knee, elbow, wrist, and ankle are the joints most commonly involved, and arthritis tends to progress to other joints as the first joints improve. Total duration of all joint involvement is less than 4 weeks, even if untreated. Arthritis is slightly more frequent in males.

Chorea may appear several weeks to months after an acute streptococcal infection, long after acute phase laboratory findings have returned to normal. Some authors consider all cases of Sydenham's chorea as rheumatic in origin. It is two to three times more common in females, and usually occurs between 7 and 14 years of age. Chorea is characterized by random, purposeless movements not limited to a single muscle group, a history of recent change in disposition or mood, inability to sustain muscular contraction, and sustained knee jerk.

Subcutaneous nodules occur only in patients with active carditis and usually appear several weeks after onset of illness. The frequency of this finding increases with the severity of carditis.

Erythema marginatum rarely occurs as a single major manifestation. When it does, it is usually during a recurrent, rather than an initial, attack. It also is commonly associated with carditis.

Fever that ranges between 38°C and 40°C, with no specific temporal pattern, occurs in 90% of patients.

Arthralgia is characterized by pain in one or more joints without evidence of redness, swelling, tenderness to touch, or limitation of motion. The larger joints are more frequently involved and arthralgia may often be migratory. In patients with monoarticular arthritis, the presence of arthralgia in other joints strengthens the diagnosis of rheumatic fever. Arthralgia must not be confused with arthritis. In addition, pain originating above, under, or near a joint must be differentiated from true arthritis or arthralgia.

DIAGNOSIS

The modified Jones criteria for guidance in the diagnosis of rheumatic fever (from the American Heart Association Council on Rheumatic Fever and Congenital Heart Disease) are listed below.

Major criteria and their incidence in 275 initial attacks (Feinstein and Spagnuolo, 1962):
- Arthritis, 76%
- Carditis, 42%
- Chorea, 8%
- Erythema marginatum, 4%
- Subcutaneous nodules, 1%

Minor criteria
- Clinical
  - Fever
  - Arthralgia
  - Previous rheumatic fever or rheumatic heart disease
- Laboratory
  - Prolonged P-R interval
  - Elevated erythrocyte sedimentation rate, elevated white blood cell count, or presence of C-reactive protein

Supporting evidence of preceding streptococcal infection; increased ASO or other streptococcal antibodies; positive throat culture for group A streptococcus; recent scarlet fever.

Diagnosis: The presence of two major, or one major and two minor, criteria indicates a high probability of the presence of rheumatic fever if supported by evidence of a preceding streptococcal infection. The absence of the latter should make the diagnosis suspect, except after a long latent period from the antecedent infection (e.g., Sydenham's chorea).

Common Errors in Diagnosis

These criteria are often misinterpreted, usually in the direction of overdiagnosis. Innocent murmurs or murmurs due to a congenital anomaly may be confusing, especially when first heard during a febrile illness. Cardiac size on x-ray may be misread because of a poor inspiratory film or if the tube-patient distance used was less than 6 feet. Diagnosing pericarditis by electrocardiographic criteria alone or using a prolonged P-R interval as evidence of carditis also results in overdiagnosis. A prominent physiological third heart sound must be differentiated from the mid-diastolic murmur associated with mitral insufficiency.

Rheumatoid arthritis can usually be distinguished by its longer course of joint involvement. In rheumatic fever, it is rare for signs and symptoms to persist in any one joint for more than 1 week, whereas this is common in juvenile rheumatoid arthritis (JRA). Fever is often the first manifestation of rheumatoid arthritis. Twice-daily temperature spikes as high as 41°C are characteristic of JRA. The rash of JRA may be found occasionally on the face, soles, or palms, whereas these sites are rarely affected in rheumatic fever. The rash of rheumatic fever rarely lasts more than a week or two, in contrast with that of JRA, which usually recurs for a year or more. The arthritis of JRA typically lasts longer than 12 weeks, in contrast to a duration of only a few weeks in rheumatic fever.

A *habit spasm,* neurogenic tic, or the fidgety, hyperactive child who cannot sit still should not be mistaken for evidence of chorea. Hyperthyroid tremors or Friedreich's ataxia may be confused with chorea. Since mitral insufficiency murmurs and a prolonged P-R interval may be found in patients with *thyrotoxicosis,* such individuals may be misdiagnosed as rheumatic fever.

A history of unequivocal rheumatic fever or evidence of preexisting rheumatic heart disease increases the likelihood that a subsequent rheumatic-like complaint is in fact due to rheumatic fever.

ELECTROCARDIOGRAPHY

Electrocardiographic evidence of developing chamber enlargement is suggestive of active carditis. Increasing degrees of atrioventricular block also suggest active carditis.

A prolonged P-R interval occurs in 35% to 40% of patients with acute rheumatic fever. This is entirely independent of the severity of carditis and cannot be used to diagnose it. Its presence bears no relation to the ultimate prognosis.

LABORATORY FINDINGS

A group A β-hemolytic streptococcal infection precedes every adequately documented attack of acute rheumatic fever. Proof of preceding streptococcal infection is usually based upon demonstration of antibodies to products of the streptococcus. Antistreptolysin O (ASO; an antibody to a potent antigenic enzyme) levels are elevated usually within 1 week, eliciting an antibody response in approximately 85% of patients following an infection with group A streptococci. An increasing ASO titer is evidence that a previous infection has occurred, even in the absence of positive throat culture.

In addition to streptolysin O, several other streptococcal antigens have been described, of which desoxyribonuclease B (DNase B) and nicotinamide adenine dinucleotidase (NADase, formerly designated DPNase) have been found to be useful in diagnosis of streptococcal infection. High antibody titers to these antigens can be demonstrated in acute rheumatic fever with the same order of frequency as elevated ASO titers. Using more than one antibody measurement (i.e., ASO, anti–DNase B, anti-NADase) gives positive evidence of antecedent streptococcal infection in over 95% of cases of acute rheumatic fever.

Recently it has been determined that a group-specific polysaccharide in the streptococcal cell wall produces an antibody response following infection. Group A carbohydrate (A-CHO) antibody rises more slowly following streptococcal infection than does ASO or anti–DNase B, and thus it is of less help in diagnosing acute rheumatic fever. However, anti–A-CHO antibody levels remain elevated longer and, more importantly, the antibody appears to remain elevated indefinitely in patients with persistent rheumatic mitral valve disease. According to some authors, the antibody therefore can be used as a diagnostic test in children with mitral insufficiency. Not widely available as yet, the value of this antibody test remains to be confirmed by further use.

MANAGEMENT

An adequate course of an antibiotic as defined in Table 35 is the only drug therapy of established value in acute rheumatic fever. The 10-year combined United Kingdom–United States study compared ACTH, cortisone, and aspi-

Table 35. Treatment of beta-hemolytic streptococcal infections

Drug	Route	Dosage	Frequency of administration
Benzathine Penicillin G	I.M.	600,000 to 1,200,000 units	Once
Penicillin	Oral	250,000 units	3 times daily × 10 days[a]
Erthromycin[b]	Oral	125 to 250 mg	4 times daily × 10 days[a]

[a] Success of oral therapy is dependent on patient cooperation. Therapy must be continued for the entire 10 days regardless of disappearance of symptoms.

[b] Recommended treatment in patients with penicillin sensitivity.

rin. Follow-up for 10 years showed no statistical difference between any of the three therapeutic groups, regardless of initial cardiac status. Another combined rheumatic fever study reported in 1960 compared cortisone in high doses with aspirin and also found no difference in outcome in terms of residual cardiac murmurs.

Dorfman, Gross, and Lorincz compared four treatment groups: 1) no treatment other than penicillin; 2) aspirin; 3) hydrocortisone in high doses for long duration; and 4) aspirin plus hydrocortisone. Their results indicated a lower incidence of significant murmurs 1 year later in the hydrocortisone-treated groups. This study has been criticized on the basis that 30% of their patients with carditis had minimal carditis, a group that rarely develops residual rheumatic heart disease regardless of therapy.

Steroids, as well as aspirin, are beneficial in alleviation of the acute inflammatory manifestations of rheumatic fever. Although steroids act more rapidly, recurrence of symptoms is more likely to occur after the drug has been discontinued. Steroids may be advisable in treatment of severe carditis because of their ability to reduce the inflammatory process in the myocardium. They are also helpful in rapidly alleviating the discomfort associated with pericarditis. Otherwise, they have no advantage over aspirin.

There is no conclusive evidence that steroids or aspirin, in high or low dosage and for long or short periods of time, have any effect on prognosis, even when treatment is begun early in the course of the disease. Residual cardiac damage can be related only to the presence of active carditis during the acute phase of the disease.

PREVENTION

Eradication of the streptococcus by adequate antibiotic treatment, prior to 9 days after the onset of the initial streptococcal infection, is effective in preventing acute rheumatic fever. Adequate penicillin therapy, as defined by the American Heart Association Committee on Prevention of Rheumatic Fever, is the treatment of choice (Table 36). If penicillin sensitivity exists, erythromycin should be given for 10 days. Sulfadiazine is not effective in preventing rheumatic fever.

Table 36. Rheumatic fever prophylaxis

Drugs	Route	Dosage	Interval
Benzathine Penicillin G	I.M.	1,200,000 units	28 days
Penicillin[a]	Oral	250,000 units	Twice daily
Sulfadiazine	Oral	500 mg	Twice daily

[a] Pencillin G, if taken before meals (i.e., fasting), is as effective as more expensive preparations.

All patients diagnosed as having acute rheumatic fever, regardless of the presence of carditis, should receive antistreptococcal prophylaxis indefinitely. This may be given as monthly injections of benzathine penicillin or as daily oral penicillin or sulfadiazine (Table 36). The oral route should be used only when full patient-parent understanding and cooperation are assured.

PATTERN OF RECURRENCES

The criteria necessary to establish a recurrence are the same as those for an initial attack (see "Diagnosis," above). Rheumatic fever is more common in individuals who have previously had an attack, with the rate being directly related to the number of previous attacks. Recurrences are also more frequent in patients who had their first attack early in life. About 75% of recurrences occur within 3 years after the initial attack.

The clinical manifestations of rheumatic fever recurrences mimic closely those of the first attack. In one study of 27 patients without carditis during their initial attack, only two developed carditis with the recurrent attack. In another study of 39 patients without carditis during their first attack, none developed carditis with the recurrent attack. All patients who had carditis during their first attack had carditis during the recurrence. In another study, however, it was found that 13 of 50 patients in whom evidence of carditis was present in the recurrence had no diagnosed carditis with their initial attack.

PROGNOSIS

Prognosis depends entirely on cardiac status (Tables 37 and 38). Neither arthritis nor chorea has significant permanent sequelae. Rheumatic carditis

Table 37. Initial cardiac status and residual rheumatic heart disease after acute rheumatic fever[a]

Initial cardiac status	Number of patients	Deaths	Percent with residual RHD
No carditis	181	0	0
Possibly significant murmur	44	0	9
Significant murmur(s), without failure or cardiac enlargement	141	1	55
Cardiac enlargement and/or congestive failure	75	11	87

[a] Adapted from Feinstein, A. R., Stern, E. K., and Spagnuolo, M. 1964. The prognosis of acute rheumatic fever. Am. Heart J. 68:817–834.

Table 38. Prognosis in relation to cardiac status at start of treatment[a]

Cardiac status at start of treatment	Incidence of heart disease after 10 years	Number of deaths from rheumatic fever in 10 years
No or questionable carditis	6%	0
Apical systolic murmur, grade 1	30%	0
Apical systolic murmur, grade 2 or 3	26%	2
Apical systolic and apical mid-diastolic murmurs	37%	2
Basal diastolic murmur with or without other murmurs	40%	1
Failure and/or pericarditis	68%	1
Preexisting heart disease	67%	13

[a] Adapted from U.S. and U.K. Joint Report on Rheumatic Disease. 1965. Circulation 32: 457–476. By permission of the American Heart Association, Inc.

does not develop in patients previously known to be free of it. However, a 20-year follow-up of patients with chorea to whom no prophylaxis was given showed that 25% developed rheumatic heart disease. If no carditis is present during the initial attack, the incidence of significant murmurs after 10 years is approximately 6% (combined U.K.-U.S. study).

The combined U.K.-U.S. study also reported that mitral stenosis was rare at the 5-year follow-up, but definitely present in 18 of 347 cases examined at 10 years, and in seven of the 19 deaths. It was most likely to occur in females with initial severe carditis.

The patient with acute rheumatic fever who has carditis alone, with no fever or heart failure, may not seek medical attention because he does not feel ill. Subsidence of the acute attack leaves this patient with cardiac damage that may only be discovered much later, often after another attack that produces further cardiac damage.

RHEUMATIC HEART DISEASE

In the child, mitral insufficiency remains the major manifestation of chronic rheumatic heart disease. Mitral stenosis generally takes at least 10 years to develop and thus is uncommon in the pediatric age range. Aortic insufficiency is usually present only in association with mitral insufficiency. When isolated aortic insufficiency occurs, it is usually mild. Aortic stenosis is not found in childhood as a result of rheumatic fever.

Physical findings in chronic rheumatic valve involvement include murmurs similar to those described earlier with regard to acute rheumatic fever. These murmurs tend to be stable on repeated examination.

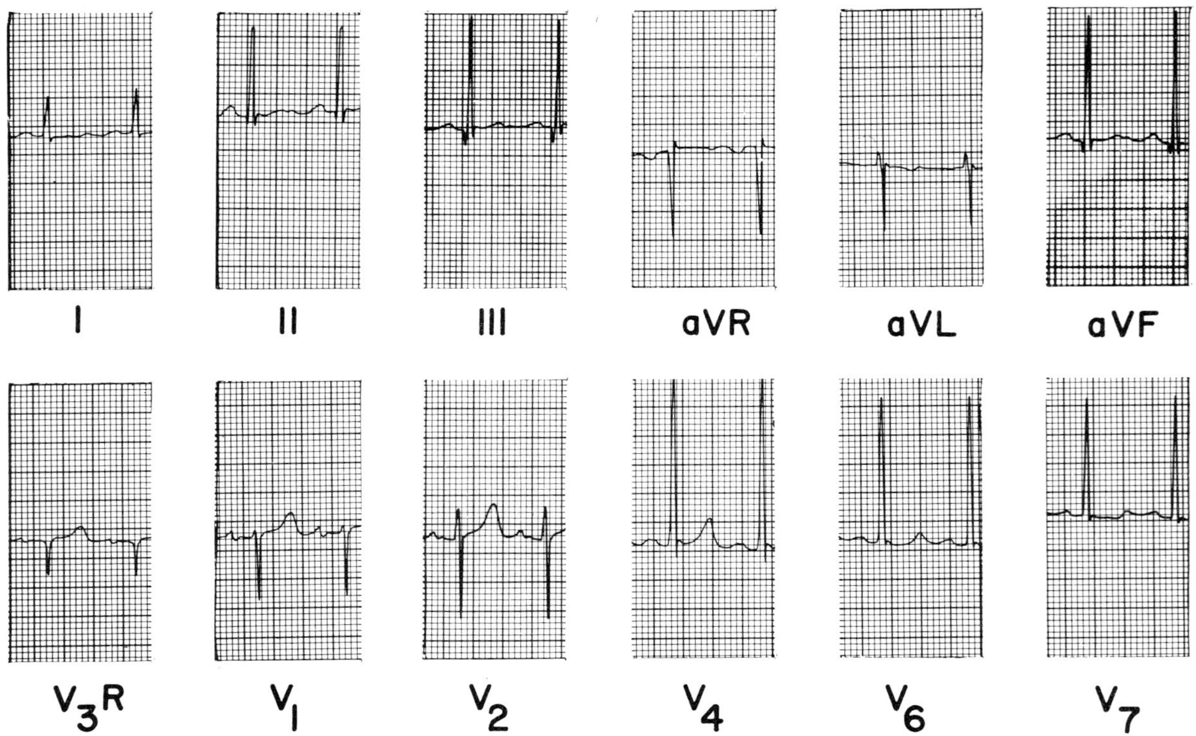

Figure 209. ECG of a 16-year-old with chronic rheumatic heart disease.

The ECG generally demonstrates left atrial enlargement and left ventricular hypertrophy, characterized by the absence of q waves in the left precordial leads together with flat T waves (Figure 209). Chest radiographs frequently reveal the shadow of the left atrial appendage, a finding not present in other forms of mitral insufficiency or left atrial volume overload lesions. Thus, in the evaluation of a patient with mitral insufficiency of undetermined etiology, radiographic evidence of left atrial appendage enlargement suggests a rheumatic etiology.

Criteria for surgical treatment in a patient with chronic rheumatic heart disease are not easily defined. Recurrent episodes of congestive heart failure with poor medical control, progressive cardiomegaly, and poor left ventricular function are suggested indications for surgery. Some investigators believe that earlier surgery may prevent myocardial deterioration. However, valve replacement in a child or even an adolescent is not an encouraging prospect.

BIBLIOGRAPHY

Diamond, E. F. 1957. Hereditary and environmental factors in the pathogenesis of rheumatic fever. Pediatrics 19:908–915.

Dorfman, A., Gross, J. I., and Lorincz, A. E. 1961. The treatment of acute rheumatic fever. Pediatrics 27:692–706.

Dudding, B. A., and Ayoub, E. J. 1968. Persistence of streptococcal group A antibody in patients with rheumatic valvular disease. J. Exp. Med. 128:1081–1098.

Feinstein, A. R., and Spagnuolo, M. 1962. The clinical patterns of acute rheumatic fever. A reappraisal. Medicine 41:279–305.

Feinstein, A. R., Stern, E. K., and Spagnuolo, M. 1964. The prognosis of acute rheumatic fever. Am. Heart J. 68:817–834.

Grossman, B. J., and Stamler, J. 1963. Potential preventability of first attacks of acute rheumatic fever in children. JAMA 183:985–988.

Kelley, M. J., Elliott, L. P., Shulman, S. T., Ayoub, E. M., Victorica, B. E., and Gessner, I. H. 1976. The significance of the left atrial appendage in rheumatic heart disease. Circulation 54:146–153.

Kuttner, A. G., and Mayer, F. E. 1963. Carditis during second attacks of rheumatic fever. Its incidence in patients without clinical evidence of cardiac involvement in their initial rheumatic episode. N. Engl. J. Med. 268:1259–1261.

Markowitz, M., and Kuttner, A. G. 1965. Rheumatic Fever: Diagnosis, Management and Prevention. W.B. Saunders Co., Philadelphia.

Shulman, S. P., Ayoub, E. M., Victorica, B. V., Gessner, I. H., Tamer, D. F., and Hernandez, F. A. 1974. Differences in antibody response to streptococcal antigens in children with rheumatic and non-rheumatic mitral valve disease. Circulation 50:1244–1251.

U.K. and U.S. Joint Report on Rheumatic Heart Disease. 1965. The natural history of rheumatic fever and rheumatic heart disease. Ten-year report of a cooperative clinical trial of ACTH, cortisone and aspirin. Circulation 32:457–476.

chapter 32

ENDOCARDIAL FIBROELASTOSIS

HISTORICAL NOTES

Although there were earlier reports of "fetal endocarditis," the first clear description of endocardial fibroelastosis was by Gross in 1941. He emphasized that the endocardial thickening was devoid of inflammatory residua. Gross thought it was best described as simple hyperplasia of endocardial fibroelastic tissue and postulated that it was a developmental defect.

Weinberg and Himelfarb, in 1943, used the term *fibroelastosis* to describe the grayish-white diffusely thickened endocardium. They noted that there was no history of maternal infection during either pregnancy in the two siblings reported. They adduced this as evidence for a developmental origin.

This entity remained the sole possession of the pathologist until Vlad, Rowe, and Keith, in 1955, documented the characteristic clinical and electrocardiographic findings of 23 necropsy-verified cases of primary endocardial fibroelastosis, thus pointing the way to antemortem diagnosis.

INCIDENCE

For undetermined reasons, endocardial fibroelastosis (EFE) has recently declined in incidence. It occurs most frequently between the ages of 2 months and 1 year. Although females predominate in some series, others report approximately equal sex distribution.

We have reported a high incidence of nonobstructive cardiomyopathy in Negroes, with most patients recovering (Figure 210). Clinically these infants are initially indistinguishable from patients with classical primary endocardial fibroelastosis. However, the different clinical course and the absence of pathologic proof of the diagnosis leave unanswered the question of whether or not these patients do in fact have primary endocardial fibroelastosis.

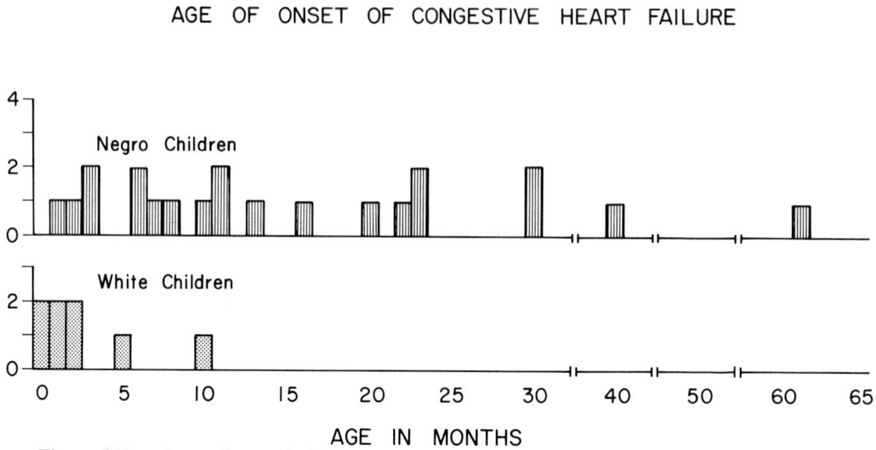

Figure 210. Age and race of children with endocardial fibroelastosis seen at the J. Hillis Miller Health Center from 1959 to 1965. (Adapted from McLoughlin, T. G., Schiebler, G. L., and Krovetz, L. J. 1966. Endocardial fibroelastosis in American Negro children: A distinct entity? Am. Heart J. 71:748.)

ETIOLOGY

Intrauterine tubercular infection was proposed by Kreysig in 1916 as a possible cause, but Gross refuted this. Recently, the concept that EFE is the aftermath of infection has been proposed by a number of authors. Although a history of mumps during pregnancy is unusual, many cases of EFE have a positive response to mumps skin-test antigen. Fruhling and co-workers noted an increased frequency of deaths due to EFE following viral (Coxsackie?) epidemics. Histologic evidence of a spectrum of progression from postinfectious myocarditis to EFE has been shown by Hutchins and Vie and confirmed by Schryer and Karnauchow; this is consistent with a common origin.

Anoxia has also been thought to cause EFE, and various revascularization operations have been advocated and tried. There is little or no evidence to support this hypothesis. Indeed, a better case can be made for hyperoxia, since EFE is found almost exclusively where endocardium is in contact with oxygenated blood.

Hereditary factors have been considered because the disease has occurred in consecutive siblings. An overwhelming percentage of the reported instances, however, occur sporadically.

EFE most probably is a *nonspecific response* to ventricular myocardial damage and subsequent dilatation. Endocardial fibroelastosis may be the end result of a number of disease processes. As in cirrhosis of the liver, the end stage may be similar for vastly different initial insults.

PATHOLOGY

In various series, 28 to 63% of EFE is found associated with congenital heart disease, most commonly coarctation of the aorta, aortic atresia, or aortic stenosis. EFE occurs only with systemic ventricular pressures in the presence of oxygenated blood. For example, it occurs in the diminutive left ventricle found in aortic atresia with open mitral valves, but not with concomitant mitral atresia.

EFE is classified as *primary* or *isolated* when no other cardiac anomaly is present. However, the mitral valve is so nearly universally involved, with resultant insufficiency or stenosis, that Moller and colleagues consider this a part of the overall picture. The aortic valve is sometimes affected, but tricuspid and pulmonic valves are only occasionally involved.

Mitral insufficiency per se may produce endocardial thickening in the left atrium. Since there is a lack of left ventricular involvement, this is not included in our definition of primary endocardial fibroelastosis.

Three forms of endocardial fibroelastosis may be seen:

1. *Dilated left ventricle* with congestive heart failure and left ventricular enlargement. This is by far the most common type (Figures 211 and 212).
2. *Hypoplastic left ventricular* cavity with pulmonary hypertension and right ventricular hypertrophy secondary to severely impaired left ven-

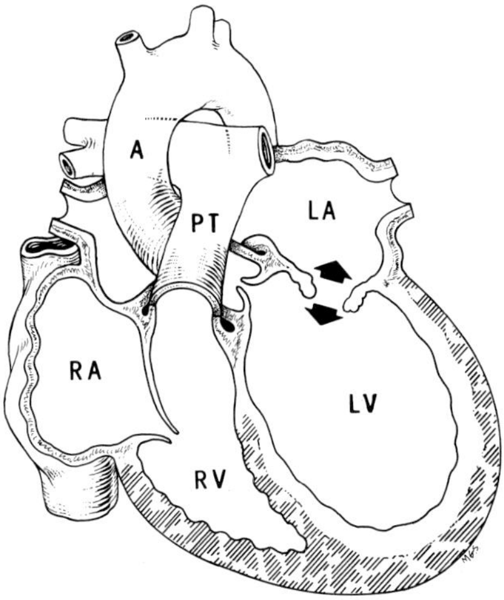

Figure 211. Schematic drawing of the intracardiac hemodynamics in endocardial fibroelastosis. The increased thickness of the left ventricular endocardium limits the contractility of the left ventricle, both in filling and emptying. The mitral valve is frequently involved in the process, resulting in mitral regurgitation. (From Elliott, L. P., and Schiebler, G. L. 1968. X-Ray Diagnosis of Congenital Cardiac Disease. Courtesy of Charles C Thomas, Publisher, Springfield, Ill.)

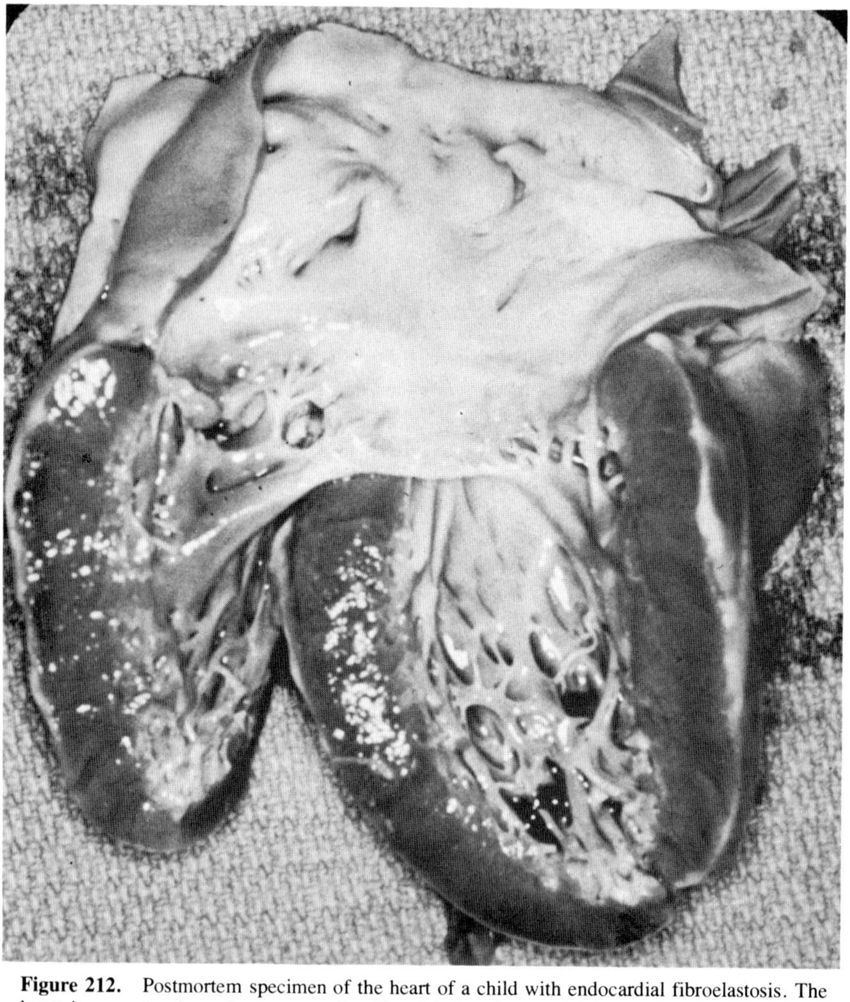

Figure 212. Postmortem specimen of the heart of a child with endocardial fibroelastosis. The heart is open to show the enormously dilated left atrium and left ventricle. The thickened endocardium appears pearly white in both of these chambers. Note the thickening of the mitral valve and the thick, short chordae tendineae.

tricular function. This "contracted" type comprises less than 5% of cases of isolated EFE.

3. *Isolated right ventricular involvement* occurs, but is also uncommon.

CLINICAL FEATURES

Since the secondary form is dominated by signs and symptoms of the primary lesion, the remainder of this chapter considers EFE without associated cardiac abnormalities, except for mitral insufficiency.

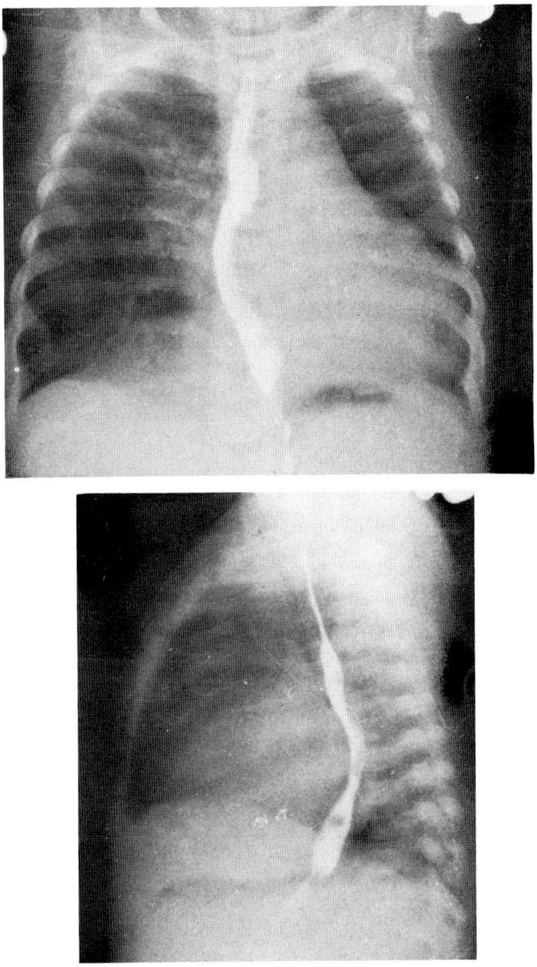

Figure 213. AP and lateral views of a 7-month-old child with endocardial fibroelastosis. There is a patch of pneumonia visible in the right upper lobe. Note also the marked degree of left atrial and left ventricular enlargement.

Congestive heart failure, manifested by hepatomegaly, tachycardia, tachypnea, and a gallop rhythm, is seen in 90% of patients. Peripheral, periorbital, and facial edema may be so striking that the initial impression is the nephrotic syndrome. Coughing spells occur in 40%. Intermittent cyanosis may occur in conjunction with severe congestive heart failure or in terminal states.

Although the typical patient has no significant murmur, those with mitral insufficiency will demonstrate a characteristic systolic murmur. Increased left ventricular activity and prominent third and fourth heart sounds are common.

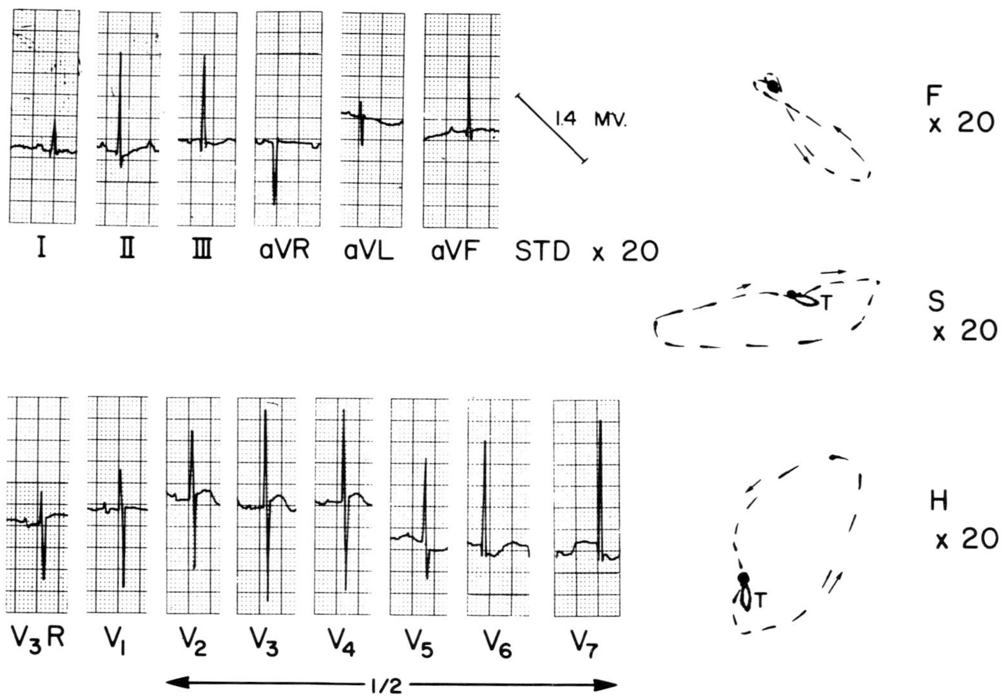

Figure 214. Typical electrocardiogram of a patient with endocardial fibroelastosis showing left ventricular hypertrophy. Note also the diphasic P waves in leads V_3R and V_1, suggesting left atrial enlargement. (From Elliott, L. P., and Schiebler, G. L. 1968. X-Ray Diagnosis of Congenital Cardiac Disease. Courtesy of Charles C Thomas, Publisher, Springfield, Ill.)

ROENTGENOGRAPHIC FEATURES

Left ventricular hypertrophy and left atrial enlargement are usually striking (Figure 213).

Pulmonary vascular markings are usually increased, because of passive venous congestion (see Figures 91 and 93). At times, this may be misread as a left-to-right shunt, but venous markings are of a more "patchy" or "puffy" nature.

ELECTROCARDIOGRAPHY

Left ventricular hypertrophy is found in 90% of patients (Figure 214). Right ventricular hypertrophy or combined ventricular hypertrophy is seen in the remainder.

Wolff-Parkinson-White syndrome, varying degrees of heart block, and paroxysmal atrial tachycardia have been reported to occur in 10% of affected children.

DIFFERENTIAL DIAGNOSIS

Myocarditis usually has a more sudden onset and accompanying fever, with rapid return to normal or progression to death. The electrocardiogram in myocarditis commonly shows lower voltage and more ST-T segment changes than are seen in EFE.

Anomalous origin of the left coronary artery from the pulmonary artery usually shows the electrocardiographic pattern of anterolateral myocardial infarction. These patients may also have EFE and mitral insufficiency, apparently secondary in nature.

Critically severe aortic stenosis in infancy may not have a murmur, thus resembling EFE. Left heart catheterization is needed for definitive diagnosis.

Glycogen storage disease of the heart can be differentiated by a steady progressive decline and macroglossia. A shorted P-R interval and biventricular hypertrophy characterized by enormous QRS voltages are seen on electrocardiogram. The diagnosis may be confirmed by a skeletal muscle biopsy that shows excess glycogen.

PROGNOSIS

The *fulminating type* accounts for about one-fourth of total cases, mostly infants under 6 weeks of age. There is an abrupt onset of tachypnea, overwhelming congestive heart failure, and circulatory collapse. Death often follows in a matter of hours, even with vigorous treatment.

The *acute type* is found in about one-half of total cases. These infants range from 6 weeks to 6 months of age. It has a slower onset and tachypnea is usually the first sign. There may be dramatic improvement with digitalis.

A more *chronic type* is seen in the remaining one-fourth of cases. These children usually present after 7 months of age, although the history may go back some time. Congestive heart failure is not as invariably present as in the other two types.

Many authors consider EFE to be primarily an autopsy diagnosis, and survivors with similar clinical findings are assumed to have had myocarditis, or other forms of nonobstructive cardiomyopathy. Others report methods of confirming the diagnosis by angiocardiography and catheterization, and suggest that some of these cases may survive for many years.

Negro children apparently have a better prognosis than white children.

MANAGEMENT

Congestive heart failure requires digitalization, diuretics, low-sodium diet, and other aids as outlined in Chapter 10.

Surgical approaches to increase myocardial oxygen supply are lacking in rationale and have high mortality rates (30 to 40%). Surgery is indicated, of course, for primary disease, such as coarctation; risk with associated EFE is increased, but not as much as formerly thought. Long-term survivors may eventually need surgery for valvar involvement.

BIBLIOGRAPHY

Black-Schaffer, B. 1957. Infantile endocardial fibroelastosis: A suggested etiology. Arch. Pathol. 63:281–306.

Hutchins, G. M., and Vie, S. A. 1972. The progression of interstitial myocarditis to idiopathic endocardial fibroelastosis. Am. J. Path. 66:483–492.

Krovetz, L. J., Maron, B. J., Morse, A., Brown, H., and Goldbloom, S. D. 1975. Prognostic implications of left ventricular function in endomyocardial disease in infants and children. J. Pediatr. 87:389–395.

McLoughlin, T. G., Schiebler, G. L., and Krovetz, L. J. 1966. Endocardial fibroelastosis and American Negro children: A distinct entity? Am. Heart J. 71:748–756.

McLoughlin, T. G., Schiebler, G. L., and Krovetz, L. J. 1968. Hemodynamic findings in children with endocardial fibroelastosis. An analysis of 22 cases. Am. Heart J. 75:162–172.

Miller, G. A. H., Rahimtoola, S. H., Ongley, P. A., and Swan, H. J. C. 1965. Left ventricular volume and volume change in endocardial fibroelastosis. Am. J. Cardiol. 15:631–637.

Morgan, A. D., McLoughlin, T. G., Bartley, T. D., and Shanklin, D. R. 1966. Endocardial fibroelastosis of the right ventricle in the newborn. Presenting the clinical picture of the hypoplastic right heart syndrome. Am. J. Card. 18:933–937.

Schryer, M. J. P., and Karnauchow, P. N. 1974. Endocardial fibroelastosis. Am. Heart J. 88:557–565.

Westwood, M., Harris, R., Burn, J. L., and Barson, A. J. 1975. Heredity in primary endocardial fibroelastosis. Br. Heart J. 37:1077–1084.

chapter 33

CHARACTERISTICS AND SPECIFIC PROBLEMS OF THE CYANOTIC CHILD

CHARACTERISTIC PICTURE

In addition to cyanosis of the mucous membranes and clubbing of the digits, the older cyanotic child often has a prominent head with large veins over the skull and over the bridge of the nose. Multiple capillary hemangiomata occur over the whole body, especially the cheeks. Suffusion of the conjunctiva, carious teeth, reddening of the tips of the digits, and numerous bruises are common. Weak, flabby muscles of the arms and legs, stunted physical growth, and an irritable personality are frequent problems.

COMMON CLINICAL PROBLEMS

These children prefer fluids and soft foods to hard foods. In fact, their diet may consist so heavily of milk and milk products that *iron deficiency anemia* occurs. Since cyanosis is not usually seen unless there is at least 3–5 g/dl of reduced hemoglobin, with anemia the level of reduced hemoglobin may be too low to produce visible cyanosis. The combination of anemia and cyanosis often produces a pale, light bluish-gray skin color.

Nearly one-half of cyanotic infants with right ventricular obstruction have *hypoxic episodes* characterized by paroxysmal hyperpnea and increased cyanosis (see Chapter 23). Often, these are accompanied by limpness and rolling back of the eyes. The dangers of these spells should not be minimized simply because they are so common. Morgan and associates have shown that nearly one out of 10 of these youngsters will have a cerebrovascular accident, and a similar proportion will die, following one or more spells. Increasing duration or increasing frequency of these spells is an indication for early surgery. Keep in mind that these spells may occur even in patients who demonstrate only mild cyanosis at rest.

Small doses of morphine, oxygen, and assumption of the knee-chest position are helpful in alleviating the spell. Acute spells can often be terminated by β-adrenergic blockage using parenteral propranolol. Since many of these patients become acidotic, a pH should be obtained. If the pH is low, it can be corrected by intravenous sodium bicarbonate. Since cyanotic patients should have a compensatory polycythemia, the finding of a normal hemoglobin or hematocrit may indicate a relative anemia. Patients having hypoxic spells in the presence of iron deficiency anemia often have fewer spells when given iron therapy, but may develop polycythemia.

Polycythemia may induce thrombocytopenia severe enough to cause significant hemorrhages. Thrombocytopenia is one of the few indications for phlebotomy, particularly prior to surgery, since it may restore platelet levels toward normal. Recurrent low-grade fevers are also common. These may also be due to polycythemia and the concomitant lowering of fluid reserve in the intravascular compartment. For the same reason, fluid intake in cyanotic children should be increased in periods of excess water loss, such as during high environmental temperatures, diarrhea, or fever, in order to reduce the risk of vascular thrombosis.

Constipation is a recurrent and annoying problem in cyanotic children, and stool softening measures should be instituted to relieve it before it becomes a battle between parent and child.

The mother may relate to the physician that the child complains of recurrent *headaches* or diffuse nonspecific *muscle cramps*. These usually disappear with palliative surgery or with correction of the defect.

BIBLIOGRAPHY

Guntheroth, W. G., Morgan, B. C., and Mullins, G. L. 1965. Physiologic studies of paroxysmal hyperpnea in cyanotic congenital heart disease. Circulation 31:70–76.

Morgan, B. C., Guntheroth, W. G., Bloom, R. S., and Fyler, D. C. 1965. A clinical profile of paroxysmal hyperpnea in cyanotic congenital heart disease. Circulation 31:66–69.

chapter 34

RHYTHM DISTURBANCES

In *normal sinus rhythm,* a P wave (atrial depolarization) precedes each QRS wave (ventricular depolarization) in a regular succession (Figure 215). *Sinus arrhythmia* is a common normal variant secondary to respiration (Figure 215). A P wave again precedes each QRS complex, but the maximum interval between QRS complexes is at least 1.5 times the minimum. The R-to-R intervals decrease with inspiration and increase with expiration, resulting in inverse variations in heart rate.

SUPRAVENTRICULAR ARRHYTHMIAS

Sinus bradycardia is a slower than normal heart rate for age (Table 39; Figure 215). It may be a result of hypothyroidism or athletic training.

Sinus tachycardia is a rapid, regular heart rate faster than normal for age (Table 39), with regularly occurring P waves. The P waves may, however, be superimposed on preceding T waves. In addition to congestive heart failure, it may be seen with hypermetabolism, as in fever or thyrotoxicosis.

Supraventricular premature beats, either atrial or nodal, are usually followed by a less than complete compensatory pause, i.e., the duration of the two cycles including the premature beat is less than the duration of two normal cycles.

Paroxysmal atrial tachycardia starts and ends abruptly. Heart rate ranges from 180 to 300 beats per minute, with completely regular QRS complexes. P waves may be difficult to distinguish because they are often superimposed on the preceding T waves (Figure 216). The pacemaker may be located in the atria or the upper AV node. After return to a normal sinus rhythm, the electrocardiogram may show ST segment and T wave changes that persist for days or even weeks (Figure 217). These changes have been attributed to myocardial ischemia during the tachycardia, because coronary flow is diminished when diastole is very short.

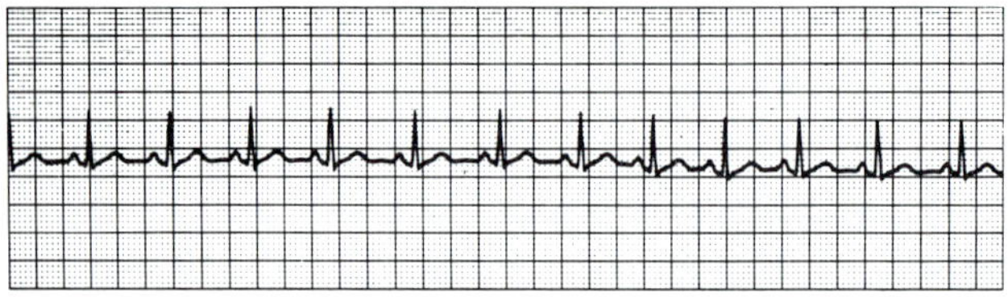

NORMAL SINUS RHYTHM-LEAD II

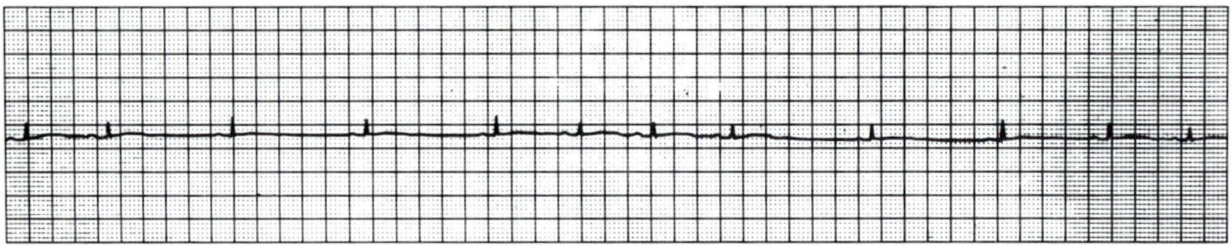

SINUS BRADYCARDIA WITH SINUS ARRHYTHMIA-LEAD II
1/2 SENSITIVITY

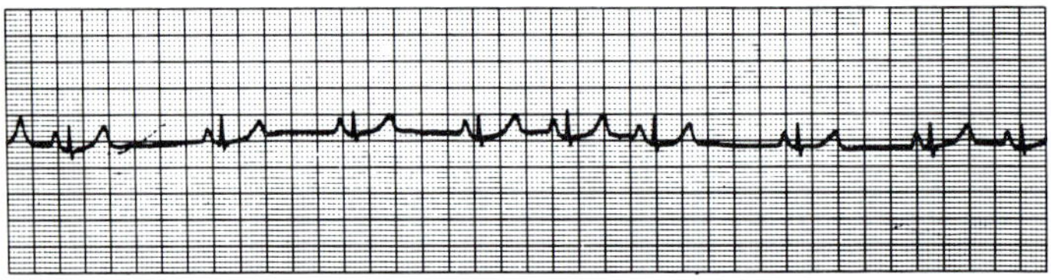

SINUS ARRHYTHMIA-LEAD II

Figure 215. (Upper strip) Shows normal sinus rhythm in an electrocardiogram taken on a normal 3-year-old girl. (Middle strip) Shows, in contrast to the one above, marked variation in rate with respiration called sinus arrhythmia. The ventricular rate slows to 50 beats per minute, sinus bradycardia. This continuous strip of lead II was taken in a 3-year-old girl with a brain tumor and multiple electrolyte problems. (Lower strip) Marked sinus arrhythmia is noted in this continuous strip of lead II. The R-R interval varies from a minimum of 0.68 sec to a maximum of 1.18 sec. Sinus arrhythmia occurs in most normal children. This particular strip was obtained from a 6-year-old girl with cyanotic tetralogy of Fallot.

This arrhythmia occurs in three forms. The acute variety is most common in male infants under 4 months. It is most prevalent in the spring, suggesting a viral etiology. Presenting symptoms include pallor, restlessness, and poor feeding. If the arrhythmia lasts more than 24 hr, congestive heart failure is common.

Another variety, also called "repetitive paroxysmal tachycardia," occurs in older children and is less frequent in pediatric practice. It consists of paroxysms of ectopic beats that are interrupted by short runs of sinus rhythm. Although it responds poorly to drug therapy, it rarely causes heart failure or significant symptoms. The prognosis is good, and many children learn to abort these transient episodes by Valsalva maneuvers.

Table 39. Heart rate and QRS axis at various stages[a]

	Heart rate		QRS axis	
Age	Mean	Range	Mean	Range
0–24 hours	120	77–155	137°	70 to 205°
1–7 days	138	100–188	125°	75 to 185°
8–30 days	162	125–188	108°	30 to 190°
1–3 months	161	115–215	75°	25 to 125°
3–6 months	149	125–215	65°	30 to 96°
6–12 months	147	115–188	65°	10 to 115°
1–3 years	130	100–188	55°	6 to 108°
3–5 years	105	68–150	62°	20 to 105°
5–8 years	102	75–150	65°	16 to 112°
8–12 years	88	51–125	62°	15 to 112°
12–16 years	83	38–125	65°	20 to 116°

[a] Modified from Ziegler, R. F. 1951. Electrocardiographic studies in normal infants and children. Courtesy of Charles C Thomas, Publisher, Springfield, Ill.

Persistent supraventricular tachycardia is rather rare. It is characterized by variable rates and abnormal P waves. This form of tachycardia may persist for many months or even years, despite therapy. Cerebrovascular accidents and congestive heart failure have been reported.

Stimulation of the vagus by pressing on the carotid sinus or eyeballs has not been effective in our experience. Eyeball pressure may cause damage and should not be used. Digoxin is the drug of choice, especially in infants who usually respond promptly. If necessary, propanalol may be added as a second drug (Table 40). In seriously ill infants, direct current countershock is a safe and reliable method. Usually 1–2 watt-sec/kg will convert the arrhythmia to normal sinus rhythm.

Atrial flutter has an atrial rate of 200–350 beats per minute. The ventricular response is regular but slower, and may be in the ratio of 1:2, 1:3, 2:3, or some other simple fraction of the atrial rate. P waves (flutter waves) are usually distinguishable even when superimposed on T waves (Figure 218).

Atrial fibrillation is characterized by continuous, irregular atrial activity at rates of 400 to 700 beats per minute, with a slower and usually grossly irregular ventricular response at rates of 110–150 beats per minute. Atrial fibrillation is rare in children and when seen is almost always secondary to congenital or acquired heart disease.

Atrioventricular heart block is found in varying degrees. In 2:1 block there are two P waves for each QRS complex (Figure 219). There may be other simple ratios of P to QRS waves, such as 3:1, 3:2, etc. In any case there is a consistent relationship of one QRS complex to the next QRS complex, with a constant time interval.

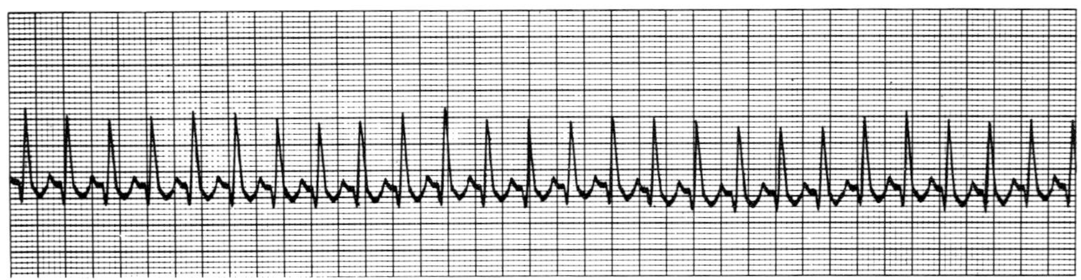

Figure 216. A continuous strip of lead II showing supraventricular tachycardia with a rate of 195 beats per minute in a 5-year-old girl with Turner syndrome and a coarctation of the aorta. Such episodes can occur with or without coexistent congenital or acquired heart disease.

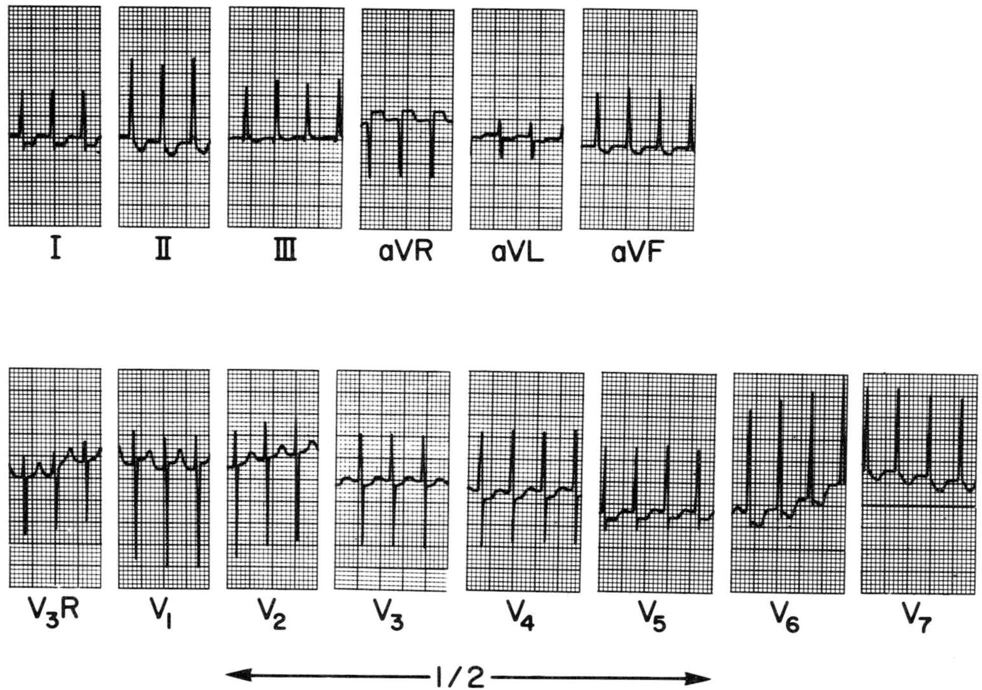

Figure 217. Electrocardiogram demonstrating a bout of supraventricular tachycardia with a rate of about 215 beats per minute. Distinct P waves are not seen. Note the ST vector directed rightward, superiorly, and slightly anteriorly, causing ST segment–T wave changes called "tachycardial ischemia." Such ST-T changes may last for several weeks after the cessation of the tachycardia. This ECG was taken on a 3-year-old boy who had recurrent bouts of tachycardia. There was no associated heart disease.

Table 40. Antiarrhythmic drugs in pediatric practice

Drug	Type of arrhythmia[a]					Contra-indications	Dosage[b]
	Supraventricular tachycardia	Atrial flutter	Atrial fibrillation	Ectopic ventricular arrhythmia	Arrhythmia secondary to digitalis toxicity		
Digoxin	++	(+)	++			Ventricular arrhythmia (Use with caution in AV block)	0.07 mg/kg, <1 year 0.06 mg/kg, 1–2 years
Diphenylhydantoin	(+)			+	++	Use with caution in AV block	2–3 mg/kg i.v.
Lidocaine	–	–	–	++	(+)	Hypotension	1 mg/kg i.v.
Propranolol	++	+	++	(+)	(+)	Congestive heart failure; AV block; obstructive lung disease	0.025–0.1 mg/kg i.v. 0.5–1 mg/kg p.o. (up to 3 mg/kg/day)
Procainamide	(+)	(+)	+	++	(+)	AV block	3–5 mg/kg i.v.
Quinidine	+	(+)	++	(+)	(+)	AV block	30 mg/kg/day p.o. (Usually divided into 5 equal doses)
Potassium salt	in cases of low serum potassium concentrations						0.3–0.5 mEq/kg/hr i.v.

[a] Symbols: ++ = drug of choice; + = moderately effective; (+) = varying degree of effectiveness; – = not effective.
[b] All antiarrhythmic drugs given i.v. must be given slowly. Diphenylhydantoin, lidocaine, propranolol, or procainamide may be repeated in the same dosage after 20 min.

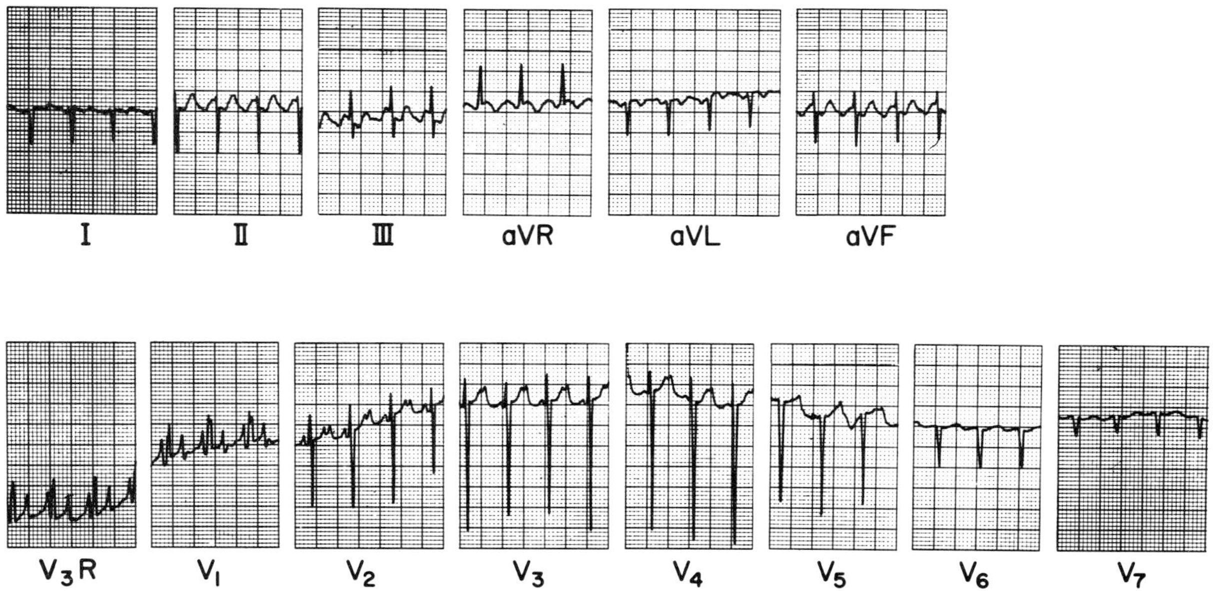

Figure 218. Auricular flutter with 2:1 conduction. Atrial waves are 300 beats per minute and ventricular complexes are 150 beats per minute. Regular contour of all wave forms is seen in all leads. Flutter (F) waves are best seen in right precordial leads where electrode is closest to right atrium. Auricular flutter is not an uncommon arrhythmia in individuals after a Blalock-Hanlon procedure (surgical creation of an atrial septal defect). This electrocardiogram was taken on a 3-year-old child with complete transposition of the great vessels.

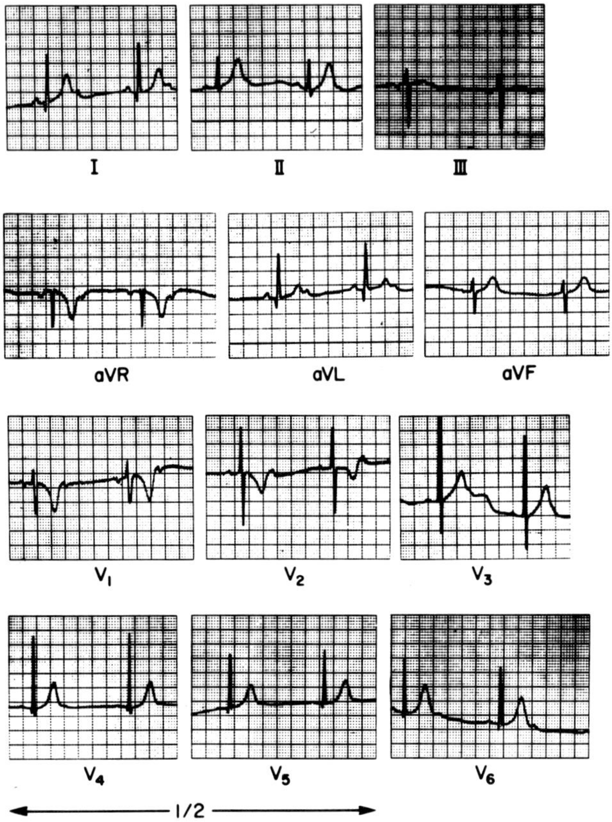

Figure 219. This electrocardiogram demonstrates 2:1 AV block with two P waves noted in constant position for each QRS complex. This was taken on a 7-year-old boy who had an endocardial cushion defect repaired. He developed this conduction anomaly postoperatively, along with residual mitral insufficiency.

Complete atrioventricular block exhibits no such regular relationship between P waves and QRS complexes. There are always many more P waves than QRS complexes. The ventricular rate is characteristically slower than normal, sometimes 50 beats per minute or less (Figure 220). If the ventricular rate does not increase with exercise, if there are Stokes-Adams attacks, or if the QRS complex is wider than 0.12 sec, insertion of a pacemaker is indicated. Recently, congenital complete heart block has been associated with maternal systemic lupus erythematosus.

VENTRICULAR ARRHYTHMIAS

A *ventricular premature beat* is a QRS complex shaped differently than the normal conducted beat and usually followed by a compensatory pause (Figure

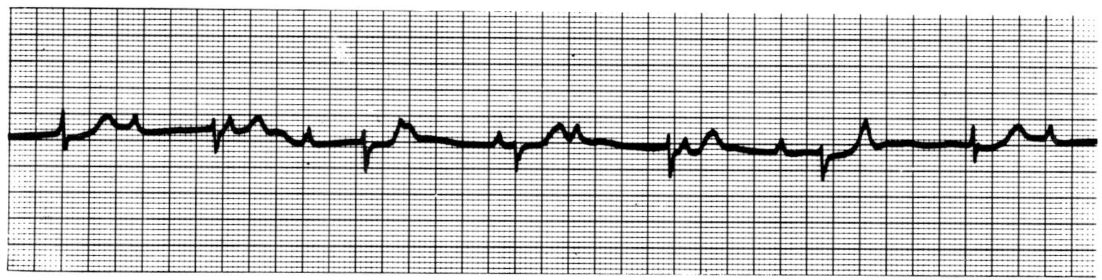

Figure 220. Complete atrioventricular block in an asymptomatic 5-year-old child without any other associated anomaly. Note in this strip of lead I the slow ventricular rate (about 54 beats per minute), and the totally irregular relationship of the small peaked P waves to the QRS complexes.

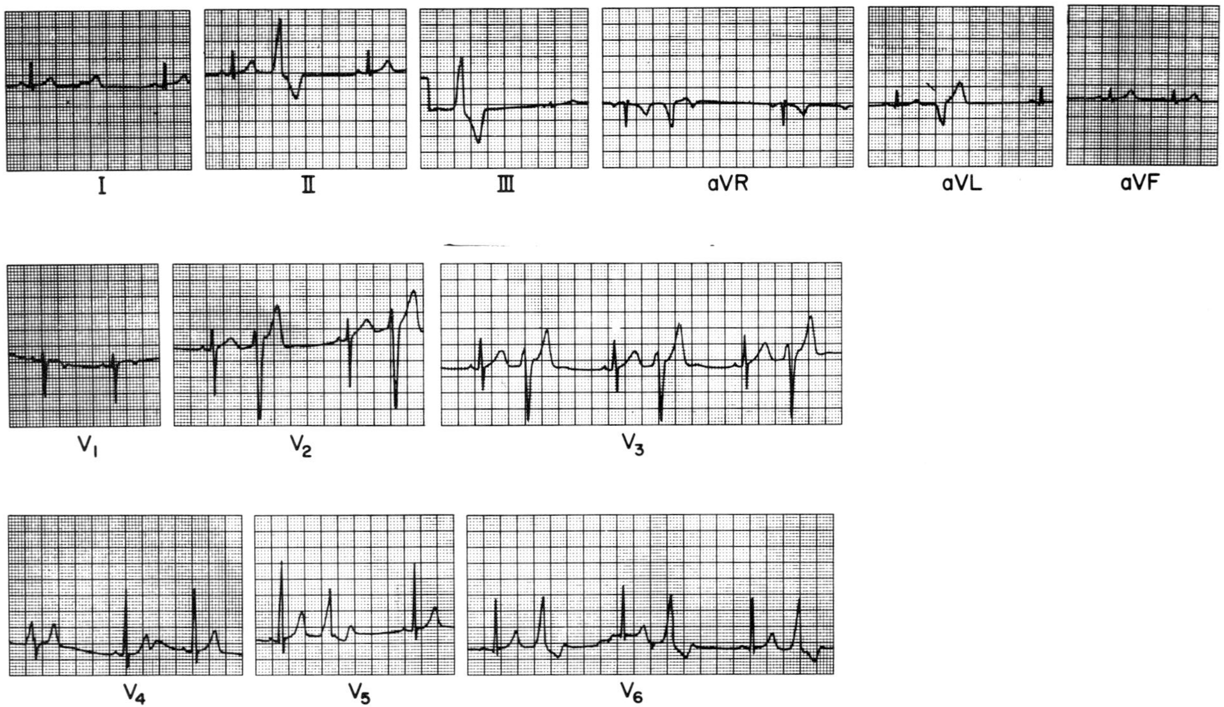

Figure 221. This electrocardiogram shows unifocal premature ventricular beats in a healthy, asymptomatic 13-year-old girl. At times there is a bigeminal pattern.

221). When the shape of the QRS complexes of the premature beats looks alike, they probably are originating from one area of the ventricular myocardium and are called unifocal. When the QRS complexes vary in shape, they are said to be multifocal in origin and carry a more serious import.

When the premature beats alternate with normally conducted beats, the rhythm is referred to as bigeminy. Frequent premature ventricular beats are not uncommon in otherwise healthy adolescents. When the frequency of premature beats decreases with exercise, the prognosis is good.

Ventricular premature beats are difficult to distinguish from *nodal premature beats* with aberrant conduction. The latter, however, commonly have an rSR′ pattern in lead V_1, whereas the former rarely do.

Ventricular tachycardia is suggested by rapidly inscribed, abnormally wide, bizarre QRS complexes with slight variations in the R-R intervals. This arrhythmia is rarely seen in children. When it occurs, it is usually paroxysmal in nature. Intravenous lidocaine (1–2 mg/kg) is useful for the emergency treatment of this disorder. His bundle electrograms are invaluable aids in determining appropriate antiarrhythmic therapy for patients with sustained or recurrent tachyarrhythmias.

Ventricular fibrillation exhibits bizarre QRS complexes fused with T waves with totally irregular R-R intervals. It usually occurs as a terminal event. Prompt electrical defibrillation may be lifesaving.

BIBLIOGRAPHY

Hernandez, A., Strauss, A., Kleiger, R. E., and Goldring, D. 1975. Idiopathic paroxysmal ventricular tachycardia in infants and children. J. Pediatr. 86:182–188.

Mantakas, M. E., McCue, C. M., and Miller, W. W. 1978. Natural history of Wolff-Parkinson-White syndrome discovered in infancy. Am. J. Cardiology 41:1097–1103.

Mody, G., Whitman, V., Edelstein, J., Liebman, J., and DeJoseph, R. B. 1976. Tachyarrhythmias and ectopic beats with aberrant intraventricular conduction in children. Pediatrics 57:691–695.

Radford, D. J., and Izukawa, T. 1977. Atrial fibrillation in children. Pediatrics 59:250–267.

Roberts, N. K., and Gelband, H. 1977. Cardiac Arrhythmias in the Neonate, Infant, and Child. Appleton-Century-Crofts, New York.

Rutkowski, M. M., Doyle, E. F., and Cohen, S. N. 1973. Drug therapy of heart disease in pediatric patients. III. The therapeutic challenge of supraventricular tachyarrhythmias in infants and children. Am. Heart J. 86:562–568.

Singh, B. N., and Hauswirth, O. 1974. Comparative mechanism of action of antiarrhythmic drugs. Am. Heart J. 87:367–382.

Yabek, S. M., and Jarmakani, J. M. 1978. Sinus node dysfunction in children, adolescents, and young adults. Pediatrics 61:593–598.

chapter 35

HYPERTENSION IN CHILDHOOD

INCIDENCE AND IMPORTANCE

Over the past two decades it has become increasingly clear that hypertension is one of the more common diseases. It is estimated that one in 10 adult Americans has elevated blood pressure. Surveys have shown that only one-half of this hypertensive population is aware of their hypertension, and less than one in four is receiving adequate treatment.

In the past much attention has been focused on recognition and treatment of "curable" hypertension, i.e., forms that are secondary to specific causes such as pheochromocytoma, Cushing syndrome, or renovascular disease (see "Secondary Hypertension," below). Recognition and proper treatment of these relatively uncommon forms of hypertension may result in dramatic shifts in blood pressure. Benign, essential hypertension has received less attention for a variety of reasons. Some physicians are still uncertain whether or not therapy with antihypertensive drugs will prevent the development of cardiovascular complications. Other physicians may not be convinced that the benefits of treatment outweigh the known side effects of currently available drugs. The potential benefits of treatment are even less clear in pediatric practice, since there is often a long latency period between discovery of elevated blood pressure in a child and the development of overt complications.

In Evans County, Georgia, 50 adolescents and young adults who had average blood pressure readings of greater than 140 mm Hg systolic or 90 mm Hg diastolic were selected for follow-up study. After 7 years, two deaths from cerebral hemorrhage had occurred and one subject had hypertensive heart disease. Sustained hypertension with cardiovascular and cerebrovascular symptoms had developed in three others, and 12 had severe but asymptomatic hypertension. Only 11 of the group had become normotensive. This and other similar studies emphasize the importance of hypertension even in the young.

SPHYGMOMANOMETRY

Measured blood pressure depends to some extent on the techniques used, such as the speed of compression and deflation of the cuff, the cuff size, the position of the arm in relation to the body, the criteria used to estimate blood pressure, the degree of apprehension of the subjects, and the amount of rest permitted the subjects before the measurements are made. Blood pressure as assessed by sphygmomanometry is also influenced by the compressibility of the intervening tissues and the elasticity of the arterial wall. At least part of the correlation of elevated blood pressure with obesity may be artifactual.

Possible Sources of Error in Measuring Blood Pressure

Equipment
- Defective sphygmomanometer, tubing, cuff, stethoscope

Use of equipment
- Instrument not at heart level
- Improper cuff size
- Overly rapid deflation
- Mercury column not at eye level

Examiner
- Hearing deficiency
- Variations in use of single or multiple determinations of blood pressure
- Variations in zero preference

Variations in condition of subject
- Presence of pain or anxiety
- Bladder distension
- Alcohol ingestion
- Infection
- Smoking
- Coffee or tea ingestion
- Drug therapy
- Fever

Environment
- Diurnal variation
- Room too hot or too cold
- Noisy room

Recommended Methods

Older children should be seated with the arm resting on a table so that it is at heart level. In infants blood pressure is usually measured in the supine position. For infants under 1 year of age the Doppler method of detecting systolic blood pressure is highly recommended. For patients over 3 years of age stethoscopic detection of Korotkoff sounds is usually best. For patients from 1 to 3 years of age the stethoscope should be used when the child will cooperate and lie quietly, whereas the Doppler method may be simpler with an uncooperative child.

For any patient, the proper size of blood pressure cuff is essential, and a variety of sizes should be available. Ideally the bladder should be large enough to encircle the arm completely and as wide as can be fitted on the upper arm. We have not encountered the "wide cuff" effect in which the recorded blood pressure is said to be artificially low. On the other hand, we have encountered false elevations of blood pressure when the cuff used was too small.

The bag should be inflated to a pressure about 15–20 mm Hg above the expected systolic. Pressures much above this level are unnecessary and may produce ischemic pain and false elevation of blood pressure. Deflation should be at a rate that allows for a drop in the reading of 2–3 mm Hg per heart beat. Systolic pressure is easily recognized as the beginning of Korotkoff or Doppler sounds and oscillation of the needle or mercury column.

Diastolic pressure may be defined as that which occurs at the point of muffling or at the cessation of sound. Muffling is easier to detect but is slightly higher than intra-arterial pressure, whereas the point of cessation of sound is too low. Comparisons of intra-arterial measurements of blood pressure with measurements by various indirect techniques have uniformly shown that the correlation with systolic blood pressure is relatively satisfactory, but that the correlation with diastolic blood pressure is poorer.

DEFINITION OF HYPERTENSION

There is a lack of agreement among investigators as to the definition of hypertension in children. Londe defines blood pressures between the 90th and 95th percentile (for age and sex) as suspicious and those above the 95th percentile as hypertensive. Lauer uses values above 140/90 mm Hg as hypertensive. Loggie classifies patients under 20 years of age with diastolic blood pressure above 90 mm Hg as being hypertensive. Furthermore, the observed increase of blood pressure with age is considered by some authors to be pathologic rather than to result from a normal aging process. Perhaps the best definition is that offered by Blumenthal's Task Force, who considered sustained blood pressure elevations (i.e., obtained on at least three separate occasions) above the 95th percentile to be abnormal. It is clear that any cut-off point represents an arbitrary decision at any age. In view of this, Blumenthal suggests that the term "high normal blood pressure" be used with the child and his parents to avoid the negative implications associated with hypertension.

An increase in blood pressure during puberty has sometimes been thought to be secondary to sexual maturation and therefore of little clinical significance. Londe and associates found that blood pressure readings were not higher in patients with more advanced sexual development, nor were there significant correlations with serum follicle–stimulating or luteinizing hormone levels in the patients studied.

In contrast to the study by Londe and associates, Shock found a distinct increase in systolic blood pressure that appeared suddenly and developed rapidly after 13½ to 14 years of age. The paper by Londe and associates raises the possibility that a blood pressure elevation seen in adolescents cannot be assumed to be related to the onset of puberty.

SECONDARY HYPERTENSION

Estimates of the prevalence of secondary forms of hypertension in childhood vary widely. Studies have shown that as little as 5% and as much as 45% of childhood hypertension is due to renal disease, vascular abnormalities, tumors, or endocrine disorders. Part of this variation is no doubt due to the difficulty in determining and defining the hypertensive population. A thorough search for all possible causes of secondary hypertension in every patient would be prohibitively expensive in relation to the number of potential cures. Fortunately, many of the causes of hypertension can be determined by relatively simple means.

Causes of Secondary Hypertension in Children

- Curable forms
  - Renal
    - Pyelonephritis
    - Hydronephrosis
    - Trauma
    - Hypoplastic kidney
    - Wilms' and other renal tumors
  - Vascular
    - Coarctation of aorta
      - Unilateral renal artery stenosis, aneurysm, arteritis, or fibromuscular dysplasia
      - Thrombosis of a renal artery
    - Adrenal
      - Neuroblastoma
      - Pheochromocytoma
      - Adrenogenital syndrome
      - Cushing's disease
      - Primary aldosteronism
    - Miscellaneous
      - Ingestion of excessive licorice
      - Administration of glucocorticoids

Incurable forms
- Renal
  - Chronic glomerulonephritis
  - Chronic bilateral pyelonephritis
  - Bilateral hydronephrosis
  - Polycystic kidneys
  - Polyarteritis nodosa
  - Systemic lupus erythematosus
- Vascular
  - Bilateral fibromuscular dysplasia
  - Generalized aortic hypoplasia
- Miscellaneous
  - Lead nephropathy (chronic)
  - Porphyria
  - Renal parenchymal damage from irradiation

History and Physical Examination

The history and physical examination can provide clues to the etiology of hypertension. For example, a history of acute flank pain or hematuria may be a valuable clue to the presence of renovascular hypertension. Angiospastic funduscopic changes (arteriolar narrowing without hypertensive sclerosis) or a bruit in the upper abdomen or flank suggest the need for further renal studies.

The child's history should be reviewed for conditions or drugs known to be associated with or predisposing to high blood pressure, e.g., renal disease, corticosteroid usage, or oral contraceptives.

A history of paroxysms of hypertension in association with head pain, pallor, palpitation, and perspiration should alert the physician to the possible presence of a pheochromocytoma. It should be be recognized that two-thirds of patients with pheochromocytomas are asymptomatic and have sustained hypertension. A history of spells, weakness, polyuria, and muscle cramps suggests possible aldosteronism.

The family history should be obtained, with emphasis on the obstetrical history of the mother (eclampsia) and familial occurrence of hypertension. Special attention should be paid to evidence of target organ damage in parents or grandparents less than 50 years old. Major target organs that are susceptible to damage from hypertensive vascular disease are the brain, heart, and kidney. Accordingly, hypertensive disease should be suspected with a history of stroke, heart attack, or kidney failure of unknown origin.

Children under 10 years of age and white teenage girls are most likely to have secondary forms of hypertension. On the other hand, a strong family history of essential hypertension suggests that no secondary cause will be found.

There are two primary objectives of the physical examination. The first is to exclude secondary causes of hypertension. Easily detected examples include neurofibromatosis, Cushing's disease, acromegaly, and coarctation of the aorta. Bruits over the abdomen or flank areas suggest major renal artery stenosis. The second objective is to detect evidence of target organ damage by funduscopic and cardiac examination. It is unlikely that secondary changes in the fundi and/or of the heart will be detectable in the asymptomatic individual with slightly elevated pressures.

Blood pressure measurements should be obtained on all first-degree relatives who are 3 years old or older. Such measurements are rarely performed in pediatric settings, but may be clinically significant, and offer an optimal approach to cost-effective detection and entry of affected individuals into the health care system.

Blood pressure values, unlike height and weight in children, will not precisely follow percentile tracks (Figures 222 and 223). There is considerable variation in most children's pressures. These charts provide a mechanism for a child's pressure to be recorded so that a pattern over a period of time may be observed.

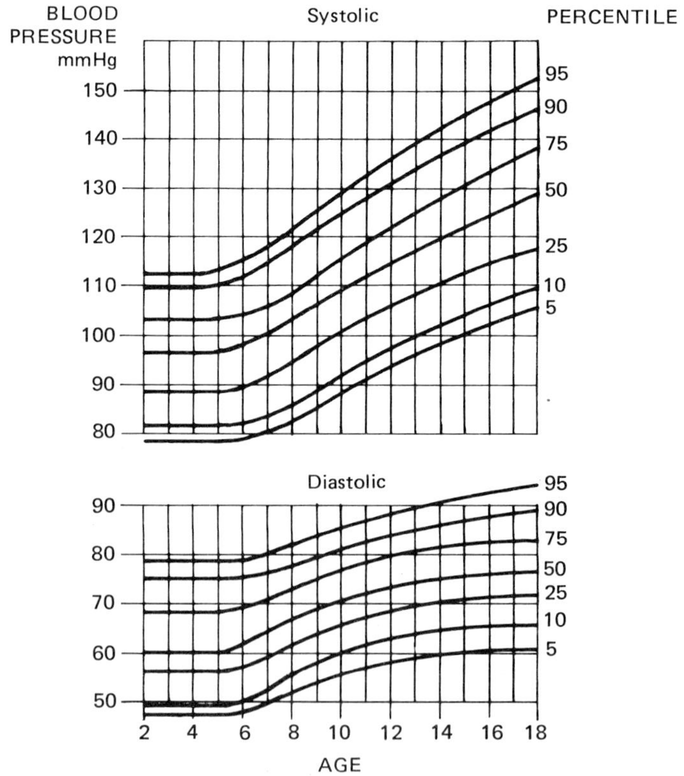

Figure 222. Percentiles of blood pressure measurement in boys (right arm, seated).

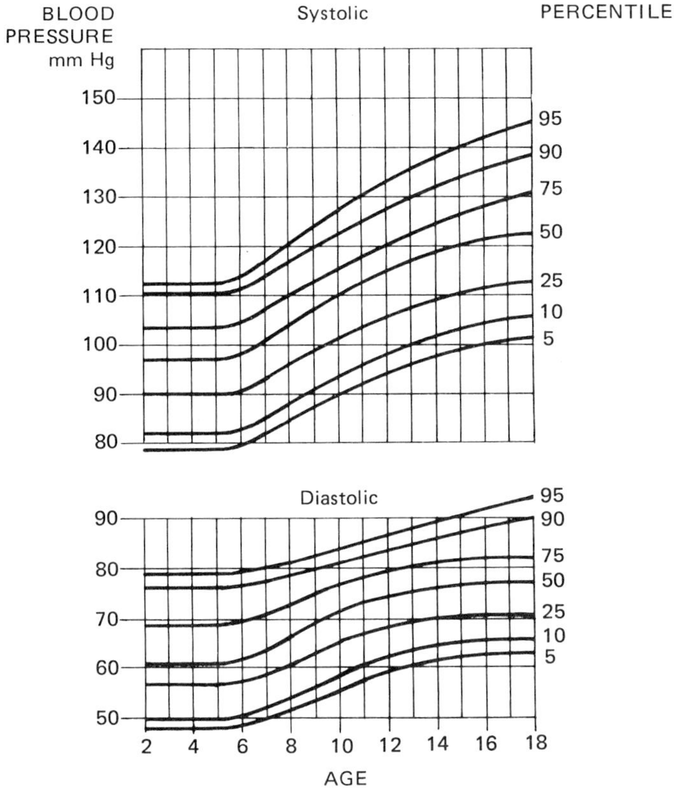

Figure 223. Percentiles of blood pressure measurement in girls (right arm, seated).

Blood pressure should always be measured in the legs as part of the initial evaluation. Palpable femoral pulses do not exclude coarctation of the aorta.

DIAGNOSTIC PROCEDURES

In hypertensive patients, in addition to the history and physical examination, a blood count and urinalysis should be done, and creatinine clearance, serum urea nitrogen, and potassium should be measured.

Hypokalemia in the absence of diuretic therapy should suggest primary aldosteronism. Low-sodium diets may mask this sign, which may be uncovered by administration of supplementary sodium chloride for 4 days.

Urinary catecholamines should be done routinely in all hypertensive children. Some authors advocate a chest x-ray and electrocardiogram as useful additional procedures.

What should a pediatrician do when he discovers an elevated blood pressure reading in a child or adolescent? First, he should repeat the blood pressure measurements on several more occasions with the child in as basal a condition as possible. Second, if repeated readings of the blood pressure continue to be elevated, he should then institute a search for the etiology and initiate appropriate treatment. Third, if the blood pressure is elevated on only a few readings, it would seem wisest to continue observation and repeat measurements of blood pressure on subsequent office visits.

LABILE HYPERTENSION

The true significance of labile hypertension is not known. The study done in Evans County, Georgia, cited above and an earlier study of hypertension among army officers would indicate that *even a single detection of an elevated blood pressure is associated with a significant increase in mortality rate*. The presence of even a single elevated blood pressure should not be dismissed in an offhand manner. Until more data are accumulated on the natural history of labile hypertension, it would seem prudent to explain the situation to the parents and to repeat blood pressure determinations at subsequent visits. Only in that way can the pediatrician be assured that the occasional elevated blood pressure reading is truly of benign origin.

MANAGEMENT

Despite the availability of many potent drugs, the success of any therapeutic regimen depends largely on the skill of the physician in exploiting the nuances of their pharmacodynamic actions. Tranquilizers and sedatives are *not* effective in lowering blood pressure and are not recommended as primary therapy. If they are given for other indications, possible interaction with antihypertensive agents must be carefully considered.

Management of most children with chronically elevated blood pressure is generally facilitated by starting with low doses of a given drug and building slowly to therapeutically effective levels. This often allows the patient to accommodate the unpleasant side effects of therapy, such as light-headedness, urinary frequency, postural hypotension, sedation, or altered bowel movement patterns.

Selection of specific drugs is dependent on many factors, including age of the patient, clinical circumstances, and potential side effects of the drug. For example, reserpine is not favored in children because of its possible deleterious behavioral effects.

The choice of treatment in the young patient is somewhat difficult. We personally think a β-blocking agent (e.g., propranolol) is the best initial drug in young patients; we then add a diuretic if necessary, and finally a vasodilator. Our reasoning is that many young patients have high renin levels and will respond to β-blockage.

Many children respond to a decrease in vascular fluid volume brought about by a reduction in dietary salt intake or by diuretic treatment; the former is extremely difficult to implement in children. Oral diuretic agents may be combined with a potassium-sparing agent if supplementation with potassium chloride or with dietary regimens proves inadequate. If a child's blood pressure remains elevated with the preceding regimens, a vasodilator agent in combination with propranolol (not currently approved by the Food and Drug Administration for use in children with hypertension) and a thiazide diuretic has proven to be very effective (Tables 41 and 42). In patients with hyperactivity of the sympathetic nervous system, guanethidine in small (5–10 mg) doses can be very effective without producing postural hypotension. It has the dual advantages of requiring only one dose per day and being relatively inexpensive.

It is worthwhile to emphasize that all categories of antihypertensive agents, including those acting on components of the adrenergic nervous sys-

Table 41. Pediatric dosage regimen for antihypertensive agents

Drug	Daily starting oral dose (mg/kg)	Dosage increment[a] interval (days)	Daily maximum oral dose	
			mg/kg	Total mg
Diuretics				
Chlorothiazide	10	14	20	1000
Hydrochlorothiazide	1	14	2	100
Chlorthalidone	1	14	2	100
Furosemide	0.5–1	14	2	[b]
Spironolactone[e]	2	14	4	200
Vasodilator agents				
Hydralazine	1	3–4	5	200
Minoxidil[c]	0.1–0.5	7	1–2	[b]
Agents acting on adrenergic nervous system				
Methyldopa	10	3–7	40	2000
Propranolol[d]	1	3–6	[b]	[b]
Guanethidine	0.2–0.5	12–14	1–2	[b]

[a] The time required to achieve a maximum therapeutic response and/or steady-state blood level varies for each drug. Consequently, daily drug dosage should be increased during the suggested time intervals. Increments carried out over a shorter time span may cause an exaggerated pharmacological response.

[b] Maximal dose for these agents has not been established in children.

[c] Experimental drug available at present time only for use in subjects refractory to conventional antihypertensive therapy. Dosage regimens for children are currently under development.

[d] Not currently approved by the Food and Drug Administration for use in children with hypertension.

[e] Potassium sparing.

Table 42. Sympathetic inhibitors

Site of action	Preparation
Central (α-stimulation)	Clonidine
Combined central reduction of sympathetic outflow plus peripheral norepinephrine depletion	Rauwolfia alkaloids Methyldopa
Ganglion blockage	Trimethaphan Pentolinium
Peripheral (postganglionic) norepinephrine depletion	Guanethidine Bethanidine
Receptor blockage	
α-receptors	Phenoxybenzamine Phentolamine
β-receptors	Propranolol

tem and those causing direct vasodilatation, tend to produce fluid accumulation. Consequently, it is generally advisable to administer a diuretic concurrently with the drug regimens discussed. Despite aggressive pharmacotherapy, it is occasionally impossible to lower a preadolescent's blood pressure to acceptable levels on an outpatient basis. In these situations, hospitalization is mandatory.

RECOMMENDATIONS OF THE TASK FORCE ON BLOOD PRESSURE CONTROL IN CHILDREN*

1. Children 3 years old and older should have their blood pressure measured annually as part of their continuing health care.
2. High blood pressure detection programs per se for children should not be established.
3. Blood pressure measurements on infants and children should be taken in a quiet environment, with the correct cuff size, and with the fourth phase Korotkoff sound used for the diastolic pressure.
4. Blood pressure measurements obtained should be recorded on appropriate blood pressure charts (see Figures 222 and 223).
5. Caution should be exercised in labeling children as hypertensive because of psychosocial and economic implications; use of the term "high normal blood pressure" is appropriate during evaluation and follow-up to avoid unnecessary negative implications.
6. Sustained blood pressure levels (obtained at least on three separate occasions) that are above the 95th percentile should be considered ab-

*Adapted from Blumenthal, S., et al., 1977 (see Bibliography).

normal, with recognition that any cutoff point represents an arbitrary decision at any age.

7. In infants and children with sustained blood pressure above the 95th percentile, a medical history should be obtained, a physical examination performed, and further tests completed (as outlined in this chapter) to determine a possible cause.
8. Children with sustained elevated blood pressure should receive a systematic long-term follow-up program, which may include hygienic counseling covering weight control, salt intake, exercise, and smoking, and antihypertensive pharmacotherapy when indicated.
9. Physicians who manage hypertensive children with pharmacotherapy should use the "stepped-care" approach, with emphasis on minimal effective dosages of appropriate agents.
10. Children at high risk of developing elevated blood pressure should be evaluated for other atherosclerotic risk factors and should be taught to observe necessary hygienic measures for lowering risk factors.

BIBLIOGRAPHY

Blumenthal, S., Epps, R. P., Heavenrich, R., Lauer, R. M., Lieberman, E., Mirkin, B., Mitchell, S. C., Naito, V. B., O'Hare, D., Smith, W. M., Tarazi, R. C., and Upson, D. 1977. Report of the task force on blood pressure control in children. Pediatrics, 59:797–820.

Heyden, S., et al. 1969. Elevated blood pressure levels in adolescents, Evans County, Georgia. JAMA 209:1683–1689.

Levy, R. L., et al. 1944. Transient hypertension: its significance in terms of later development of sustained hypertension and cardiovascular renal disease. JAMA 126:829–833.

Londe, S., Bourgoignie, J. J., Robson, A. M., and Goldring, D. 1971. Hypertension in apparently normal children. J. Pediatr. 78:569–577.

Londe, S., and Goldring, D. 1976. High blood pressure in children: problems and guidelines for evaluation and treatment. Am. J. Cardiol. 37:650–657.

Londe, S., Johanson, A., Kronemer, N. S., and Goldring, D. 1975. Blood pressure and puberty. J. Pediatr. 87:896–900.

Moss, A. J., and Adams, F. H. 1963. Index of indirect estimation of diastolic blood pressure. Am. J. Dis. Child. 106:364–367.

Shock, N. W. 1944. Basal blood pressure and pulse rate in adolescents. Am. J. Dis. Child. 68:16–22.

Strong, C. G. 1977. Editorial: Surgically correctable causes of hypertension. Mayo Clin. Proc. 52:585–586.

chapter 36

ATHEROSCLEROSIS IN CHILDHOOD

HISTORICAL NOTES

Virchow postulated in 1862 that lipid infiltration into the arterial wall was the prime cause of atherosclerotic lesions. This hypothesis was fortified in 1913 by Anitschkow, who demonstrated that a diet with unnaturally high cholesterol levels induced atherosclerosis in rabbits and that correction of the diet caused the lesions to regress. Gofman and colleagues, in 1950, described a method for characterizing the lipoproteins of blood serum by ultracentrifugation. Fredrickson, Levy, and Lees (1967) suggested a system for classifying the hyperlipoproteinemias using Roman numerals I through V.

INCIDENCE

Atherosclerosis may be seen during childhood as a result of certain very rare disorders such as progeria and some of the genetic mucopolysaccharidoses (see Chapter 41). Accelerated vascular aging may also accompany juvenile diabetes or hypothyroidism.

Genetically transmitted hyperlipidemias are also encountered in childhood. Of the five recognized varieties (Table 43), only types II and IV are important in childhood. Although it is estimated that only 1%–5% of the overall population has genetic hyperlipidemia, this group accounts for approximately one-third of the coronary artery disease manifested clinically before 50 years of age.

Type I hyperlipoproteinemia occurs in childhood as abdominal colic. Eruptive xanthomas on the abdomen, buttocks, and mucous membranes, as well as lipemia retinalis, are present. This disorder has not been found to predispose to early vascular disease. The characteristic symptoms and the turbidity of the plasma both respond promptly to complete removal of dietary fat.

Type II, the most common of the hyperlipoproteinemias, is also known as familial hyper-β-lipoproteinemia, familial hypercholesterolemia, and famil-

Table 43. The Frederickson-Lees classification of hyperlipoproteinemias

Type	Lipoprotein abnormality	Prevalence[a] 0–19 years (percentage)	Clinical features			
			Coronary arteries	Peripheral arteries	Xanthomas	Other
I	Chylomicrons elevated	0	0	0	0	Abdominal pain
IIa	β-lipoproteins elevated	67	+	?	+	Aortic stenosis
IIb	β- and pre-β-lipoproteins elevated	3				
III	Abnormal β-lipoproteins	1	+	+	+	
IV	pre-β-lipoproteins elevated	28	+	+	0	Often obese
V	Chylomicrons + pre-β-lipoproteins elevated	1	?	?	0	

[a] Based on 90 children seen by Neill, C. A., Ose, L., and Kwiterovich, P. O., Jr. 1977. Hyperlipidemia: Clinical clues in the first two decades of life. Johns Hopkins Med. J. 140:171. Copyright, Johns Hopkins University Press, 1977.

ial xanthomatosis. As these names imply, it is characterized by elevated serum cholesterol levels and an increased β-lipoprotein band on electrophoresis. Patients with the rare homozygous form of this disorder usually develop xanthomas on the extensor tendons of the hand, the Achilles tendon, and the tibial tuberosities early in life. Clinically evident coronary artery disease may also occur in early childhood, often by 10 years of age.

Type III is a rare disorder inherited as an autosomal recessive. It occurs primarily in obese adults with glucose intolerance.

Type IV is often associated with obesity, hyperuricemia, glucose intolerance, and premature coronary arteriosclerosis. It may be secondary to diabetes mellitus, hyperthyroidism, dysglobulinemia, obstructive liver disease, or the nephrotic syndrome.

Type V has all of the clinical manifestations of Type I except that it occurs in adults.

RISK FACTORS

A number of factors have been associated with premature coronary artery disease. The most important appears to be *hypertension,* which greatly accelerates vascular aging, especially when associated with elevated cholesterol levels. Cigarette smoking, excess intake of animal fats, obesity, and lack of exercise have all been linked to an increased risk of coronary heart disease. Moderate consumption of coffee and alcohol, marital status, and family size (possible indicators of emotional stress) are apparently unrelated to excess risk.

Personality factors have been postulated as a risk factor by Friedman and Rosenman, who suggested that the "Type A" personality has an increased rate of myocardial infarction. The Type A individual is described as having a sense of time urgency manifested by rapid speech, walking, and eating, and impatience with the rate at which most events take place. They also frequently try to do two or more things simultaneously and have difficulty trying to relax. One obvious difficulty with attempts to prove (or disprove) personality or stress linkages to a disease is that such profiles are rarely pure. Also, Type A personalities tend to smoke more and have poorer health habits.

Correlations of risk with *exercise* levels have also been difficult to prove. In any given category some workers are more active than others and many have additional risk factors. Exercise programs often show a higher initial rate of sudden deaths, especially among middle-aged, previously sedentary males. There is some evidence that fit and active people are spared the complications of atherosclerosis. The amount of long-distance running or similar activity needed for such protection is uncertain but would appear to be equal to running several miles each day. Lower levels of exercise may make the runners or joggers feel better, but we do not know if they offer any protection against ischemic heart disease.

The National Heart and Lung Institute reported "The idea that regular physical exercise decreases the danger of death or disability from coronary atherosclerotic disease is based on a number of assumptions, some proven and some of questionable validity. . . . But there is no convincing data to indicate that exercise will, in fact, decrease either the rate of development of atherosclerosis, or prevent its complications."

Tobacco has been incriminated as a risk factor, but no direct proof has been provided to show that cigarette smoking is in itself atherogenic.

Diabetes mellitus also appears to be a risk factor. It is difficult to implicate the associated hypertriglyceridemia itself, since, although blood sugar levels may be well controlled in the diabetic patient, the atherosclerotic process may continue to advance. Probably some undisclosed diabetic factor causes the premature atherosclerosis.

Obese subjects have shown a modest excess of coronary disease in most studies. This increased disease may be due not to excess weight as such but to two complications of obesity—diabetes and hypertension.

A major advance in risk identification was made by Goldstein et al., who demonstrated that 50% of survivors of acute myocardial infarction under 60 years were *hyperlipemic* when studied approximately 3 months after the attack. One-half of this group were found to be from families with genetically dominant hyperlipemias. Two disorders characterized by Goldstein, familial hypercholesterolemia and familial mixed hyperlipidemia (increased cholesterol and triglycerides), were associated with premature coronary artery disease in family members.

Measurements of high density lipoprotein (HDL) fractions by either ultracentrifugation or by selective lipoprotein precipitation are generally available and useful to clinicians. Elevation of HDL cholesterol is inversely correlated with coronary artery disease and levels of HDL are widely variant in childhood. Therefore, evaluation of pediatric hypercholesterolemia should include determinations of both low and high density lipoprotein cholesterol. Measuring only one type may be one reason for reports of individuals with hypercholesterolemia but without heart disease.

DIET AND HEART DISEASE

Many of the current dietary recommendations on lipids were based on experimental findings in animals given diets to which their species are not naturally accustomed. Extrapolation of these data to humans assumes human diets have an equally deleterious effect when used for a longer time span.

A predominant role of genetic factors in the determination of plasma lipids is not supported by study of population groups. Most hypercholesterolemia is not due to familial hyperlipoproteinemias or to polygenic traits. Rather, current evidence suggests that the level of plasma cholesterol is determined by the intake of dietary cholesterol, saturated and polyunsaturated fat, and total calories. Many investigators believe that the development, progression, and regression of atherosclerosis are closely, if not causally, related to the resultant plasma cholesterol level.

In four dietary modification trials, there were significant lowering of plasma cholesterol and suggestive, but not unequivocal, reduction in coronary artery disease. The relatively small clinical trials to date may have failed to detect a substantial effect on coronary heart disease, since they began in adults whose atherosclerosis was advanced and probably irreversible.

Possibly too much emphasis has been placed on lipids as a cause of atherosclerosis; only 20% of patients admitted to a coronary care unit has an ''abnormal'' serum lipid profile. However, in all fairness lipid values now considered ''normal'' might actually be too high, because within the usual range of cholesterol values there is a fivefold range of risk proportional to the level. Two well-designed recent studies showed that, although niacin or clofibrate reduced cholesterolemia by 15%–20%, neither drug had a measurable effect on the pattern of coronary heart disease during the 5 years of observation. Since the effect of drugs on cholesterolemia is about twice that achieved by rigorous dietary modification, dietary modification alone is unlikely to do as well. Furthermore, several cholesterol-lowering drugs have been abandoned because of adverse reactions, including more deaths in the treated than in the control groups.

The Cordays caution that most changes in mortality from heart disease should be attributed not solely to a change in lifestyle, but also to the fact that people are now living to an age when pathologic lesions and symptoms of atherosclerosis become clinically evident. The late Isadore Snapper taught in 1940 that atherosclerosis was not a clinical problem in China because the Chinese ate a nonatherogenic diet. We now learn that there is a high incidence of coronary disease in China. While there has been no documented change in the general diet, life expectancy was less than 33 years at the time Snapper lived in China, but now the population survives to an average age of 56 years.

To present another side to this controversy, epidemiological studies have suggested that a reduction both in serum cholesterol intake and in the incidence of heart disease occurs when saturated fat intake is lowered. Similarly, one might cite the reduction in myocardial infarction in a Finnish mental hospital study, where greatest benefit was obtained in hypercholesterolemic young males.

Mortality from coronary heart disease has been on the decline since 1964. This decrease has been most marked in the 35–54-year-old age group, where a 27% decrease in coronary mortality occurred between 1963 and 1975. In 1964, the Surgeon General of the Public Health Service warned of the health hazards of smoking. A few months later the American Heart Association recommended a change in the general American diet, limiting intake of saturated fat and cholesterol. Effective antihypertensive therapy also became available shortly after this. There has also been an increased public awareness of the need to seek earlier care for hypertension. In many communities mobile coronary care units were organized. Between 1963 and 1975 there was a decrease of 57% in the per capita consumption of animal fats and oils and an increase of 44% in vegetable fats and oils. Smaller decreases were reported for tobacco, milk, butter, and eggs. It is of course impossible to determine which, if any, of these factors has been responsible for the decline in coronary and cerebrovascular mortality rates.

RISK FACTOR INTERVENTION IN CHILDHOOD

Intimal thickening of the coronary arteries may begin before birth and progress through a latent period until it produces clinical manifestations in middle age. Once these changes produce clinical manifestations they apparently cannot be reversed. Most persons treated for coronary heart disease are 50 years old or older when the disorder first becomes evident. Whyte has used the Framingham experience to calculate the advantage to be expected if cholesterolemia were reduced for 20 years, by whatever means. His calculations show that there would be only a tiny advantage in young adult males, and none in men past 55 years of age.

At present, there is no conclusive evidence that correction of single risk factors will prevent atherosclerotic heart disease. Quoting again from the National Heart and Lung Institute report: "Despite evidence that combinations of risk factors increase the risk of atherosclerosis and its complications there is, as yet, no conclusive evidence that intervention with respect to normalizing these risk factors will reduce the risk of atherosclerosis."

If changes in diet are able to affect the course of the disease, this probably should be started in the pediatric age group. However, the benefits of major dietary alterations are still unproved and risks are unknown. For instance, the use of fat-free milk has been challenged because dietary practices that cause relative hypocholesterolemia during the first few months of life may lead to abnormal development of the brain and nervous system. Before large scale intervention is attempted, studies are needed to determine whether measures to alter the diets of infants are safe or if long-term dietary changes are potentially harmful.

RECOMMENDATIONS

For the present it would appear advisable to identify and treat the 5 to 10% of children with plasma cholesterol levels over 220 mg/dl. In these children, high blood pressure and obesity should be treated, if present, and smoking discouraged. Measurements of serum cholesterol and triglycerides should be obtained from all first degree relatives of adults with premature myocardial infarction. This is advisable even if the relatives are asymptomatic and clinically healthy. Lipoprotein typing should be an integral part of the routine evaluation of infants and young adults who have a threatening family history of early coronary heart disease in first degree relatives.

About one in 500 children is heterozygous for hypercholesterolemia, and at serious risk of premature cardiovascular disease. For these patients, vigorous attempts should be made to lower serum cholesterol by dietary and pharmacological means.

Finally, we agree with Kannel, who stated: "Until more data on the efficacy of preventive measures becomes available, the practicing physician must decide for himself whether sufficient rationale for intervention exists. He must weigh the hazards against the potential benefits. . . . If he elects to proceed on the incomplete evidence available, he can take comfort in the fact that the measures advocated are good health practices and have other benefits. Who can seriously argue with the general merit of a program that advocates maintenance of lean body weight, a less rich diet, physical fitness, giving up cigarettes, and control of hypertension, diabetes, and hyperlipidemia?" Most physicians would agree that there is no harm in advising any patient to follow a prudent diet and lifestyle. Physicians often must make decisions in the absence of absolutely conclusive scientific proof. A reasoned resolution of the diet/heart controversy is not currently possible.

BIBLIOGRAPHY

Corday, E., and Corday, S. R. 1975. Prevention of heart disease by control of risk factors: The time has come to face the facts. Am. J. Cardiol. 35:330–338.

Editorial. 1974. Can I avoid a heart attack? Lancet 1:605.

Gluck, C. J., Mattson, F., and Bierman, E. L. 1978. Diet and coronary heart disease: another view. N. Engl. J. Med. 298:1471–1474.

Goldstein, J. L., Hazzard, W. R., Schrott, D. G., Bierman, E. L., and Motulshy, A. G. 1972. Trans. Assoc. Am. Physicians 85:120–138.

Kannel, W. B. 1974. Prevention of coronary heart disease by control of risk factors (questions and answers). JAMA 227:338.

Mann, G. V. 1977. Diet-Heart: End of an Era. N. Engl. J. Med. 297:644–650.

National Heart and Lung Institute Task Force on Arteriosclerosis. 1971. Arteriosclerosis: A Report of the National Heart and Lung Institute Task Force on Arteriosclerosis, National Institute of Health, Vol. II. U.S. Government Printing Office, Washington, D.C.

Neill, C. A., Ose, L., and Kwiterovich, P. O., Jr. 1977. Hyperlipidemia: Clinical clues in the first two decades of life. Johns Hopkins Med. J. 140:171–176.

Schubert, W. K. 1973. Fat, nutrition and diet in childhood. Am. J. Cardiol. 31:581–587.

Walker, W. J. 1977. Changing United States lifestyle and declining vascular mortality: cause or coincidence? N. Engl. J. Med. 297:163–165.

chapter 37

INFECTIVE ENDOCARDITIS

The term bacterial endocarditis has been supplanted by the more technically correct "infective endocarditis," since the responsible agent may be a bacteria or a fungus. Infective endocarditis is usually differentiated into acute and subacute varieties. This classification, based primarily on duration, has some clinical significance, since acute bacterial endocarditis generally lasts less than 6 weeks and is caused by a different spectrum of bacteria. However, clear differentiation is not always possible, and at present there appears to be increasing overlap in the organisms encountered in each group. Classification is particularly difficult when acute bacterial endocarditis is superimposed on a preexisting cardiac lesion. From a clinical standpoint, it would appear preferable to classify infective endocarditis as to whether or not there is underlying cardiac pathology.

HISTORICAL NOTES

Although there were descriptions of what would appear to have been bacterial endocarditis as early as 1554 by Fernel, clear distinction between rheumatic and bacterial endocarditis is credited to Matthew Baillie, in 1797. William Senhouse Kirkes in 1852 first attributed systemic emboli to vegetations on the heart valve. By 1870, bacteriology had progressed far enough so that Winge and Keiberg were able to recognize microorganisms in valvar vegetations at necropsy.

In 1885, Osler analyzed 109 cases of malignant endocarditis and recognized that healed rheumatic valvulitis was a frequent precursor. Horder, in 1905, described a method for obtaining blood cultures and had grown a streptococcus from blood in such a case. Leo Loewe, in 1943, successfully treated seven cases of bacterial endocarditis with the then new drug, penicillin.

INCIDENCE

Infective endocarditis constitutes between 0.5% and 2% of autopsy material in a number of hospitals. It accounts for between five and 34 of each 10,000 hospital admissions. These admission rates have decreased at some but not all large centers over the past 40 years, and apparently have been affected little by antibiotics.

The mean age of incidence has increased in recent years and now lies between 50–54 years. A slight excess of males over females has been reported. Infective endocarditis is uncommon in the first decade of life. Before 2 years of age it is rare and, when seen, is usually of the acute variety attacking normal valves, especially the tricuspid.

The highest incidence of infective endocarditis occurs between January and March.

PATHOGENESIS

Over 90% of affected patients have evidence of underlying heart disease. The most common cardiac problem is rheumatic in origin. The relative importance

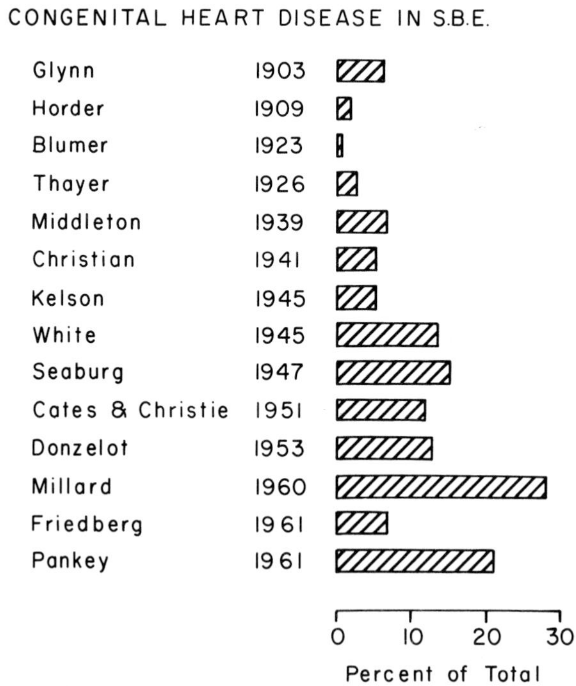

Figure 224. Incidence of congenital heart disease in various large series of bacterial endocarditis. The relative importance of congenital heart disease has been increasing, probably as a result of a declining incidence of rheumatic heart disease.

of congenital heart disease has been increasing recently, and ranges from 12% to 28% in recent series (Figure 224).

The most common congenital cardiac anomalies underlying infective endocarditis are ventricular septal defect, tetralogy of Fallot, patent ductus arteriosus, and a bicuspid aortic valve (Table 44). Although atrial septal defect (secundum) is the fifth most common congenital heart anomaly, it is very rarely seen with infective endocarditis.

Acute infective endocarditis develops from a septic focus and results in metastatic infection at many sites, one of which is the heart. *Streptococcus viridans* endocarditis is usually dental in origin, even when no recent extraction or poor dental hygiene is detectable (Table 45). *Streptococcus viridans* is regularly present in the mouth, and a transient bacteremia has been shown to follow dental extractions, rocking a tooth in its socket, and even chewing paraffin. Other minor surgical procedures also followed by transient bacteremia include tonsillectomy (28%–38%), bronchoscopy (15%), and sigmoidoscopy.

Transient bacteremias occur frequently in all individuals and are usually of little clinical significance. Disturbed blood flow, such as occurs with valve damage or left-to-right shunts, is frequently accompanied by sterile platelet fibrin thrombi at the site of endothelial damage. In the presence of a sufficient inoculum of bacteria, circulating agglutinins may cause the bacteria to clump and adhere to a sterile platelet-fibrin deposit, which favors multiplication of the bacteria.

Focal embolic glomerulonephritis, previously thought to result from multiple small emboli, is now considered a hypersensitivity vasculitis. It is also likely that the arthralgia and arthritis seen in some patients are a result of the

Table 44. Incidence of congenital heart anomalies associated with infective endocarditis

		Type of anomaly[a]						
Report	Year	VSD	PDA	BAV	TOF	COA	PS	ASD
Abbott	1926	13	21	9	0	7	5	2
Gelfman	1942	13	4	11	2	1	5	0
Cates	1951	22	11	7	0	1	2	1
Cutler	1958	7	8	0	10	3	2	1
Blumenthal	1960	3	1	0	5	3	1	0
Friedberg	1961	1	1	1	2	1	0	0
Vogler	1962	15	7	3	7	1	1	0
Subtotals		74	53	31	26	17	16	4

[a] Key: VSD = ventricular septal defect; PDA = patent ductus arteriosus; BAV = bicuspid aortic valve; TOF = tetralogy of Fallot; COA = coarctation of the aorta; PS = pulmonic stenosis; ASD = atrial septal defect.

Table 45. Noncardiac underlying disease in patients with infective endocarditis[a]

	Incidence
Post-dental extraction infection	6%
Urologic infection	5%
Previous infective endocarditis	9%
Addiction	4%
Diabetes	7%
Postoperative infection	
Cardiac surgery	9%
Noncardiac surgery	2%
Miscellaneous	14%
None	42%

[a] After Cherubin, C. E., and Neu, H. C. 1971. Infective endocarditis at the Presbyterian Hospital in New York City from 1938–1967. Am. J. Med. 51:83.

deposition of circulating immune-complex components in the synovia. Osler's nodes, Janeway lesions, Roth spots, subungual hemorrhages, and even petechiae are now thought to be manifestations of an allergic vasculitis involving small arteries.

PROPHYLAXIS

The current recommendations of the American Heart Association for all patients with known heart disease are:

1. One hour before surgery or dental work, give 1,200,000 units of procaine penicillin I.M. or penicillin V 500 mg orally. Follow this with:
   One tablet of penicillin V 250 units orally, 4 hours after surgery and four times a day for 3 days (12 doses); *or*
   Procaine penicillin 600,000 units I.M. daily for 2 days.
2. If the patient is allergic to penicillin or has been on long-term oral penicillin for prevention of recurrent rheumatic fever, give:
   Erythromycin 500 mg or 20 mg/kg orally, 4 hours preoperatively; *then*
   Erythromycin 250 mg or 10 mg/kg/dose, four times a day for 3 days.

CLINICAL FEATURES

Fever and malaise are almost invariably present. In the absence of fever, the presence of subacute bacterial endocarditis is quite unlikely, *unless there is associated renal involvement.* Approximately *40% of Vogler and Dorney's patients never developed any manifestations of infective endocarditis other than fever and malaise*. This makes it incumbent on the physician to obtain blood cultures in patients with known heart disease and fever of unknown origin.

Recent weight loss is also a common complaint. Symptoms of respiratory tract infection ranging from sinusitis to pleuritic chest pains are found in an additional 20% of patients. The remaining patients will present primarily with petechiae, hematuria, and evidence of embolization.

A significant murmur, due to the underlying cardiac disease, is often heard. When the picture is complicated by severe congestive heart failure, however, the murmur may be soft and not easily appreciated. A changing murmur is often mistakenly considered to be characteristic of subacute bacterial endocarditis; it was in reference to acute endocarditis that this sign was described. When the murmur does change in subacute bacterial endocarditis, it is an unequivocal event and usually *consists of the development of a new murmur*.

Splenomegaly is found in approximately one-half of patients and hepatomegaly in about one-third. Congestive heart failure is present in approximately one-third of patients, and approximately one-third will have petechiae, especially in nailbeds or conjunctiva. Osler's nodules, which are "ephemeral spots of a painful nodular erythema," are extremely rare in the pediatric age group. Except for congestive heart failure, arterial emboli are the most frequent complications of infective endocarditis. According to Weinstein and Schlesinger, the clinically detected incidence of these emboli has decreased from between 70% and 97% before antibiotic therapy to between 15% and 35% at present. Splenic and/or renal emboli have been discovered in about one-half of fatal cases, but are less often recognized clinically.

Embolic phenomena occur relatively late in the course of the disease. A splenic infarct may be detected by listening for a friction rub over the spleen. Renal infarction is accompanied by pain, and urinalysis will show albuninuria, red cells, casts, or white cells. It is frequently unappreciated that bacterial endocarditis may present with neurological manifestations. Major cerebral emboli occur in nearly one-third of patients with infective endocarditis. In one series, 20% of patients were believed initially to have neurological problems. The most frequent signs of neurological disease are hemiplegia or hemiparesis, meningitis, cranial nerve palsies, and ocular hemorrhages.

LABORATORY FINDINGS

A low hemoglobin concentration is found in over one-half of patients. The white blood cell count is extremely variable and is clearly elevated in approximately three-fourths of the cases. The latex fixation test is sometimes positive in endocarditis.

S. viridans is by far the most common organism in the pediatric age range, being present more than 60% of the time. Postoperative patients are more apt to have *Staphylococcus aureus* or enterococci as the infecting organism. *Staphylococcus epidermidis* has become more common, related almost entirely to its occurrence following cardiac surgery. Enterococci and *S. epidermidis* are found in diabetic patients three to five times more frequently than in nondiabetic patients. Patients with urologic infection and endocarditis will have an enterococcus about one-third of the time. Although septicemia today is commonly caused by Enterobacteriaceae, gram-negative bacteria are infrequent as etiologic agents for infective endocarditis. Failure to identify the causative organism, despite two or more blood cultures, ranged from 4% to 25% in recent series.

It is important to realize that even a single blood culture gives a high percentage of positive results. In Cates and Christie's series, 82% of the positive cultures were positive in the first attempt. If the culture is going to be positive, it is rare that it will not be detected in the first few cultures. Since the bacteremia is continuous, it is not necessary to obtain blood cultures at the time of temperature elevations.

MANAGEMENT

Treatment should begin as early as possible, before the vegetations are covered by a thick fibrin-platelet shield. As a general rule, we attempt to secure five blood cultures within the first 24 hr, but do not delay treatment while awaiting results of the cultures.

The more typical the case of bacterial endocarditis, the sooner the correct diagnosis will be made. On the other hand, the most favorable outcome will be in those patients who are treated prior to the onset of many of the manifestations of the disease. In Friedberg's study seven of the 10 deaths occurred in patients who had symptoms for more than 4 months before diagnosis and treatment. Furthermore, congestive heart failure and/or cerebral embolism occurred in only 13% of those with symptoms of less than 2 weeks duration, and in 17% of those with symptoms of 2 to 4 weeks duration, but in 30% of those with symptoms that had been present for more than 4 weeks. If a patient has fever of unknown origin with an elevated ESR, mild anemia, a murmur, and some petechiae, treatment should be started without waiting for the isolation of the causative organism.

A treatment schedule for various organisms is given in Table 46. Bacteriostatic drugs should never be used alone, but should be supplemented by bactericidal drugs. Plate dilution tests are recommended for proper selection of antibiotics. Dosage can be best evaluated by in vitro bacterial testing of the patient's serum against the organism cultured.

Table 46. Therapy for bacterial endocarditis

Organism	Drug	Dose
Streptococcus viridans	Penicillin	1–5 million[a] units i.v. q6h for a minimum of 3 weeks
	Streptomycin	1 g q12h for 2 weeks
Enterococci	Penicillin	20–40 million units i.v. daily for 4–6 weeks
	Streptomycin[b]	1.0 g q12h for 3 weeks, then 1.0 g daily for 3 weeks
Staphylococci	Methicillin or oxacillin	6–12 g/day i.v. for 6 weeks i.v. for 6 weeks

[a] Dosage dependent on sensitivity of organism.
[b] If not sensitive to streptomycin, use kanamycin or gentamicin.

Since penicillin is often the drug of choice, the problem of the patient who is sensitive to penicillin is most important. It is vital to take an accurate history. Many times, a diagnosis of penicillin sensitivity proves to have been made on tenuous grounds. If the previous reaction was unequivocal, then cephalothin or vancomycin should be used.

When no organism is cultured, treatment should be based on several considerations. Since *S. viridans* is the most likely causative organism, penicillin should be included in the treatment of any bacterial endocarditis in this category. This is particularly true if the disease has followed dental or oral surgery. If gastrointestinal or genitourinary surgery preceded the onset of bacterial endocarditis, then suspicion should rest on an enterococcus or a coliform organism. The staphylococcus organism occurs most commonly after intracardiac surgery or skin infections. If the infected site is on prosthetic material, it must be removed.

There has been a recent trend to treat patients with oral penicillin. We prefer parenteral treatment initially and oral penicillin during the last 2 to 3 weeks of treatment *only if the organism is extremely sensitive to penicillin.*

After the recommended course of therapy is completed, it is wise to obtain repeated blood cultures, and to discontinue therapy only if three consecutive blood cultures are negative.

RESULTS OF TREATMENT

In the preantibiotic era, the spontaneous cure rate of bacterial endocarditis was about 0.5%. Sulfonamide therapy increased the cure rate to approximately

5%. The cure rate in the early antibiotic era was approximately 60% and later increased to an average of 80%. There has been relatively little improvement in overall survival rates during the last 20 years, largely because we are treating older, more precariously ill patients year by year (Figure 225).

Table 47 lists major causes of death in various series. One of the major reasons for onset of congestive heart failure is rupture of a heart valve or chordae tendineae.

Morgan and Bland reported on later complications of bacterial endocarditis. The mean annual death rate in their study averaged 5%–7%. These findings were in accord with the earlier studies of Cates and Christie, who found the death rate to be 4% per annum.

Congenital heart disease is significantly more frequent in patients with multiple episodes of subacute bacterial endocarditis than in those with single episodes. Patients with congenital heart disease also have an apparently greater rate of reinfection than patients with other types of heart disease. Whether this apparent increased susceptibility is due to special hemodynamic alterations or to a longer period at risk is undetermined. We recommend surgical closure of even small VSD's after one episode of subacute bacterial endocarditis, since we estimate that the risk of death for such patients is higher

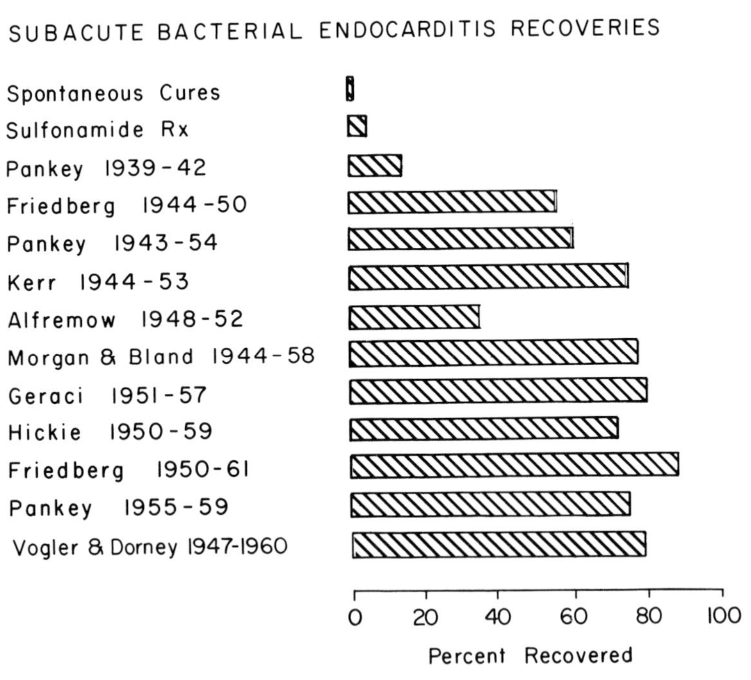

Figure 225. Summary of short-term hospital cures of subacute bacterial endocarditis. Note that in the more recent series the cure rate seems to have stabilized at about 80%.

Table 47. Major causes of deaths associated with bacterial endocarditis

Report	Year	Total patients	Number of deaths	Percentage	Cause[a]				
					CHF	Emb	Uremia	CH	RI
Anderson and Keefer	1948	457	149	32	33	22	3	5	53
Friedberg	1950	148	50	34	29	13	6	0	6
Cates and Christie	1951	408	108	24	50	13	14	10	25
Morgan and Bland	1959	175	56	32	32	21	5	6	0
Friedberg	1961	87	10	11	5	4	1	0	0
Vogler and Dorney[b]	1962	38	8	21	4	2	0	1	1

[a] Key: CHF = coronary heart failure; Emb = embolism; CH = cerebral hemorrhage; RI = resistant infection.
[b] Series included only patients with congenital anomalies.

than operative mortality. Admittedly, however, not all pediatric cardiologists agree with this approach.

BIBLIOGRAPHY

Blumenthal, S., Griffiths, S. P., and Morgan, B. C. 1960. Bacterial endocarditis in children with heart disease. A review based on the literature and experience with 58 cases. Pediatrics 26:993–1017.

Cherubin, C. E., and Neu, H. C. 1971. Infective endocarditis at the Presbyterian Hospital in New York City from 1938-1967. Am. J. Med. 51:83-96.

Diamond, E. F. 1973. Quiet clues to bacterial endocarditis in children. Resident and Staff Physician (Dec.):28–32.

Kaplan, E. L., et al. 1977. (American Heart Association Committee Report): Prevention of bacterial endocarditis. Circulation 56:139A–143A.

Levinson, M. E., Kaye, D., Mandell, G. L., and Hook, E. W. 1970. Characteristics of patients with multiple episodes of bacterial endocarditis. JAMA 211:1355–1357.

Morgan, W. L., and Bland, E. F. 1959. Bacterial endocarditis in the antibiotic era with special references to the later complications. Circulation 753–765.

Wann, L. S., Dillon, J. C., Weyman, A. E., and Feigenbaum, H. 1976. Echocardiography in bacterial endocarditis. N. Engl. J. Med. 295:135–139.

Washington, J. A. 1975. Blood cultures: principles and techniques. Mayo Clin. Proc. 50:91–98.

Weinstein, L., and Schlesinger, J. J. 1974. Pathoanatomic, pathophysiologic and clinical correlations in endocarditis. N. Engl. J. Med. 191:832–837, 1122–1126.

chapter 38

BRAIN ABSCESS IN ASSOCIATION WITH CONGENITAL HEART ANOMALIES

HISTORICAL NOTES

This complication of congenital heart lesions has been recognized for many years. The association was first reported by Farre in 1814.

INCIDENCE

Brain abscess occurs in about 2% of cases of cyanotic congenital heart lesions. Approximately 10% of cases of brain abscess are associated with a cardiac anomaly.

Brain abscess is extremely rare under the age of 2 years. Approximately one-half of all cases occur between 2 and 10 years of age.

The sex incidence is equal.

PATHOLOGY

Two predisposing factors are usually found.

1. *Right-to-left shunt,* which allows bacteria direct access to the brain. The shunt negates the filtering effect on blood of passage through the lungs. Although all cases have a right-to-left shunt, clinically apparent cyanosis need not be present.
2. *Underlying brain damage.* Bacterial contamination alone is not usually sufficient to cause an abscess. Animal experiments have shown that direct inoculation of bacteria into the carotid artery will not cause a brain abscess. In children with cyanotic congenital heart disease, it is thought

that cerebral phlebitis, related to small repeated thromboses, is responsible for causing the initial predisposing damage.

The abscess may occur in any part of the brain. Brain abscess is rarely associated with infectious endocarditis in spite of the presence of bacteremia in the latter. The source of the infection is determined in only 40% of cases of brain abscess.

The most frequently cultured organism is *Streptococcus hemolyticus,* followed by the staphylococci. Hemophilus influenzae, pneumococci, actinomycetes, and coliform organisms have also been isolated.

In the majority of cases, the associated heart anomaly is tetralogy of Fallot, reflecting the predominance of this anomaly among cyanotic congenital heart disease patients over 3 years of age.

CLINICAL FEATURES

Usually there is a *gradual onset* lasting 7 to 10 days, which consists of such general signs as fever, lethargy, and anorexia. A history of a preceding infection elsewhere in the body can often be elicited. Although most patients will have fever and leucocytosis, bacteria are rarely grown from blood or cerebrospinal fluid cultures.

In the early stages, diagnosis may be difficult. Symptoms and signs of *increased intracranial pressure*, headache (frequently localized over the site of the abscess), vomiting, impairment of sensorium, and behavior changes may not be present until late in the course of the disease.

Convulsions, frequently focal in nature, are prominent presenting complaints. Other focal neurological abnormalities may also appear, including visual field deficits and motor and sensory disturbances.

Slowing of the pulse, depressed respirations, and an enlarged pupil on the ipsilateral side are grave signs, indicating brain stem compression.

DIAGNOSTIC PROCEDURES

Any child over 2 years of age with cyanotic heart disease and cerebral symptoms should be considered as having a brain abscess until proven otherwise. Since the lesion is usually of short duration, plain skull films are rarely helpful. In chronic cases, suture separation will be seen. The electroencephalogram will help to localize the site of tbe abscess by showing characteristic slow wave activity in the affected region. Echoencephalography may indicate a shift of the midline structures. Computerized axial tomography is now the definitive method for defining a brain abscess. When clinical evidence of increased intracranial pressure is present, a lumbar puncture carries risks of herniation and brain stem compression. A lumbar puncture should be performed only when specifically indicated in the individual patient.

TREATMENT

Prognosis is related to rapidity in diagnosis and treatment. Mortality is significant and about one-half of survivors have residual neurological damage. Antibiotic therapy should be initiated as soon as the diagnosis is considered, but the value of this is uncertain once abscess formation has begun. The treatment is neurosurgical and repeated aspirations are generally satisfactory.

Prevention is accomplished by anatomic correction of the cardiac anomaly prior to age 2, when feasible.

BIBLIOGRAPHY

Calkins, R. A., and Ball, W. E. 1967. Cerebral abscess and cyanotic congenital heart disease. Lancet 87:403–410.

Fischbein, C. A., Rosenthal, A., Fischer, E. G., Nadas, A. S., and Welch, K. 1974. Risk factors for brain abscess in patients with congenital heart disease. Am. J. Cardiol. 34:97–102.

Matson, D. D., and Salam, M. 1961. Brain abscess in congenital heart disease. Pediatrics 27:772–789.

Raimondi, A. J., Matsumoto, S., and Miller, R. A. 1965. Brain abscess in children with congenital heart disease Int. J. Neurosurg. 23:588–595.

chapter 39

DISEASES OF THE PERICARDIUM

ACUTE PERICARDITIS

Historical Notes

Pericarditis was first described in the Middle Ages, before most other forms of heart disease were known or understood. Laennec, in 1819, in discussing acute pericarditis noted that "there are few diseases attended by more variable symptoms, or of more difficult diagnosis, than this."

Incidence

Pericarditis is found in 4%–5% of postmortem examinations. The age distribution by type is given in Table 48.

Clinical Features

The most characteristic feature of acute pericarditis is the friction rub—a grating, superficial extracardiac sound of high frequency and varying inten-

Table 48. Relative incidence of pericarditis by age groups

Type	Under 2 years	2–5 years	5–10 years	Over 10 years	Total cases
Rheumatic	0	6	56	67	129
Rheumatoid	2	6	0	0	8
Septic	30	11	17	9	67
Tuberculous	1	3	3	0	7
Idiopathic (acute, benign)	0	7	5	1	13

sity. In its classical form, this rub consists of three distinct components (Figure 226). When the ventricles contract, the damaged pericardial surfaces slide against each other, producing the systolic component of the friction rub. When the ventricles relax, the injured pericardial surfaces again slide against each other, and this sound is the early diastolic component of the friction rub. In late diastole, when the atria contract, the atrial component of the friction rub is produced.

Any one of these three components may be present alone, or they may exist in any combination. The diagnosis is most definitive when all three components are noted. Effusions often accompany pericarditis in children, and fluid may separate the adhering surfaces and cause the rub to disappear. The cardiac sounds themselves are difficult to hear in the presence of the friction rub.

Pain may be mild, severely pleuritic in nature, or oppressive in older children, and is commonly aggravated by respiration, cough, or motion. Precordial pain is not as frequent a feature of pericarditis in children as it is in adults. This may reflect the less accurate histories offered by young children or the lower level of attention paid to symptoms in the pediatric age range.

Roentgenographic Examination

With the development of a pericardial effusion, the cardiac borders enlarge and a pear-shaped silhouette is produced. When a marked increase in cardiac shadow occurs within less than a month, it is almost always due to a pericardial effusion.

Electrocardiogram

Elevation of the ST segment may best be recognized by serial electrocardiograms, especially in left precordial leads. T waves often become flattened, and

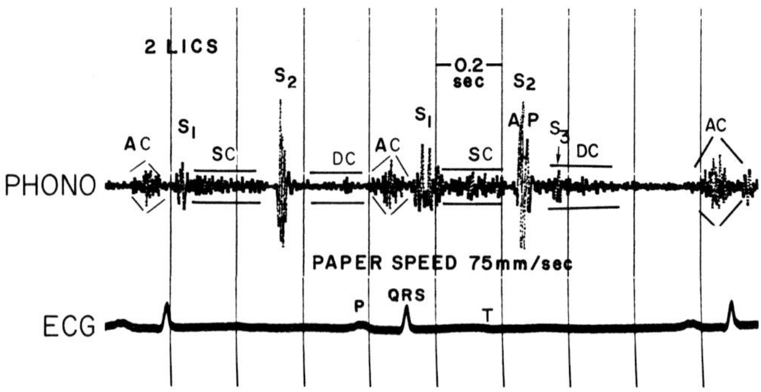

Figure 226. Electrocardiogram of a 12-year-old girl with lupus erythematosus and a pericardial friction rub. Three components of the friction rub may be distinguished: (1) a systolic component (SC) concomitant with ventricular contraction; (2) a diastolic component (DC) associated with ventricular relaxation; and (3) an atrial component (AC) with atrial contraction.

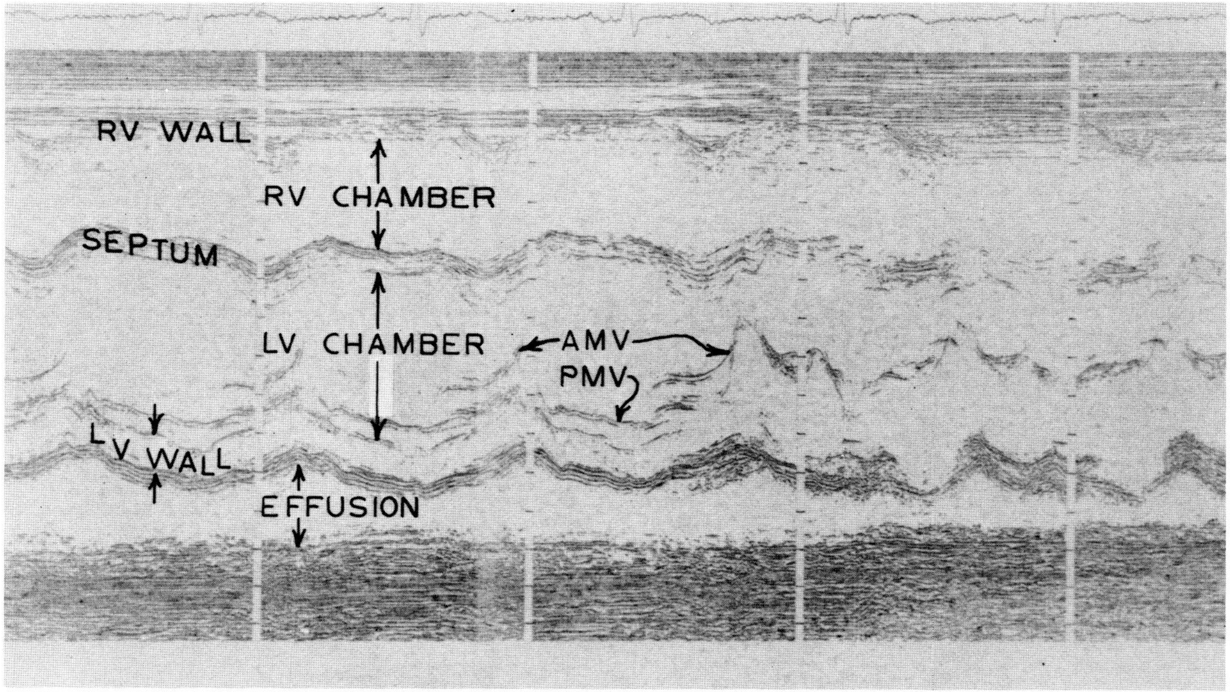

Figure 227. Echocardiogram of a patient with pericardial effusion. The extra reflection behind the posterior wall of the left ventricle is the pericardium.

even inverted. The amplitudes of the QRS and T waves are frequently diminished in the presence of pericardial effusion.

Echocardiography

The visceral and parietal layers of the pericardium are normally 1–2 mm apart at the peak of the anterior motion of the posterior ventricular wall. In the presence of a significant pericardial effusion, the parietal pericardium becomes flatter and more distinctly separate from the visceral pericardium (Figure 227).

Differential Diagnosis

Once acute pericarditis has been detected, the underlying etiology must be discovered as quickly as possible, since the treatment for the various forms differs markedly. As in all pediatric problems, age is of considerable importance in establishing the correct etiology (Table 49).

Pericarditis in a child under 2 years of age should be considered as *septic* until proven otherwise. Septic pericarditis is especially likely in a child who develops signs of congestive heart failure or shows a sudden increase in cardiac silhouette during the course of a bacterial infection. In one series, associated illnesses were present in 24 out of 25 patients with acute bacterial pericarditis.

Rheumatic pericarditis is generally accompanied by arthritis, erythema multiforme, subcutaneous nodules, or typical murmurs. (For detailed description of clinical features see Chapter 31.)

Pericarditis also commonly occurs following *surgical operations* where the pericardium has been opened.

When *rheumatoid arthritis* is the underlying etiology, there is high fever that

Table 49. Frequency of various types of pericarditis in 312 children[a]

	Frequency
Rheumatic	45%
Purulent	24%
Idiopathic (acute, benign)	11%
Rheumatoid	6%
Tuberculous	3%
Viral (Coxsackie)	1%
Constrictive	1%
Miscellaneous	9%

[a] Modified from data in Keith, J. D., Rowe, R. D., and Vlad, P. 1978. Heart Disease in Infancy and Childhood, 3rd ed. Macmillan Publishing Company, Inc., New York.

is unaffected by salicylates and transient arthritis that is eventually followed by more typical joint swellings.

Uremic pericarditis is usually obvious because of the underlying nephritis.

Acute benign idiopathic pericarditis is diagnosed largely by exclusion. The peak incidence seems to occur in the fall and the spring of each year. The onset may be insidious, with nonspecific malaise, or abrupt, with chills, fever, and sharp substernal or precordial chest pains.

Treatment

Obviously the underlying disease must be the primary focus of therapy. Therapy for rheumatic fever is outlined in Chapter 31. Early diagnosis and treatment of septic pericarditis are mandatory since progressive and lethal tamponade may occur rapidly. Septic pericarditis is best treated when the organism has been cultured directly from the pericardial fluid aspirate. Various antibiotics can be tested for sensitivity and the proper drug given in suitable doses.

PERICARDIAL EFFUSION

Some degree of effusion invariably accompanies most varieties of acute and chronic pericarditis. Rapid accumulation of 100 ml of effusion or more may produce tamponade. Muffled heart sounds, narrowed arterial pulse pressure, and rapidly increasing cardiac size are strongly suggestive of effusion. The tendency to disappearance of the radial pulse at the end of inspiration (Kussmaul's sign) is a valuable finding when present. Pulsus paradoxicus is an exaggeration of the normal respiratory variation. A drop of 15 mm Hg or more in systolic blood pressure at the end of inspiration confirms this finding. In the event of rapidly accumulating pericardial fluid, pericardiocentesis may be a lifesaving procedure.

CHRONIC CONSTRICTIVE PERICARDITIS

When the pericardium becomes thickened, inelastic, and sometimes calcified, it limits the diastolic flow of the ventricles. This is extremely rare in the pediatric age range. The clinical picture mimics that of severe right-sided heart failure. Pericardiectomy is the procedure of choice, but still carries a significant mortality rate.

POSTPERICARDIOTOMY SYNDROME

This syndrome is most likely a delayed response to surgical incision of the pericardium. The clinical picture is that of fever and chest pains, with or without a friction rub. Symptoms usually start 2 to 3 weeks after surgery.

Treatment consists of bed rest until the physical and roentgenographic signs of pleural or pericardial disease have disappeared. Aspirin will usually alleviate the precordial pain and discomfort.

BIBLIOGRAPHY

Engle, M. A., McCabe, J. C., Ebert, P. A., and Zabriskie, J. 1974. The postpericardiotomy syndrome and antiheart antibodies. Circulation 49:401–406.

Joyner, C. R., Jr., Herman, R. J., and Reid, J. M. 1967. Reflected ultrasound in the detection and localization of pleural effusion. JAMA 200:399–402.

Okoroma, E. O., Perry, L. W., and Scott, L. P., III. 1975. Acute bacterial pericarditis in children: Report of 25 cases. Am. Heart J. 90:709–713.

Shabetai, R., Fowler, N. O., and Guntheroth, W. G. 1970. The hemodynamics of cardiac tamponade and constrictive pericarditis. Am. J. Cardiology 26:480–489.

chapter 40

NEUROLOGIC DISORDERS MANIFESTING CARDIAC ABNORMALITIES

MUSCULAR DYSTROPHIES

Duchenne's pseudohypertrophic muscular dystrophy is transmitted as a sex-linked recessive disease in about 90% of cases. Initial symptoms usually occur during the first year of life. The disease is rapidly progressive, leading to total disability and death in adolescence.

Electrocardiographic abnormalities have been reported in as many as 90% of cases. These include right ventricular conduction delay, right ventricular hypertrophy, deep q waves in left precordial leads, prolonged Q-T intervals, and primary ST segment and T wave changes. Labile sinus tachycardia is a frequent finding. Premature ventricular contractions, occasionally multifocal in origin, and paroxysmal ventricular tachycardia may occur. Congestive heart failure is uncommon in children.

Pathological and biochemical findings in cardiac muscle are similar to those found in skeletal muscle. Fat and connective tissue are increased with disappearance of muscle cells. The remaining muscle cells vary greatly in size, with some being atrophied and others hypertrophied. The endocardium may be slightly thickened and endocardial fibroelastosis has been reported. One investigator has identified a noninflammatory arteriopathy of the arteries to the SA and AV nodes, with degeneration of nodal fibers. This is suggested as a possible cause of the frequent arrhythmias, as well as the occurrence of sudden death.

Limb-girdle dystrophy occurs predominantly in young adult males, and is usually inherited as an autosomal recessive. These patients may have systemic hypertension and congestive heart failure. Electrocardiographic abnormalities occur in two-thirds of cases, and are similar to but less severe than those seen in the Duchenne type. The most common are right ventricular hypertrophy, right ventricular conduction delay, and T wave changes.

Fascioscapulohumeral dystrophy is transmitted as a dominant, affecting both sexes. Cardiac abnormalities are not commonly seen in this form.

Myotonic dystrophy, another hereditary myopathy usually transmitted as a dominant, is primarily a disease of adult males. It is characterized by dystrophy of facial, neck, and lower extremity musculature, and myotonic reaction of the muscles.

The heart may show diffuse fibrosis with some hypertrophied, as well as atrophied, muscle fibers. The changes in cardiac muscle are similar to those in skeletal muscle.

Electrocardiographic abnormalities are seen in three-fourths of patients. First degree heart block, ventricular conduction delay, atrial fibrillation and flutter, atrioventricular dissociation with Stokes-Adams attacks, myocardial ischemia, and even myocardial infarction have been reported.

FRIEDREICH ATAXIA

This hereditary disorder occurs equally in both sexes. Ataxia of gait begins in childhood or early youth and progresses slowly. Scanning dysarthria typically occurs later. Deep tendon reflexes may be absent and a Babinski sign may be present. High arched feet (pes cavus or ''Friedreich foot'') and deformities of the great toes are characteristic.

Electrocardiographic abnormalities, especially arrhythmias, occur in up to 90% of patients. Premature atrial and ventricular contractions, atrial fibrillation, and atrial flutter are the most frequent arrhythmias. T wave inversion in leads aVR, V_5, and V_6 at rest that disappears with exercise is especially common. Heart failure is rare in patients under 10 years of age, but ECG abnormalities are often present in early childhood.

Cardiac involvement frequently is either the primary cause or a contributing cause of death, which occurs at an average age of 30 years. The heart shows muscle fiber hypertrophy, interstitial fibrosis, focal degeneration, and (rarely) active necrosis. A small vessel arteriopathy has been identified that involves arteries to sinoatrial and atrioventricular nodes as well as other small coronary arteries.

FAMILIAL PERIODIC PARALYSIS

This condition is probably inherited as a dominant trait, with diminished penetrance in the female. Occasional, sporadic nonfamilial cases also occur. The age at onset is 7 to 21 years in 90% of cases. The hypokalemic type, the most common, is thought to be due to a defect in carbohydrate metabolism in the muscle fiber, leading to acute and severe shifts of potassium into the cell. These cause an abrupt fall in plasma potassium concentration and electrocardiographic signs of potassium deficiency.

Typically, this disorder is characterized by acute transient paralysis of proximal musculature of the extremities and the trunk with complete freedom from symptoms between attacks. Attacks may be provoked by exercise or a high carbohydrate intake, usually occur at night and last 6 to 24 hr. Severity of attacks is extremely variable and death may occur.

Bradycardia and the electrocardiographic changes of hypokalemia (see Chapter 7) may be seen during an attack. Cases of familial periodic paralysis have been described with cardiac arrhythmias, including premature ventricular contractions and supraventricular tachycardia. While these cases otherwise resemble the hypokalemic type, serum potassium is not necessarily depressed during an attack.

Treatment consists of oral or parenteral administration of potassium (1 mEq/kg).

FAMILIAL DYSAUTONOMIA (RILEY-DAY SYNDROME)

This dysfunction of the autonomic nervous system is inherited as an autosomal recessive and occurs almost exclusively in Ashkenazic Jews. Decreased lacrimation, "crying without tears," is the most constant sign. Instability of temperature, blotching of the skin, excessive sweating, insensitivity to pain, muscular incoordination, and emotional lability are other manifestations.

Patients may have supraventricular tachycardia and transient hypertension, as well as orthostatic hypotension.

MYASTHENIA GRAVIS

This disease, predominantly seen in females, usually has its onset in late adolescence and has a high incidence of electrocardiographic abnormalities. These include flat to inverted T waves, ST segment depression (especially after exercise) and various arrhythmias, such as premature atrial and ventricular contractions and sinus tachycardia. In some cases, the electrocardiographic abnormality can be eliminated by the administration of neostigmine.

Myocardial lesions are often seen at necropsy. Interstitial fibrosis scattered through the myocardium, atrophic myocardial fibers, focal necrosis, and, on occasion, frank myocarditis have all been reported.

CEREBRAL ARTERIOVENOUS FISTULA

This may cause heart failure in the newborn. In such cases, a loud bruit can be heard on auscultation of the head.

RELATIONSHIP OF THE CENTRAL NERVOUS SYSTEM AND THE CARDIAC CONDUCTION SYSTEM

Electrocardiographic abnormalities may occur secondary to acute primary brain damage in man. For example, it has been noted that inversion of T waves and elevation of the ST segment may be seen following subarachnoid hemorrhage (due to rupture of a berry aneurysm) and that these changes frequently will revert to normal within a few days. It is also possible to produce electrocardiographic abnormalities by experimental stimulation of the brain. In the cat, electrical stimulation of the hippocampal formation and medial nuclei of the amygdala can produce ST segment and T wave changes, with prolonged Q-T interval. Repeated stimulation may result in complete heart block and ventricular fibrillation. In such animals, transection of the spinal cord at the midcervical level will restore the electrocardiogram to normal within a few seconds. Pathologic examination of the hearts of these animals reveals no abnormalities. Experiments such as these help to provide a rational basis for the association of neurologic lesions and electrocardiographic abnormalities.

BIBLIOGRAPHY

Boyer, S. H., Chisholm, A. W., and McKusick, V. A. 1962. Cardiac aspects of Friedreich's ataxia. Circulation 25:493–505.

Heymsfield, S. B., McNish, T., Perkins, J. V., and Felner, J. M. 1978. Sequence of cardiac changes in Duchenne muscular dystrophy. Am. Heart J. 95:283–294.

James, T. N., and Fisch, C. 1963. Observations on the cardiovascular involvement in Friedreich's ataxia. Am. Heart J. 66:164–175.

Kohn, P. M., Tucker, H. J., and Kozokoff, N. J. 1965. The cardiac manifestations of myasthenia gravis with particular reference to electrocardiographic abnormalities. Am. J. Med. Sci. 249:561–570.

Perloff, J. K., deLeon, A. C., Jr., and O'Doherty, D. 1966. The cardiomyopathy of progressive muscular dystrophy. Circulation 33:625–648.

Petkovich, N. J., Dunn, M., and Reed, W. 1964. Myotonia dystrophica with A-V dissociation and Stokes-Adams attacks. A case report and review of the literature. Am. Heart J. 68:391–396.

Porter, R. W., Kamikawa, K., and Greenhoot, J. H. 1962. Persistent electrocardiographic abnormalities experimentally induced by stimulation of the brain. Am. Heart J. 64: 815–819.

Van der Hauwaert, L. G., and Dumoulin, M. 1976. Hypertrophic cardiomyopathy in Friedreich's ataxia. Br. Heart J. 38:1291–1298.

Welsh, J. D., Lynn, T. N., and Haase, G. R. 1963. Cardiac findings in 73 patients with muscular dystrophy. Arch. Intern. Med. 112:199–206.

chapter 41

CONNECTIVE TISSUE DISORDERS MANIFESTING CARDIAC ABNORMALITIES

LYSOSOMAL STORAGE DISEASES (Genetic Mucopolysaccharidoses)

Lysosomal storage diseases, which result in accumulation of macromolecular compounds (mucopolysaccharides and glycoproteins) in connective tissue, result in multisystem degenerative disorders. Individuals affected with the various forms of the mucopolysaccharidoses excrete excess amounts of acid mucopolysaccharide in the urine, particularly dermatan sulfate, heparan sulfate, and keratan sulfate. A characteristic of lysosomal storage diseases is the occurrence of multiple *phenotypic* forms associated with deficiency of each of the lysosomal enzymes.

As a group these disorders may be classified as Hurler-like disorders and include the mucolipidoses, mucopolysaccharidoses, and abnormalities of glycoprotein metabolism (see Table 50). The most common form of this disorder, and the best known, is the Hurler syndrome, which is inherited as an autosomal recessive trait. It is characterized by coarse facies, dwarfism with skeletal abnormalities, mental retardation, and early death from cardiovascular complications (Figure 228). The second most common form is the Hunter syndrome, inherited as an X-linked recessive disorder. Affected males show many similarities with the Hurler syndrome, but the corneas are clear, and the prognosis is slightly better. Defective lysosomal catabolism of mucopolysaccharides and glycoproteins results in deposition of abnormally large amounts of these materials in the liver and spleen, causing hepatosplenomegaly, in the brain, causing hydrocephalus and mental retardation, in cartilage, causing

Table 50. Characteristics of the genetic mucopolysaccharidoses

Type	Genetic features	Biochemical features	Cornea	Mental retardation	Cardiovascular features[a]	Other clinical features
I (Hurler syndrome)	Autosomal recessive	Chondroitin sulfate B, heparitin sulfate	Early clouding	+	Hypertension MR, MS, CVD, LVD	Grave manifestations
II (Hunter syndrome)	X-linked recessive	Chondroitin sulfate B, heparitin sulfate	Clear	±	AR, LVD	Milder course
III (Sanfilippo syndrome)	Autosomal recessive	Heparitin sulfate			0	Mild somatic, severe central nervous system effects
IV (Morquio syndrome)	Autosomal recessive	Keratosulfate	Cloudy	±	AR	Severe distinctive bone changes
V (Scheie syndrome)	Autosomal recessive	Chondroitin sulfate B	Cloudy	±	AR	Stiff joints, coarse facies
VI (Maroteaux-Lamy syndrome)	Autosomal recessive	Chondroitin sulfate B	Cloudy	0	MR, LVD	Severe osseous changes

[a] Key: AR = aortic regurgitation; CVD = coronary vascular disease; LVD = left ventricular dysfunction; MR = mitral regurgitation; MS = mitral stenosis.

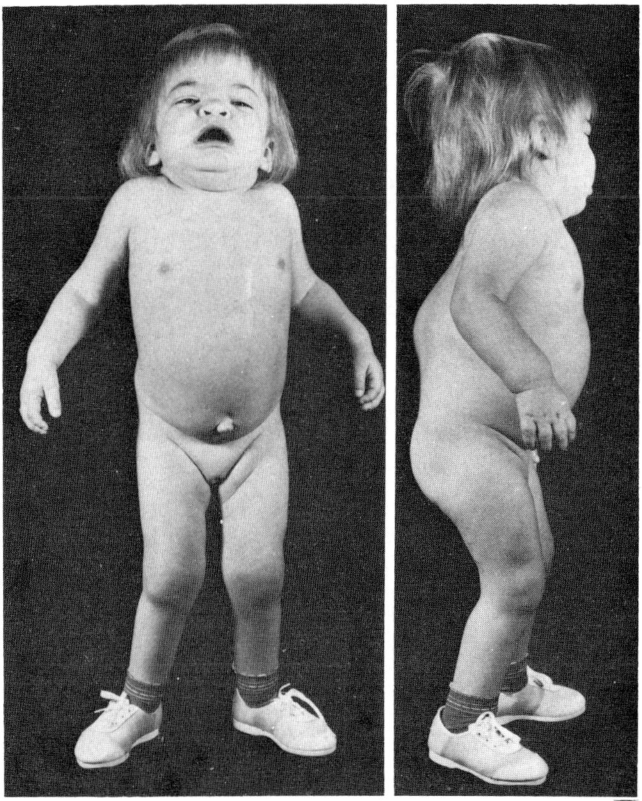

Figure 228. Two views of a 3-year-old child with Hurler syndrome. These individuals are short and have marked hypertelorism, bushy eyebrows, low hairlines, and large brachycephalic skulls with prominent foreheads. Lips are thick and the tongue is broad and deeply fissured. There is a prominent gibbus (projection in the thoracolumbar area of the back). Contractures of the major joints may be severe and produce clawlike hands. Severe peripheral vasoconstriction with cyanosis may be seen. These physical features are reproduced so faithfully that individuals with this syndrome often look like siblings.

skeletal abnormalities, in the cornea, causing corneal clouding, and (of a special pertinence) in the heart and great vessels.

Cardiovascular Pathology

Thickened and nodular valves are commonly found. The frequency of involvement is similar to that seen in rheumatic heart disease, i.e., the mitral and aortic valves are most commonly affected. Thickening of the intima of pulmonary artery and aorta and evidence of peripheral and coronary artery disease are commonly seen at necropsy. Endocardial and epicardial thickening have been reported. Interestingly enough, no congenital heart defects have been documented.

Cardiovascular Examination

Systemic hypertension is common, and occasionally is severe. With systemic hypertension, the aortic component of the second sound is accentuated.

The apex beat may be difficult to palpate and the heart sounds, particularly the first, are softer than normal. While these would suggest left ventricular dysfunction, clinically evident congestive heart failure is a late manifestation.

The electrocardiogram and chest x-ray reflect the underlying pathology and most commonly show evidence of left atrial enlargement and left ventricular hypertrophy. Electrocardiographic evidence of coronary artery disease has not been documented.

Prognosis

The average age at death of the Hurler syndrome is about 7 years, with three-fourths of affected children dying before the age of 12. The few who survive the second decade (Figure 229) most likely have the sex-linked variety (Type II). α-L-Iduronidase deficiency is manifest clinically in three forms: the Hurler syndrome, with life expectancy between 6 and 10 years; the Scheie syndrome, with near normal life expectancy; and the Hurler-Scheie compound, with life expectancy in the twenties.

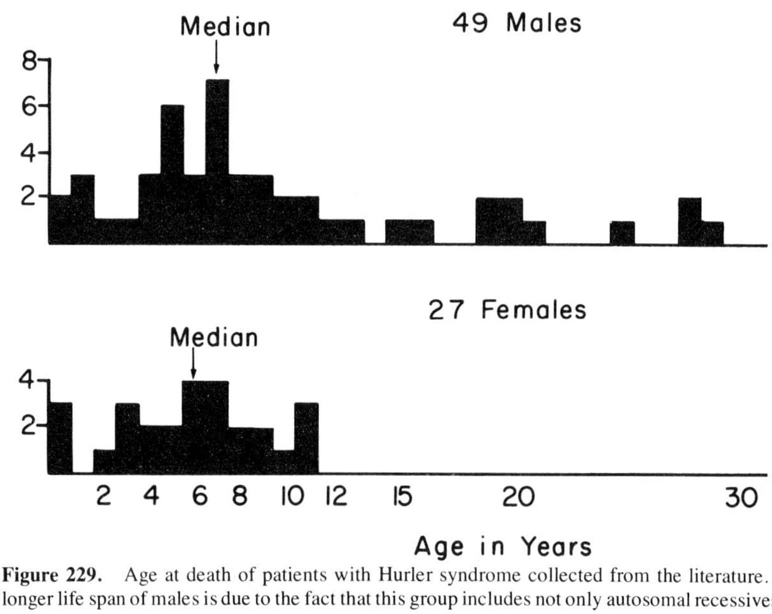

Figure 229. Age at death of patients with Hurler syndrome collected from the literature. The longer life span of males is due to the fact that this group includes not only autosomal recessives but also the milder sex-linked Hunter syndrome. (From Krovetz, L. J., Lorincz, A. E., and Schiebler, G. L. 1965. Cardiovascular manifestations of the Hurler syndrome: Hemodynamics and angiocardiographic observations in 15 patients. Curriculum 31:132. By permission of the American Heart Association, Inc.)

About one-half of affected patients succumb to the effects of heart disease: 30% develop congestive heart failure and the other 20% die suddenly, presumably as a result of arrhythmias. Respiratory infections and obstructed airways are also common causes of death.

Treatment

No specific treatment is currently available.

MARFAN SYNDROME

This disorder of connective tissue was first reported in 1896. There is no sex or racial predominance. The disorder is transmitted as an autosomal dominant trait and is inherited from an affected parent in 85% of the cases. In the remaining 15% the disorder occurs as a result of a new dominant mutation. Severely affected children more often are the result of a new dominant mutation and occur as a sporadic case in the family. New mutations resulting in dominantly inherited disorders such as the Marfan syndrome are associated with older age of the fathers.

Marfan syndrome is characterized by certain clinical features (Figure 230). There is also increased urinary excretion of hydroxyproline and sulfated acid mucopolysaccharides, particularly chondroitin sulfuric acid A.

Cardiovascular Pathology

The majority of affected individuals have cardiac involvement. Cystic medial necrosis of the aorta and pulmonary arteries is frequent. The accompanying dilatation of aortic and pulmonic artery sinuses, with resultant dilatation of the valve rings, produces regurgitation. Dissecting aneurysms of the ascending aorta and of the pulmonary artery are common. The Marfan syndrome accounts for one-fifth of all dissecting aneurysms occurring before 40 years of age.

Redundancy, thickening, and nodularity of the aortic, tricuspid, and mitral valves are the result of fibromyxomatous deposits, which cause valvar insufficiency. Fibroelastosis of the endocardium, upward displacement of the coronary ostia, and aneurysms of the mitral valve also occur. Congenital cardiovascular lesions, of which coarctation of the aorta is the most common, are reported to occur in more than 10% of cases.

Cardiovascular Examination

The pulmonic component of the second sound is often strikingly accentuated. This is thought to be due to dilation of the sinuses, which brings the pulmonic valve closer to the chest wall. Other findings depend on the underlying cardiac lesion, with aortic insufficiency being the most frequent.

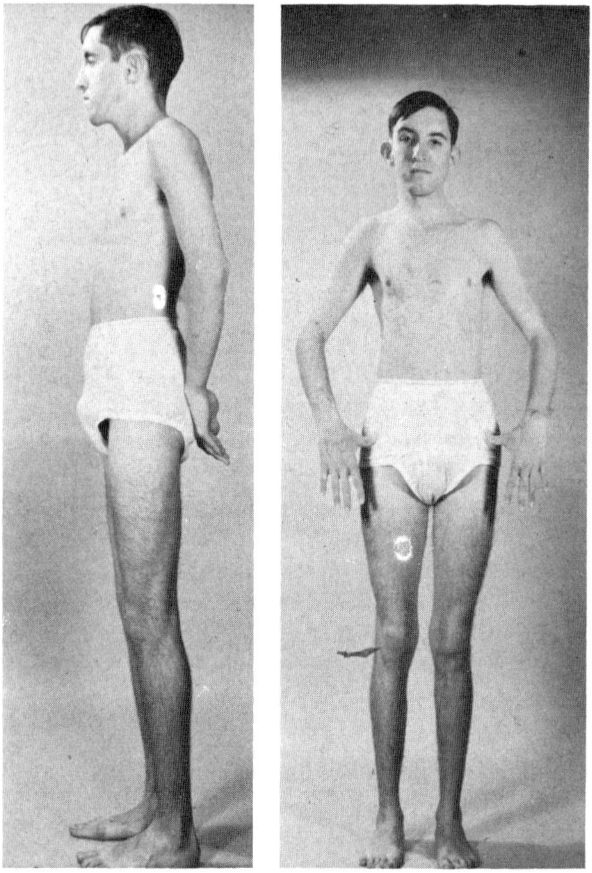

Figure 230. Seventeen-year-old male with features characteristic of Marfan syndrome—elongated extremities, absence of subcutaneous tissue, frail muscular development, scoliosis, aortic insufficiency, and a cleft palate. (Adapted from Taylor, W. J. 1966. "Genetics and the Cardiovascular System." In J. W. Hurst and R. B. Logue (eds.), The Heart: Arteries and Veins. Blakiston, New York. Used with permission of McGraw-Hill Book Company.)

HOMOCYSTINURIA

There is a variable degree of mental retardation in this condition, although normal or near normal intelligence is not uncommon. The presence of ectopia lentis and skeletal changes cause frequent confusion with the Marfan syndrome (Table 51). Cardiovascular lesions of homocystinuria consist mainly of thromboses in medium-sized arteries, especially the coronaries, the renals, and the main branches of the aorta. Damage to vessels, as in venipuncture or following arteriography, may precipitate thrombosis. The specific diagnosis is made by the demonstration of homocystine in the urine.

Table 51. Comparison of homocystinuria with the Marfan syndrome

	Homocystinuria	Marfan syndrome
Inheritance	Recessive	Dominant
Skeletal abnormality	Osteoporosis, fractures, occasional arachnodactyly	Arachnodactyly and loose-jointedness more striking
Pectus excavatum or carinatum	Frequent	Frequent
Ectopia lentis	Present	Present
Vascular disease	Dilation with thrombosis in medium-sized arteries and veins	Dilation and/or dissection of aorta
Skin	Malar flush, livedo reticularis	Striae distensae
Mental retardation	Frequent	Absent

The importance of this rare inborn error of metabolism is that it is potentially curable via vitamin therapy in a number of instances and remaining patients who are not vitamin responsive may be treated with dietary therapy. The most common form of this disease occurs secondary to a deficiency of cystathionine synthetase. Approximately one-half of patients with this disorder will have sufficient enhancement of residual enzyme activity by pyridoxine to essentially cure the disorder. Those patients who are nonresponsive to pyridoxine may be treated with a low methionine diet.

ELLIS–VAN CREVELD SYNDROME (Chondroectodermal Dysplasia)

This disorder is inherited as an autosomal recessive trait and occurs with a high incidence among the Old Order Amish. The general features of this syndrome include swarfism that results from a chondrodystrophy characterized by a symmetrical shortening of the limbs, most noted proximally, ectodermal dysplasia involving the teeth and nails, and polydactyly of the hands and feet.

Congenital heart defects, usually ventricular septal defect, atrial septal defect, or a single atrium, occur in over one-half of affected patients. Anomalous pulmonary venous drainage, patent ductus arteriosus, and transposition of the great arteries have also been reported.

MORQUIO-ULLRICH SYNDROME

This is inherited as an autosomal recessive and may be considered as another form of mucopolysaccharidosis, because large amounts of keratosulfate are excreted in the urine. This syndrome is characterized by knock-knees, pigeon breast, short neck, inability to fully extend the elbows, half-crouching stance (due to flat vertebral bodies), and diffuse clouding of the cornea. By the time these patients reach adolescence, some will demonstrate aortic regurgitation.

EHLERS-DANLOS SYNDROME

There are currently eight recognized forms of the Ehlers-Danlos syndrome. Recently described rare forms of this disorder occur as autosomal recessive traits secondary to deficiency of enzymes involved in collagen processing. Most, however, are the results of an autosomal dominant mutation. The disorder is primarily a connective tissue abnormality characterized by looseness of collagen bundles. This results in hyperextensible joints and abnormally stretchable skin (so-called India rubber man) that is fragile and bruises easily.

Coagulation defects such as diminished plasma thromboplastin component and diminished plasma thromboplastin antecedent have also been found. The great vessels have low tensile strength and rupture of the aorta or a larger artery may occur. Mitral insufficiency has been reported to occur in this syndrome.

BIBLIOGRAPHY

Husson, G. S., and Parkman, P. 1961. Chondroectodermal dysplasia (Ellis-Van Creveld syndrome) with a complex cardiac malformation. Pediatrics 28:285–292.

Kelly, T. E. 1976. Hurler-like disorders in infancy. Clin. Perinatol. 3:115–132.

Kelly, T. E. 1979. Lysosomal storage diseases. In Kelley, T. E. (ed.), Textbook of Rheumatology. W. B. Saunders Company, Philadelphia.

Krovetz, L. J., Lorincz, A. E., and Schiebler, G. L. 1968. Cardiovascular and manifestations of the Hunter-Hurler syndrome. In A. J. Moss and F. H. Adams (eds.), Heart Disease in Infants, Children and Adolescents, Chapter 41. Williams and Wilkins, Baltimore.

Krovetz, L. J., and Schiebler, G. L. 1972. Cardiovascular manifestations of the genetic mucopolysaccharidoses. In Birth Defects, Vol. VIII, No. 5, pp. 192–196. Williams and Wilkins, Baltimore.

McKusick, V. A. 1966. Heritable Disorders of Connective Tissue, 3rd ed. C.V. Mosby, St. Louis.

McKusick, V. A., Egeland, J. A., Eldridge, R., and Krusen, D. E. 1964. Dwarfism in the Amish. I. The Ellis-Van Creveld syndrome. Bull. Johns Hopkins Hosp. 115:306–336.

McKusick, V. A., Neufeld, E. F., and Kelly, T. E. 1978. The mucopolysaccharidoses and mucolipidoses. In Stanbury, Wyngaarden, and Fredrickson (eds.), Metabolic Basis of Inherited Disease, pp. 1282–1307. McGraw-Hill Book Company, New York.

Renteria, V. G., Ferrans, V. J., and Roberts, W. C. 1976. The heart in the Hurler syndrome. Am. J. Cardiol. 38:487–501.

Schieken, R. M., Kerber, R. E., Ionasescu, V. V., and Zellweger, H. 1975. Cardiac manifestations of the mucopolysaccharidoses. Circulation 52:700–705.

annotated reference list

Barratt-Boyes, B. G., Neutze, J. M., and Harris, E. A. 1973. Heart Disease in Infancy: Diagnosis and Medical Treatment. Williams & Wilkins Company, Baltimore. (Proceedings of a symposium at Green Lane Hospital in February, 1972.)

Edwards, J. E., Carey, L. S., Neufeld, H. N., and Lester, R. G. 1965. Congenital Heart Disease: Correlation of Pathologic Anatomy and Angiocardiography. W. B. Saunders Co., Philadelphia. (Two profusely illustrated volumes.)

Edwards, J. E., Dry, T. J., Parker, R. L., Burchell, H. B., Wood, E. H., and Bulbulian, A. H. 1954. An Atlas of Congenital Anomalies of the Heart and Great Vessels. Charles C Thomas, Publisher, Springfield, Ill. (Diagrams, x-rays, and pathology specimens of common and rare diseases presented in a concise format.)

Fishman, A. P., and Richards, D. W. (Eds.) 1964. Circulation of the Blood: Men and Ideas. Oxford University Press, New York. (Twelve fascinating chapters in the history of cardiovascular physiology centered on the men whose original ideas give impetus to this field.)

Friedman, W. F., Lesch, M., and Sonnenblick, E. H. 1973. Neonatal Heart Disease. Grune & Stratton, New York. (Like most multiple authored volumes, the writing is spotty. Chapters on embryology, etiology, perioperative management, and noninvasive techniques are particularly fine.)

Hamilton, W. F., and Dow, P. (Eds.) 1962. Handbook of Physiology. Section 2: Circulation. Williams & Wilkins Company (distributors for the American Physiological Society), Baltimore. (Three volumes. A comprehensive reference of cardiovascular physiology, each chapter written by an acknowledged expert in his field. Fundamentals of electrophysiology, cardiac control, and congenital heart pathophysiology are particularly pertinent.)

Keith, J. D., Rowe, R. D., and Vlad, P. 1978. Heart Disease in Infancy and Childhood, 3rd ed. The Macmillan Publishing Company, Inc., New York. (Scholarly, yet easily readable, this is the outstanding reference book in the field.)

Nadas, A. S. 1972. Pediatric Cardiology, 3rd ed. W. B. Saunders Company, Philadelphia. (A reference emphasizing the personal experiences of a skilled clinician.)

Ray, C. D. 1974. Medical Engineering. Year Book Medical Publishers, Inc., Chicago. (An encyclopedia of information on instrumentation, electrocardiography, techniques, etc.)

Rowe, R. D., and Mehrizi, A. 1968. The Neonate with Congenital Heart Disease. W. B. Saunders Company, Philadelphia. (Emphasizes physiology and diagnosis in this critical time period.)

Rudolph, A. M. 1974. Congenital Diseases of the Heart: Clinical-physiologic Considerations in Diagnosis and Management. Year Book Medical Publishers, Inc., Chicago. (Particularly interesting discussions of cardiac catheterization techniques and the pathophysiology of cardiac defects.)

index

f indicates figure; *t* indicates table.